MEDICAL COMPLICATIONS IN CANCER PATIENTS

Monograph Series of the European
Organization for Research on Treatment of Cancer
Volume 7

MONOGRAPH SERIES OF THE EUROPEAN ORGANIZATION FOR RESEARCH ON TREATMENT OF CANCER

The Monograph Series of the EORTC deals with selected topics related to cancer treatment. Volumes are usually, but not necessarily, based on the proceedings of an EORTC symposium. The responsibility of the Editorial Advisory Board is to approve the subject of each monograph; the Board does not review individual manuscripts.

Medical Complications in Cancer Patients

Monograph Series of the
European Organization for Research on
Treatment of Cancer
Volume 7

Editors

J. Klastersky, M.D.
Chief, Department of Medicine
Institut Jules Bordet
Brussels, Belgium

M. J. Staquet, M.D., M.S.
Director, EORTC Data Center
Institut Jules Bordet
Brussels, Belgium

Raven Press ■ New York

Raven Press, 1140 Avenue of the Americas, New York, New York 10036

Great care has been taken to maintain the accuracy of the information contained in the volume. However, Raven Press cannot be held responsible for errors or for any consequences arising from the use of the information contained herein.

Library of Congress Cataloging in Publication Data

Main entry under title:

Medical complications in cancer patients.

(Monograph series of the European Organization for Research on Treatment of Cancer; v. 7)
Includes index.
1. Cancer—Complications and sequelae. I. Klastersky, Jean. II. Staquet, Maurice. III. Series: European Organization for Research on Treatment of Cancer. Monograph series of the European Organization for Research on Treatment of Cancer; v. 7. [DNLM: 1. Neoplasms—Complications. W1 M0559U v. 7 / QZ200 M4885]
RC262.M42   616.99'407   80-20951
ISBN 0-89004-519-4

Preface

Cancer therapy has greatly changed during the past years, owing to the increasing use and efficacy of chemotherapy. Previously, the medical aspects of cancer therapy were primarily restricted to the problems that the cancer patient shares with any other seriously sick patient and to the management of complications related to radiotherapy or surgical treatments that were often aggressive and/or extended.

Now the medical oncologist must use an increasing number of chemotherapeutic agents, often in combination, and must face the multiple side effects and the significant morbidity that result from their use. Since many patients can be cured or significantly improved by chemotherapy, it is essential to lower to an acceptable limit the inconveniences that might result from it.

There is a complex interrelationship in the cancer patient among the manifestations linked to the tumor itself or its abnormal secretions, the diseases afflicting the patient in addition to the tumor, especially those that become common with increasing age, and the iatrogenic morbidity primarily related to cancer chemotherapy. It has become increasingly necessary that the medical oncologist be aware of the need to consider these interrelated influences equally at all times.

Therefore, the medical complications in cancer patients have become of major concern to all physicians who are faced with the comprehensive management of the cancer patient. In this volume, we meet the problem following a system/organ-oriented approach. This is deemed appropriate because clinical signs and symptoms remain the basic guides to most clinical problems in medicine. This is why cardiac, pulmonary, renal, neurologic, gastrointestinal, and cutaneous manifestations related to cancer and/or its therapy are discussed in individual chapters. In addition, endocrine manifestations of tumors and important nutritional aspects in cancer patients are discussed. Special attention is paid to the prevention and therapy of chemotherapy-induced bone marrow failure. Bleeding and infections, common morbid manifestations in cancer patients, are extensively discussed in this respect, including considerations on hematopoietic reconstitution. Another area covered is the psychological aspect of cancer diagnosis, including cancer patient terminal care and the management of pain.

The roles of cancer and of its therapy in the different body systems are analyzed. The roles of the tumor or of its therapy may be more or less important, depending on the clinical syndromes presented by the cancer patient. These are summarized in this volume: Infection is most often the consequence of therapy, while endocrinologic manifestations usually reflect the activity of the tumor itself. Nonetheless, the purpose of this book is to present the cancer patient as the entity presenting himself or herself to the clinician and in whom the natural history of the tumor is modified by the underlying clinical conditions and by cancer therapy. It is the role of the physician to sort out the various possible causes for the clinical signs and symptoms presented by the patient and to propose adequate treatments. Any approach not based on a comprehensive approach to the cancer patient would be biased toward a single and narrow aspect of cancer medicine.

Because our work is aimed at a global approach to the cancer patient, this volume will be useful to internists and oncologists alike; its purpose is to provide a system-oriented review of the morbid manifestations that can be observed in cancer patients whatever the causes may be. The editors believe that only such a comprehensive approach can be beneficial to both physicians and patients.

J. Klastersky
M. J. Staquet

Acknowledgments

The EORTC Foundation will receive all royalties from sales of this book. The authors freely gave their time and received no remuneration. We are extremely grateful to all of them.

Contents

Contributors

R. A. Abrams
Section on Hematology/Flesh Oncology
Medical College of Wisconsin
Milwaukee, Wisconsin 53226, U.S.A.

J. Aisner
Cell Component Therapy Section
National Cancer Institute
University of Maryland Hospital
Baltimore, Maryland 21201, U.S.A.

J. J. Body
Department of Medicine
Institut Jules Bordet
1000 Brussels, Belgium

J. J. Bonica
Department of Anaesthesiology
School of Medicine
University of Washington
Seattle, Washington 98195, U.S.A.

A. Borkowski
Department of Medicine
Institut Jules Bordet
1000 Brussels, Belgium

Y. A. Carpentier
Department of Surgery
Hôpital Saint Pierre
Brussels, Belgium

A. Coune
Department of Medicine
Institut Jules Bordet
1000 Brussels, Belgium

P. A. Daly
Cell Component Therapy Section
National Cancer Institute
University of Maryland Hospital
Baltimore, Maryland 21201, U.S.A.

L. J. Deftos
Endocrine Section
University of California
San Diego Veterans Administration
    Medical Center
La Jolla, California 92161, U.S.A.

A. B. Deisseroth
Experimental Hematology Section
Pediatric Oncology Branch
National Cancer Institute
Bethesda, Maryland 20205, U.S.A.

R. De Jager
Department of Medicine
Institut Jules Bordet
1000 Brussels, Belgium

B. P. First
Endocrine Section
University of California
San Diego Veterans Administration
    Medical Center
La Jolla, California 92161, U.S.A.

M. H. Gault
Dialysis Unit
Health Sciences Center
Memorial University of Newfoundland
St. Johns, Newfoundland A1B 3V6,
    Canada

J. Hildebrand
Department of Medicine
Institut Jules Bordet
1000 Brussels, Belgium

B. S. Kaplan
Nephrology Service
The Montreal Children's Hospital
Montreal, Quebec H3H 1P3, Canada

J. Klastersky
Department of Medicine
Institut Jules Bordet
1000 Brussels, Belgium

J. Knaack
Institute of Pathology
McGill University
Montreal, Quebec, Canada

M. J. Krant
University of Massachusetts Medical
Center
Worcester, Massachusetts 01605, U.S.A.

A. S. Levine
Infectious Disease Section
Pediatric Oncology Branch
National Cancer Institute
Bethesda, Maryland 20205, U.S.A.

F. M. Muggia
Division of Oncology
New York University Medical Center
New York, New York 10016, U.S.A.

C. Muquardt
Department of Medicine
Institut Jules Bordet
1000 Brussels, Belgium

M. Piccart
Department of Medicine
Institut Jules Bordet
1000 Brussels, Belgium

E. Pollard
Department of Medicine
University of Texas at San Antonio Health
Science Center
San Antonio, Texas 78284, U.S.A.

M. Rozencweig
Department of Medicine
Institut Jules Bordet
1000 Brussels, Belgium

C. A. Schiffer
Cell Component Therapy Section
National Cancer Institute
University of Maryland Hospital
Baltimore, Maryland 21201, U.S.A.

S. C. Schimpff
Section of Infection Research
Baltimore Cancer Research Program
National Cancer Institute
University of Maryland Hospital
Baltimore, Maryland 20201, U.S.A.

H. Y. Vanderpool
Institute for the Medical Humanities
University of Texas Medical Branch
Galveston, Texas 77550, U.S.A.

D. D. Von Hoff
Department of Medicine
University of Texas at San Antonio Health
Science Center
San Antonio, Texas 78284, U.S.A.

J. C. Wade
Section of Infection Research
Baltimore Cancer Research Program
National Cancer Institute
University of Maryland Hospital
Baltimore, Maryland 20201, U.S.A.

J. Waldenström
Allmänna Sjukhuset
Malmö, Sweden

R. B. Weiss
Clinical Investigations Branch
Cancer Therapy Evaluation Program
National Cancer Institute
Bethesda, Maryland 20205, U.S.A.

J. K. V. Willson
Medicine Branch
Clinical Oncology Program
National Cancer Institute
Bethesda, Maryland 20205, U.S.A.

Medical Complications in Cancer Patients,
edited by J. Klastersky and M. J. Staquet.
Raven Press, New York © 1981.

Clinical and Biological Implications of Paraneoplasia

Jan Waldenström

Allmänna Hospital, Malmö, Sweden

The term paraneoplasia, or paramalignancy, is of recent date, but the phenomenon itself has been known and discussed for several centuries. The fact that patients with malignant tumors lose weight and appetite, develop fever, become anemic, and feel miserable is nothing new. Still we do not know anything crucially causal about the basis of these general symptoms. It is possible that an analysis of other, more special results of tumor metabolism will help us understand these more fundamental mechanisms. It seems as if the majority of symptoms with a known cause that are also reversible after radical treatment of a malignant tumor could be traced to one special group of substances, i.e., polypeptides (19).

ECTOPIC HORMONES

Several authors have been active in developing the concept of ectopic hormone production by malignant cells. Albright was probably the first to suggest that an increase in serum calcium, as we sometimes see in patients with malignant tumors, might be caused by some substance produced by the tumor. At that time it was taken for granted that metastases to bone liberated calcium through destruction, but Albright and Reifenstein (1) stressed the point that a high serum calcium level could also be found in patients who had no skeletal tumors.

The first authors who showed that removal of a carcinoma normalized the serum calcium values were Plimpton and Gellhorn (13). In their patient with an ovarian carcinoma, a relapse of hypercalcemia was seen together with the development of metastases. The term ectopic hormone production was coined by Liddle and his group when they described and studied the occurrence of Cushing's syndrome in patients with tumors arising from nonendocrine tissue. This is the key observation for understanding these processes. These authors (9) showed that the tumor cells produced adrenocorticotropin (ACTH) or ACTH-like substances that stimulated the adrenal complex. Work along these lines has produced very interesting results clinically, and the number of examples illustrating the connection between hormonal activity and cancer cells is large.

1

In spite of the fact that specific activity which manifests biologically or by immunological reactivity has been established, the discussion regarding the true nature of the molecules is still lively. Regarding the hypercalcemic factor, most authors seem to accept the fact that parathormone, possibly with various structural modifications and also occurring as "big" PTH, is the hypercalcemia-producing factor. On the other hand, such studies have initiated very interesting research regarding the importance of other substances for understanding calcium homeostasis. The prostaglandins seem to play an important part in some of these situations, but it is still impossible to prove their role in cancer hypercalcemia. This is partly due to the difficulties connected with quantitative determination of these molecules and their metabolites. The effects of substances such as aspirin and indomethacin, known inhibitors of prostaglandin synthesis, are also used as arguments in this discussion. Several authors believe that steroids may be involved, especially in hypercalcemia connected with mammary carcinoma. Extensive and critical analyses of sera from such hypercalcemic patients seem to have proved convincingly that PTH-like polypeptides are the most common cause. Analyses of such sera and also of sera containing ectopic ACTH have been valuable in the establishment of molecular heterogeneity among these hormones. This seems to have taught us that "big big," "big," and small molecules may occur, which is also important for understanding normal hormone production (2).

OTHER POLYPEPTIDE HORMONES

A number of other polypeptide hormones are produced by malignant cells, and most are not ectopic. They are formed by cancer cells arising from tissues that are normal producers of such hormones. Our knowledge regarding the products of the pancreatic islet cells would be meager if we had not had the opportunity to study patients with tumors from specific cell types. Beta-cell tumors producing insulin as a topical product are well known. During the last decade the number of products from alpha-cell tumors has increased remarkably. First among these tumors were the hypergastrinomas belonging to the Zollinger-Ellison syndrome with intractable gastric and duodenal ulcerations that healed after the removal of the tumor. Some of these tumors also produced severe diarrhea, and the diarrheogenic factor vasoactive intestinal polypeptide (VIP) has been isolated in these patients.

[The reader who has a feeling for the meaning of words must have a natural reaction against such terrible constructions as insulinoma, glucagonoma, or VIPoma! For the sake of biological clarity, however, these expressions are valuable. Hence these illogical constructions have come to stay.]

The alpha cells produce a factor that may be regarded as an antagonist to insulin, i.e., glucagon. The syndrome that results from the overproduction of this polypeptide was recently described (14). Its recognition at an early stage of the disease leads to complete postoperative cure of all the symptoms. The effects of glucagon on carbohydrate metabolism are well known, but another symptom deserves special mention. It has been found that the amino acid levels in these patients are very low. Intravenous infusions of solutions containing amino acids have an almost miraculous effect on the condition of the skin in these patients, who suffer from widespread, chronic, debilitating, migratory, necrotizing dermatosis and also have a smooth, sore, bright red tongue (8). All these symptoms disappear after a few days if amino acid levels in the blood are increased. This means that the condition of the patients, as far as the skin is concerned, may become normalized preoperatively. Removal of a single tumor may give complete and lasting cure. Even if metastases are present, effects may be obtained by using a new antitumor agent that is specially effective in several types of alpha-cell tumors, i.e., streptozotocin. The reason this antibiotic should be more or less specific in this type of tumor is a problem that seems well worth investigating.

Another polypeptide hormone that may be produced by islet cell tumors is somatostatin. Recently a "somatostatinoma" was diagnosed and treated successfully. With the aid of fluorescent antibodies, it was possible to determine that the D-cells in the pancreatic islets contain somatostatin. The name means that this factor is in a way a negative, inhibiting, static hormone. It not only inhibits endocrine functions regarding somatotropin in the anterior pituitary, but also influences insulin, glucagon, pancreatic polypeptide, and the cholecystokinin–pancreozymin system, with effects on many metabolic functions. The fact that it does not have any "positive" effects makes the clinical diagnosis much more difficult. As a matter of fact, it is possible to obtain a reliable diagnosis only through quantitative determinations of the hormone in the serum. The basis for clinical suspicion is vague, consisting of dyspepsia, mild diabetes, and gallstones. As these symptoms are very common, it is clear that patients may have this triad without suffering from this very rare tumor. At the present moment it appears that no more than six cases have been diagnosed, and only one of the patients was successfully operated on and has remained asymptomatic during a follow-up of 2.5 years (3,6).

A recent publication reviews the syndrome, with a thorough study on a cooperative patient. To date, this review is the best basis for further information. The patient had multiple metastases and is now being treated with streptozotocin.

It is interesting that so many of these hormone-producing tumors excrete several active polypeptides. Somatostatinomas have also been found to produce calcitonin (two cases) and ACTH (one case). Such findings may be explained in several ways. It is well established that there are many homologies between several of the gastrointestinal hormones, e.g., secretin, glucagon, and VIP or cholecystokinin and gastrin. Another important finding is connected with the pituitary ACTH system. Big ACTH with a molecular weight of 31,000 contains normal ACTH with 39 amino acids. Within this molecule, the first 18 amino acids correspond to melanocyte simulating hormone (alpha-MSH). No less than 91 amino acids in another part of big ACTH constitute a "beta-lipotropin" (beta-LPH). This was first discovered by Li, who gave it the name beta-LPH. It contains beta-MSH and beta-endorphin consisting of 30 amino acids. A small but important part of this body peptide is the pentapeptide met-enkephalin. It is thus possible that large polypeptide molecules are formed first, and through the activity of intra- or extracellular proteases smaller fragments are set free. These may have different activities from the "mother" polypeptide.

A third possibility that must be taken seriously is that malignant cells have a tendency to derepress several independent polypeptide-forming systems in the same cell (17). Recent investigations have shown that many cancer patients have several unrelated active polypeptides in their blood. The number of ectopic nonactive, and therefore not determined, foreign polypeptides may be large.

B-LYMPHOCYTE IMMUNOGLOBULINS

I mentioned these instances of topic hormone production because they have taught us much about the biology and pathophysiology of certain cells, even though they are rare. Much more common and therefore more important from the practical point of view are such connections as immunoglobulin production by the descendants of B-lymphocytes. Practically all our knowledge regarding the structure of immunoglobulins has come from analysis of such products.

Unique in this field is the connection between one special type of myeloma and allergy. It was found that a patient with myeloma, observed at the Academic Hospital in Uppsala, Sweden, produced in pure form an immunoglobulin molecule that did not belong to the four types already established. At the same time, allergologists in the United States had found that the allergic reagin must be a special type of immunoglobulin that could be obtained only in minute quantities from very large amounts of serum from allergic patients. It was established that the myeloma globulin was of the same type, and antiserum against immunoglobulin E (IgE) was produced. With the aid of such antisera, the amount of allergic reagins that were IgE could be determined in the blood from patients with varying diseases. It may well be said that the availability of pure IgE, produced by a limited number of myeloma patients, gave a firm biochemical basis to allergology. Such experiments of nature—when a special clone of cells secretes a special product—have contributed much to the understanding of obscure biological mechanisms.

CARCINOID TUMORS

One of the most spectacular paraneoplastic syndromes is connected with metastasizing carcinoid tumors. Short intensive flushes with hyperperistalsis and diarrhea constitute the classical syndrome. Sometimes these patients also have signs of bronchoconstriction. The most surprising finding is the pulmonary and tricuspid valve lesions that develop after many years. It is quite clear that 5-hydroxytryptamine is responsible for a number of these symptoms. Carcinoid heart disease must be regarded as a biochemically induced valvular heart disease (16). Rare instances have been described with carcinoid tumors arising in the stomach. These patients have a much more long-lasting bright red and blotchy flush (18). This symptom is connected with itching, and it is clear that the mediator is histamine released from the tumor. The signals on the skin as well as the general clinical picture are different in these two types of argentaffinoma (19).

Some of these patients develop signs that have been interpreted as indicating pellagra. Workers at the National Institutes of Health (U.S.A.) performed metabolic studies on these patients and showed that a very large part of the tryptophan pool is converted to 5-hydroxytryptamine (5-HT). It is therefore diverted from the normal pathway that leads to formation of pellagra-preventing factors (niacin). This is thus a unique example of tumor "parasitism," when the neoplastic cells consume an essential factor and thereby injure the patient. This has of course been hypothesized for years but proof is lacking to date. I am certain that the possibility of such mechanisms should be considered in other situations in oncology.

Two tumor sites are of special interest in this connection. It has been found that carcinoid tumors of the lung are not rare. Sometimes they produce the typical syndrome with flushing and valvular heart disease. The fact that these valvular changes are located in the left heart speaks strongly in favor of the assumption that blood coming directly from the tumor to the heart contains an active principle which influences the endocardium.

The other situation in which a primary carcinoid tumor is found is with teratoma of the ovary. These patients have a complete syndrome, probably because the tumor products enter the inferior vena cava and are taken directly to the right heart. We have seen patients who no longer had clinical symptoms after extirpation of the tumor because they had no liver metastases. The biochemical findings also became normal, with a remarkable drop in hydroxyindole acetic acid. Initially the cardiac decompensation seemed to improve, but eventually both of our patients died from decompensated heart disease just like other patients who have carcinoid tissue in their liver metastases. We have seen one patient who had a very large hepatic tumor that was resected and had a long-lasting remission (19).

ANTIBODIES TO COAGULATION FACTORS

An interesting paraneoplastic situation is the development of specific antibodies against some coagulation factor. Such anticoagulants, active *in vivo* by causing bleeding, as well as *in vitro,* have long been known to be present in patients suffering from autoimmune disease, especially systemic lupus erythematosus (SLE). During the last few years some such inhibitors acting against factor VIII in hemophilia have also been described. Recently acquired von Willebrand's disease has been found in patients with lymphatic leukemia or lymphoma. The specific antibody has been an IgG in two cases and an IgA in two. In all four observations the immunoglobulin was monotypical, but the mode of action was rather complicated. An interesting example of this situation was recently published by Zettervall and Nilsson (20).

DISCUSSION

Do we have reason to believe that many of the enigmatic connections between tumors and very special clinical signals will be clarified in the future? A few such examples may be cited. Acanthosis nigricans is one of the classical paraneoplastic phenomena. It has a strong association with tumors in the gastrointestinal tract but has also been seen in conjunction with other cancers. Some years ago we had a patient with an astounding degree of acanthosis (10). After removing a number of mediastinal and hilar metastases containing squamous cell carcinoma, the skin lesions completely disappeared and have not reappeared during an observation time of 4 years. It may be guessed that this tumor could produce an epithelial cell growth factor. Such substances are known to be polypeptides. Large amounts of this factor, which is otherwise difficult to produce, might be isolated from the excreta of such patients. The same could be true about other, similar factors.

Osteoarthropathy is known to occur with cancer of the lung. In rare instances extirpation of other cancers have also been successful in curing these changes. Ten years ago we reported some investigations of such patients with reversal after a successful operation of the lung tumor (15). We believed that increased levels of growth hormone might have been responsible for the changes in bone and soft tissue of the hands that in many ways resemble the changes seen in acromegaly. At present, it seems that increases in growth hormone are not obligatory in this syndrome. It is probable that other growth factors (e.g., somatomedin) may be responsible. This would be easy to investigate if a typical patient is found and the serum is analyzed by a competent biochemist.

The relationship of malignant tumors to the function of blood-forming organs has been of great interest for many decades. Normochromic anemia with a low serum iron and a normal or low transferrin level is a characteristic of tumor anemia; it is also found in other chronic diseases, however, and is therefore nonspecific. It seems probable that cancer anemia is caused by some substance(s) that inhibits the erythron. Stimulators of erythropoiesis are well-known products of tumors, especially those arising in the kidney. Erythropoietin has been the subject of extensive and well-organized attempts at isolation, but without much success; it is one of the most elusive active substances in medicine. It seems reasonable to assume that pooled urine specimens from patients with renal tumors producing erythropoietin might be the most promising source for the preparation of this substance. Furthermore, the fact that nonrenal tumors may produce excessive erythropoietin is probably important to the understanding of erythropoietin formation. The relation between renal cancer cells, the epithelial lining of cerebellar cysts, and the smooth muscle in uterine myoma seems enigmatic. All three conditions are connected with polyglobulinemia, which may be reversed after operative treatment.

We may well discuss if erythropoietin should be regarded as a "hormone" active on the erythropoietic stem cell in a manner similar to the way pituitary tropins influence their target cell. Erythropoietin may also be compared to the fetal inducers, i.e., substances that induce the transformation of one type of cell to another. It is probable that one of the so-called thymic hormones that induce T-cell formation from a lymphatic stem cell is a similar substance.

There are tumors associated with marked thrombocytosis and others associated with extreme eosinophilia. In both of these instances specific poietins have been discussed. We know little about such substances in regard to platelets. We do know, however, that thrombocytosis is reversible after extirpation of the tumor. Recent work by Mahmoud and his group demonstrated the existence of eosinophilopoietin (7). This substance appears to be a polypeptide with a molecular weight in the range of 186 to 1,357. It is digested by pronase and practically inactivated by heat. Probably the excessive eosinophilia seen in some cancer patients is caused by this or similar substances. It has no eosinophilotactic activity, but work in Austen's laboratory demonstrated that comparatively simple peptides have a strong attractive influence on eosinophilic cells. It is therefore probable that eosinophilia in cancer patients may also be caused by the presence of such factors, especially when there is eosinophilia in the blood and in the tumor.

The fact that some of the tumor products are not so much ectopic as asynchronous (i.e., they represent a return to fetal production) is also an important factor in paraneoplasia. Fetuin is one such substance of great practical importance as a tumor signal (19).

It is well known that fetal liver cells produce a special protein that migrates on electrophoresis between albumin and α_1-globulin. This protein has been called α-fetoprotein, and with the aid of specific antibodies its presence can be demonstrated in the serum of adult patients with malignant hepatoma. The connection between this substance and the type of liver tumor is obscure, and about one-third of patients with malignant hepatoma lack an increase in the protein. It is also remarkable that aflatoxin hepatoma does not induce formation of α-fetoprotein, whereas other carcinogens may cause hepatomas that do. No differences in histology have been found.

There are similar examples that are still more enigmatic. Several years ago we saw a patient with a carcinoma of the lung who had severe intractable anemia and no less than 35% fetal hemoglobin in his red cells (11). Hypothetically, the tumor may produce a substance that "turns on" the synthesis of the fetal chain in globin. If this substance exists and could be recognized, this could mean much for the treatment of two of the most widespread global diseases: thalassemia and sickle cell anemia. Increased production of fetal hemoglobin could become a valuable aid in improving the anemia in these patients.

There are other interesting reversals to fetal conditions seen in carcinoma patients. One of the most astounding is the development of the "monkey face" in patients with tumors. This is explained by the fact that fetal hair (typical lanugo) grows all over the body including ears and forehead (5). As yet nobody has observed reversal after successful operation, but it does not seem far-fetched to assume a specific lanugo-promoting factor or inducer.

The examples quoted have mostly been polypeptides; a great many others may be found. In a few instances complete protein molecules have also been observed, but it is striking that single gene products are so common. This may offer a clue to tumorigenesis. We know that the greatest part of the complete genome is repressed, i.e., nonactive. The question is if all these polypeptide-synthesizing systems are dead or dormant. In the latter case they may be awakened, derepressed (17).

We have already discussed parallels with fetal physiology and the activity of inducers. Developmental biology *(Entwicklungsmechanik)* may perhaps offer some arguments for this discussion. Gurdon, an eminent experimental zoologist working in Oxford and Cambridge, performed interesting experiments in this connection (4). He showed that a nucleus from a somatic cell, if transferred to the enucleated cytoplasm of an egg from the same frog species, could induce the development of a whole fertile animal. This experiment must prove that the complete genome in every body cell is in a dormant state that can be derepressed under favorable conditions. It therefore seems probable that individual genes could be derepressed in cancer cells and start synthesizing fortuitously diverse polypeptides. As a matter of fact, recent work has shown that a great many cancer patients have numerous foreign polypeptides in the blood that can be discovered with the aid of sensitive radioimmunoassay methods.

REFERENCES

1. Albright, F., and Reifenstein, E. C. (1948): *Parathyroid Glands and Metabolic Bone Disease,* p. 93. Williams & Wilkins, Baltimore.
2. Benson, R. C., Jr., Riggs, R. C., Pickard, B. L., et al. (1974): Radioimmunoassay of parathyroid hormone in hypercalcemic patients with malignant disease. *Am. J. Med.,* 56:821–826.
3. Ganda, O. P., and Soeldner, J. S. (1977): "Somatostatinoma": follow-up studies. *N. Engl. J. Med.,* 297:1352–1353.
4. Gurdon, J. B. (1974): *The Control of Gene Expression in Animal Development.* Harvard University Press, Cambridge, Mass.
5. Hegedus, S. I., and Schorr, W. F. (1972): Acquired hypertrichosis lanuginosa and malignancy. *Arch. Dermatol.,* 106:84–88.
6. Krejs, G. J., et al. (1979): Somatostatinoma syndrome: biochemical, morphologic and clinical features. *N. Engl. J. Med.,* 301:285–292.
7. Mahmoud, A. A. F., Stone, M. K., and Kellermeyer, R. W. (1977): Eosinophilopoietin: a low molecular weight peptide stimulating eosinophil production in mice. *Trans. Assoc. Am. Physicians,* 90:127–134.
8. Mallinson, C. N., Bloom, S. R., Warin, A. P., et al. (1974): A glucagonoma syndrome. *Lancet,* 2:1–5.
9. Meador, C. K., Liddle, G. W., Island, D. P., et al. (1962): Cause of Cushing's syndrome in patients with tumors arising from "nonendocrine" tissue. *J. Clin. Endocrinol.,* 22:693–703.

10. Möller, H., Eriksson, S., Holen, O., and Waldenström, J. G. (1978): Complete reversibility of paraneoplastic acanthosis nigricans after operation. *Acta Med. Scand.,* 203:245–246.
11. Nyman, M., Skölling, R., and Steiner, H. (1970): Acquired macrocytic anemia and hemoglobinopathy—a paraneoplastic manifestation? *Am. J. Med.,* 48:792–797.
12. Parsons, J. A., editor (1976): *Peptide Hormones.* University Park Press, College Park, Maryland.
13. Plimpton, C. H., and Gellhorn, A. (1956): Hypercalcemia in malignant disease without evidence of bone destruction. *Am. J. Med.,* 21:750–759.
14. von Schenck, H., Thorell, J. I., et al. (1979): Metabolic studies and glucagon gel filtration pattern before and after surgery in a case of glucagonoma syndromes. *Acta Med. Scand.,* 205:155–162.
15. Steiner, H., Dahlbäck, O., and Waldenström, J. G. (1968): Ectopic growth-hormone production and osteoarthropathy in carcinoma of the bronchus. *Lancet,* April 13:783–785.
16. Waldenström, J. G. (1958): Clinical aspects of carcinoid tumours. In: *Modern Trends in Gastro-Enterology,* pp. 92–100. Butterworths, London.
17. Waldenström, J. G. (1970): Maladies of derepression: pathological, often monoclonal, derepression of protein forming templates. *Schweiz. Med. Wochenschr.,* 100:2197–2206.
18. Waldenström, J. G. (1976): Carcinoid tumours. In: *Bockus: Gastroenterology, 3rd Ed.,* pp. 473–480. Saunders, Philadelphia.
19. Waldenström, J. G. (1978): *Paraneoplasia. Biological Signals in the Diagnosis of Cancer.* Wiley, New York.
20. Zettervall, O., and Nilsson, I. M. (1978): Acquired von Willebrand's disease caused by a monoclonal antibody. *Acta Med. Scand.,* 204:521–528.

Medical Complications in Cancer Patients,
edited by J. Klastersky and M. J. Staquet.
Raven Press, New York © 1981.

Ectopic Hormone Production by Nonendocrine Tumors

A. Borkowski, C. Muquardt, and J. J. Body

Medical Service and Henri Tagnon Laboratory of Clinical Investigation, Department of Endocrinology, Tumor Center, Jules Bordet Institute, Free University of Brussels, 1000 Brussels, Belgium

The finding that "nonendocrine" tumors are capable of secreting polypeptide hormones was a major development in endocrinology during the last 20 years. This new field was investigated at first and most thoroughly in Cushing's syndrome resulting from the "ectopic" secretion of adrenocorticotropic hormone (ACTH) (3,6). However, most if not all polypeptide hormones can be secreted ectopically, including antidiuretic hormone (ADH), parathyroid hormone (PTH), human placental lactogen (hPL), and chorionic gonadotropin (hCG) (5,7). Similarly, most tumors are capable of ectopic hormone secretion, although some appear more prone to produce these syndromes: oat cell carcinomas of the lung, islet cell carcinomas of the pancreas, carcinoids, epithelial thymomas, and medullary carcinomas of the thyroid. The tumors are usually malignant, but some benign tumors (e.g., pheochromocytomas producing a Cushing's syndrome) also secrete ectopic hormones. The polypeptide secreted ectopically may be the final hormone [e.g., ACTH (chemical, immunological, and biological identity)] or its precursor [e.g., big ACTH (convertible to ACTH by trypsinization)] (5). It may be a hormone secreted by normal endocrine glands or one secreted by the placenta and thus found exclusively in pregnant women under normal conditions. Consequently, the finding of a placental hormone in the blood of nonpregnant subjects is thought to be abnormal and specific for a tumor. The placental hormones are thus viewed as "qualitative" tumor markers, in contrast to the other hormones, which can be suspected of being ectopic only when their secretion exceeds the normal and which are qualified therefore as "quantitative" tumor markers (2,8,9). Finally, some ectopic humoral syndromes reveal the existence of a still unknown or undefined humoral factor, as in the hypophosphatemic osteomalacia associated with mesenchymal tumors or in the hypercalcemia without bone metastases or PTH secretion associated with lymphomas.

The ectopic secretions of polypeptide hormones are of great clinical interest. They are frequent; for instance, Cushing's syndrome is found in 2.8% and inappropriate antidiuresis in 8% of lung oat cell carcinomas, and nonmetastatic hypercalcemia is found in 15% of lung squamous cell carcinomas. Their metabolic consequences may be more malignant than the tumor itself. The patient may die from hypokalemic alkalosis and diabetes mellitus (Cushing's syndrome), nonmetastatic hypercalcemia and dehydration (pseudohyperparathyroidism), or dilutional hyponatremia (Schwartz-Bartter syndrome)—whereas the tumor itself is localized and curable. Certain slow-growing tumors of mesenchymal origin, hidden for instance in the retroperitoneum, may manifest first by intractable hypoglycemia.

When the humoral syndrome precedes the diagnosis of the tumor, the presence of an ectopic secretion can be demonstrated by various means. Functional tests reveal the absence of feedback regulation, as in Cushing's syndrome due to ectopic ACTH secretion. Selective catheterizations reveal the absence of hypersecretion in the venous effluent from the glands which normally secrete the hormone, as in pseudohyperparathyroidism with high PTH concentration in peripheral blood. On the other hand, the hypoglycemia due to nonpancreatic tumors is characterized by low serum insulin levels. The demonstration that a humoral syndrome is produced by "nonendocrine" tissues is of course very important in such circumstances; it will avoid unnecessary surgery, e.g., a neck exploration for pseudohyperparathyroidism. It can also initiate the search for a small or hidden tumor within the mediastinum, retroperitoneum, or pelvis, sometimes enabling an early diagnosis. On the other hand, when the metabolic consequences are more malignant than the tumor itself, their symptomatic treatment may be life-saving or prolong comfortably the life of the patient (5).

PRESENT INVESTIGATION

We have been particularly interested in the ectopic hormone secretions as early markers of tumors. With this purpose in mind, we chose to investigate a placental protein hormone, human chorionic gonadotropin (hCG) (4). hCG is thought to be a "qualitative" tumor marker (8), its detection in the blood of men or nonpregnant women being pathognomonic of ectopic secretion. Ectopic secretion, in turn, is viewed as specific for tumor: Only tumor cells—because they are more undifferentiated and because they presumably represent reversion to an earlier embryonic phase—are thought to be the site of a genetic derepression allowing ectopic secretion.

We investigated, prospectively, hCG and its free β subunit in the plasma of 414 patients with malignant tumors and in 99 patients with various benign diseases (4). Because of the selection of the patients admitted in our institution, these benign diseases were benign tumors and benign conditions associated with tissue hyperplasia, e.g., fibrocystic hyperplasia of the breast, ovarian cysts, uterine fibromas, endometrial hyperplasias, chronic adenitis, cirrhosis of the liver, and perforated colic diverticulitis or duodenal ulcers. With a sensitivity of 1.6 ng/ml we found hCG in 16% of our patients with malignant tumors. Somewhat unexpectedly, and unlike Braunstein et al. (2), whose study was not prospective, we did not find any clear-cut difference of frequency according to the histology (except for choriocarcinomas which obviously form a distinct entity). Still more unexpectedly, we found hCG as frequently in the benign diseases as in the malignant tumors. However, the benign and malignant conditions differed from each other in that the plasma concentrations of hCG were significantly higher ($p <$ 0.005) in the malignancies and the highest plasma concentrations (> 50 ng/ ml) were specific for malignancy. Our data were consistent to some extent with the work of Vaitukaitis et al. (9), who showed that hCG can be found in the blood of nonpregnant individuals with some benign diseases of the gastrointestinal tract. This lack of specificity according to histology and the finding of hCG in patients with benign tissue hyperplasia suggested to us, as proposed by Vaitukaitis (7), a common anomaly—perhaps enhanced cellular proliferation—as the source of hCG. On the other hand, the lower plasma concentrations in the patients with benign diseases might indicate some quantitative correlation between plasma hCG and cell turnover. We wondered therefore whether still lower plasma concentrations would be found in normal nonpregnant subjects (1). Plasma hCG could then be a sensitive marker of normal cell turnover, and the so-called ectopic secretion found in tumors would simply be a quantitative deviation from normal.

There were several difficulties in identifying and measuring hCG in the plasma of normal subjects. First, if hCG was present, its concentrations were very low. Second, the large amounts of plasma proteins might interfere nonspecifically in the radioimmunoassay of hCG (9). Third, there is a substantial crossover in antigenicity between hCG and the other glycoprotein hormones, particularly human luteinizing hormone (hLH), which has the most similar structure (9). We overcame these difficulties by extracting large volumes of plasma and by purifying hCG on a DEAE-Sephadex A-50 column from hLH and the bulk of the plasma proteins. We identified hCG in the final residue by its characteristic dose-response curves in a specific radioimmunoassay and calculated its concentration in the initial plasma after correction for the losses.

With a sensitivity of up to 2 pg/ml, we found and could measure hCG in the plasma of 12 of 16 blood donors: The median concentration was 19 pg/ ml (i.e., 100 times less than the corresponding hLH concentration); the range of concentrations was < 2 to 361 pg/ml. We were able to further characterize this immunologic hCG from a pool of plasma obtained from 13 healthy male subjects by gel filtration on Sephadex G-100. hCG from normal subjects was found to be identical to standard hCG; it was quite different from hLH; it was not asialo-hCG (the carbohydrate-free molecule) either. Interestingly, there was no correlation between hCG and hLH concentrations in plasma: This is compatible with a different regulation and thus a different site of origin for these two hormones. In other words, in normal nonpregnant subjects hCG might be secreted not by the pituitary gland but, as in patients with tumors, by the peripheral tissues. The tumors, by magnifying or exaggerating this "ectopic" secretion, would reveal a normal function of "nonendocrine" tissues.

Our finding of hCG in normal nonpregnant subjects might be of more general significance. Such a small "ectopic" secretion need not to be unique to hCG; it could take place for any other protein hormone but remain unsuspected because it is undistinguishable from the much greater secretion by the corresponding endocrine gland. Furthermore, if the so-called ectopic secretion of protein hormones is a normal phenomenon, the concept of genetic derepression to explain the "ectopic" secretion by tumors of "nonendocrine" tissues is no longer necessary. The "ectopic" protein hormones might have a local role in controlling cell function, and their production might reciprocally be submitted to a local regulation.

CONCLUSION

Our observations about hCG—in patients with "nonendocrine" tumors at first, in normal nonpregnant subjects thereafter—could be an illustration of Liddle's statement 10 years ago about endocrine glands (5): "Several of the earliest insights into the functions of endocrine glands came from observations that tumors of these glands were associated with characteristic clinical abnormalities, and only later was it shown that nontumorous glands produced hormones that, in excess, could mimic the metabolic abnormalities associated with the tumors." According to our data, normal "nonendocrine" tissues might similarly be engaged in the production of protein hormones.

REFERENCES

1. Borkowski, A., and Muquardt, C. (1979): Human chorionic gonadotropin in the plasma of normal, nonpregnant subjects. *N. Engl. J. Med.,* 301:298.
2. Braunstein, G., Vaitukaitis, J., Carbone, P., and Ross, G. (1973): Ectopic production of human chorionic gonadotropin by neoplasms. *Ann. Intern. Med.,* 78:39.
3. Christy, N. P. (1961): Adrenocorticotrophic activity in plasma of patients with Cushing's syndrome associated with pulmonary neoplasms. *Lancet.,* 1:85.
4. Dosogne-Guérin, M., Stolarczyk, A., and Borkowski, A. (1978): Prospective study of the α and β subunits of human chorionic gonadotropin in the blood of patients with various benign and malignant conditions. *Eur. J. Cancer,* 14:525.
5. Liddle, G. W., Nicholson, W. E., Island, D. P., Orth, D., Abe, K., and Lowder, S. (1962): Clinical and laboratory studies in ectopic humoral syndromes. *Recent Prog. Horm. Res.,* 25:283.
6. Meador, C. K., Liddle, G. W., Island, D. P., Nicholson, W. E., Lucas, C. P., Nuckton, J. G., and Luetscher, J. A. (1962): Cause of Cushing's syndrome in patients with tumours arising from "nonendocrine" tissue. *J. Clin. Endocrinol. Metab.,* 22:693.
7. Rees, L. H., and Ratcliffe, J. G. (1974): Review article: Ectopic hormone production by nonendocrine tumours. *Clin. Endocrinol.,* 3:263.
8. Rosen, S., Weintraub, B., Vaitukaitis, J., Sussman, J., Hershman, J., and Muggia, F. (1975): Placental proteins and their subunits as tumor markers. *Ann. Intern Med.,* 82:71.
9. Vaitukaitis, J., Ross, G., Braunstein, G., and Rayford, P. (1976): Gonadotropins and their subunits: basic and clinical studies. *Recent Prog. Horm. Res.,* 32:289.
10. Yalow, R. S., and Berson, S. A. (1973): Characteristics of "big ACTH" in human plasma and pituitary extracts. *J. Clin. Endocrinol. Metab.,* 36:415.

Medical Complications in Cancer Patients,
edited by J. Klastersky and M. J. Staquet.
Raven Press, New York © 1981.

Coagulopathies in Patients with Tumors

André Coune

Department of Internal Medicine and Henri Tagnon Laboratory of Clinical Investigation,
Jules Bordet Institute, 1000 Brussels, Belgium

This chapter is devoted to a review of several hemostatic disorders encountered in patients with tumors, the pathogenesis of which is related to a quantitative or a qualitative modification of one or more components of the coagulation and fibrinolysis systems. Disorders resulting from a primary change in the number and/or function of the blood platelets are discussed in another chapter. The association between a recurrent or a migratory thrombophlebitis and a tumor was mentioned by Trousseau in 1865 (67), and the occurrence of hypofibrinogenemia with a concomitant bleeding diathesis was reported in a case of disseminated prostatic carcinoma in 1930 (35). It is especially during the second half of this century, however, that several derangements of the hemostatic balance were recorded in patients with tumors. The presence of hemostatic troubles in patients with a malignancy seems to be rather frequent as shown by a recent study where 98% of the investigated patients had at least one abnormal coagulation test (62).

A classification of the coagulopathies according to the associated clinical findings is of limited interest because there is no constant specific relation between the primary disease, the clinical manifestations of the coagulopathy, and the abnormalities of the hemostatic factors. A classification of the coagulopathies based on the modifications of the latter factors is used in this review (Table 1). In order to facilitate the discussion of the possible pathogenic mechanisms and the usual laboratory tests for diagnosis, abbreviated pathways for normal blood coagulation are depicted in Fig. 1.

DISSEMINATED INTRAVASCULAR COAGULATION

Disseminated intravascular coagulation (DIC) is known under several denominations: consumption coagulopathy, defibrination syndrome, intravascular coagulation with fibrinolysis syndrome. As the pathophysiologic mechanisms of this coagulation disorder are not clearly delineated, none of these denominations can be considered satisfactory. However, it is well demonstrated that it is never a primary disease, but is initiated by the basic disease of the patient—in the present situation a neoplasm generally at a disseminated state—and/or by a

TABLE 1. *Coagulopathies in patients with tumors*

Fibrinogen consumption
 Disseminated intravascular coagulation
  Acute
  Chronic
 Primary fibrinolysis
  Tumor-associated
  Drug-associated

Increase in certain blood clotting factors

Circulating blood clotting inhibitors
 Against fibrin polymerization
 Against other steps of the coagulation process

Reduced or abnormal synthesis of blood clotting factors
 Acquired dysfibrinogenemia
 Deficiency in vitamin K-dependent factors
 Deficiency due to liver disease
 Deficiency due to cytotoxic chemotherapy

Isolated blood clotting factor deficiency

Thrombosis without consumption coagulopathy
 Dysproteinemic syndromes
 Drug-associated

---

secondary disease due to the basic illness, e.g., an infection with septic shock. The syndrome is characterized by the formation of fibrin thrombi, the consumption of specific plasma proteins and blood platelets, and the activation of fibrinolytic proenzymes (47). When symptomatic, the coagulopathy may present clinical signs ranging from localized or diffuse bleeding to unique or multiple vascular and/or valvular thromboses. Moreover, in some patients there may be, in the absence of any clinical sign of abnormal hemostasis, clear-cut laboratory evidence of a generalized hemostatic disorder (32). Such a situation is considered to indicate a well-compensated consumption coagulopathy that may nevertheless evolve into a clinically evident decompensated state under the influence of various trigger mechanisms.

Incidence

Reported data in the literature on the frequency distribution of the syndrome as related to its various etiologies differ according to the type of study performed and to the characteristics of the patient population in each hospital. In a retrospective series of 118 cases from a large Israeli medical center, the coagulopathy was related to cancer and leukemia in 6.8% of the patients (61), whereas in a prospective study of 45 cases from the Massachusetts General Hospital the syndrome was attributed to the same causes in 31% of the patients (18). On the other hand, a prospective study performed in 108 patients with various neoplasms (62) showed an incidence of consumption coagulopathy of 68%. It

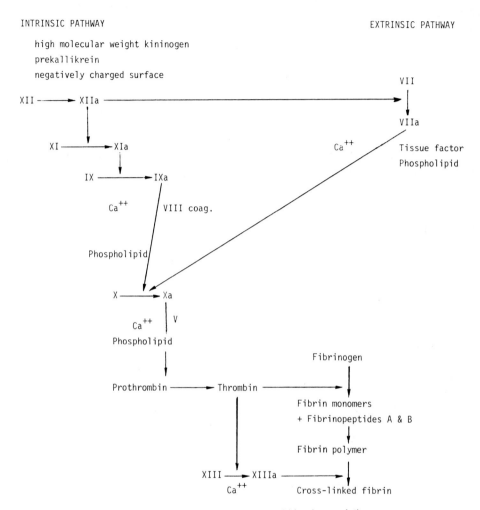

FIG. 1. Abbreviated pathways for normal blood coagulation.

is interesting to mention that in a major cancer center such as Memorial Sloan-Kettering Cancer Center a retrospective review of the medical records and coagulation laboratory data over a 3-year period provided only 89 cases of consumption coagulopathy (1), but it is probable that many cases of chronic coagulopathy were overlooked.

Clinical Presentation

When the compensation mechanisms of the organism are overwhelmed, the mode of presentation of the coagulopathy is the acute clinical form. In contrast, even incomplete compensation results in a chronic or subacute clinical form of the syndrome.

Acute Coagulopathy

The acute form of coagulopathy probably occurs less frequently than the chronic form in patients with solid tumors, but its spectacular mode of presentation usually results in its much earlier recognition (19). As no series exclusively constituted of acute cases in patients with a malignancy has been published, no adequate description of this form of coagulopathy is available. However, the few reported studies of cases from several etiologies as well as the study from the Memorial Sloan-Kettering Cancer Center where 66% of the cases had a low plasma fibrinogen level provide important clinical data (1).

The patient with an acute coagulopathy presents, within a period of a few hours to a few days, a rapid deterioration of his performance status, and a severe hemorrhagic diathesis ranging from multisite oozing to life-threatening bleeding develops. In at least 50% of cases, the skin is the site of the hemorrhage, but bleeding frequently occurs in the gastrointestinal tract and less frequently in the urinary tract, mucosae, body cavities, and central nervous system. The dermatologic manifestations are in fact the most prominent ones, appearing as flat or raised petechiae, purpura, wound bleeding, subcutaneous hematomas, acral cyanosis, and even acral gangrene (19,47). In contrast, thrombotic complications are rather infrequent in this form of coagulopathy, occurring in fewer than 10% of cases. In addition to the several features of a hemorrhagic diathesis, there may be other symptoms and clinical signs indicating dysfunction of several organs. It was previously considered that these manifestations were directly related to the coagulopathy, but more recent data suggest that many are in fact due to the primary disease or to the complication that triggered the coagulopathy, e.g., septic shock (19). Nevertheless, it is still possible that the deposition of fibrin microthrombi in the microvasculature is responsible for the dysfunction of some organs, as the impaired renal function noted after the onset of DIC in 39% of the patients in the Memorial Sloan-Kettering Cancer Center series (1) and as the generalized brain dysfunction syndrome described in 10 patients from the same hospital (17).

An acute coagulopathy may abruptly appear in acute leukemias, especially of the promyelocytic type (57). Its rapid diagnosis is very important because its hemorrhagic manifestations may be wrongly considered as due only to the central thrombocytopenia induced by the leukemia. In some of these patients, the manifestations of the hemorrhagic diathesis seem to be related to the lysis of the malignant cells induced by an effective chemotherapy (42).

Chronic Coagulopathy

The chronic form of coagulopathy is characterized by fluctuation over a period of months of the clinical signs and laboratory features of a low-grade consumption coagulopathy. Most of the information concerning this syndrome is provided by a recent review of 182 retrospectively collected cases (58). It should be stressed that at least 90% of these cases are associated with a malignant tumor already at a disseminated stage. Nevertheless, a chronic consumption coagulopathy may be related to a nonmalignant tumor, e.g., a multiple congenital hemangioma (1) or a hemangiomatous transformation of the spleen (60). The clinical manifestations are more proteiform than those of the acute form. Thrombophlebitis is seen at least once in 67% of the patients, whereas a hemorrhagic diathesis is present in 41%. Migratory episodes are recorded in 78% of the patients with venous thromboses. In a few cases this sign even precedes the clinical signs of a neoplasm. Arterial emboli that may affect any organ are evident in 25% of the patients; when occurring as microemboli in a large limb muscle, they may result in pain and tenderness, suggesting the presence of a venous thrombosis. In 10% of cases, the triad of venous thrombosis, hemorrhagic diathesis, and arterial embolism is simultaneously or sequentially observed. Patients with the longest clinical course have the highest chances of developing the various clinical manifestations of the syndrome. Postmortem examinations in 42 of 45 patients with arterial emboli have shown the presence of a nonbacterial thrombotic endocarditis in 74% of cases. The valvular lesions involve both left heart valves equally, whereas the tricuspid valve is involved in only a small percentage of cases. No bacterial colonization of the valvular lesions has been noted.

Another feature of the chronic form of consumption coagulopathy is the microangiopathic hemolytic anemia that may result in a clinical picture suggestive of Moschowitz's syndrome. In a series of 12 cases associated with a malignancy, each of the patients had a mucinous adenocarcinoma (9).

For many years it was considered that migratory thrombophlebitis, one of the clinical signs most frequently associated with chronic consumption coagulopathy, was especially suggestive of the presence of a carcinoma of the pancreas. In more recent studies, clinical signs due to this form of coagulopathy have been observed in a great variety of malignant tumors (58). However, lung cancer, prostate cancer, and acute promyelocytic leukemia are the neoplasms most frequently associated with this syndrome. Patients whose cancer is associated with a coagulopathy have a shorter survival than patients without a coagulopathy. Finally, it must be remembered that a neoplasm that occurs as frequently as breast cancer in women is rarely associated with a consumption coagulopathy.

Pathology

Although both forms of the consumption coagulopathy may be accompanied by thromboses of large vessels, the pathological hallmark of the syndrome is considered to be the formation of fibrin microthrombi, especially in the kidney, probably because of its well-developed microvasculature (54). However, there is no evident relationship between the duration and intensity of the coagulopathy and the number of these thrombi. In about one-third of cases, no thrombi at all are found at postmortem examination. Their absence is commonly attributed to local activation of the blood fibrinolytic activity that may induce the disappearance of the fibrin deposits, but some authors consider that fibrin deposition may in fact occur in extravascular sites (45).

Laboratory Diagnosis

At the present time there is no unequivocal routine procedure for diagnosing an intravascular coagulation process. Although chronic coagulopathies may exist without major alteration of the usual hemostatic tests, most cases of acute coagulopathy are characterized by modification of several hemostatic parameters. The following abnormalities are considered of value for screening: a prolonged prothrombin time (at least 3 sec over control), a decreased plasma fibrinogen concentration, and a decreased platelet count (19). In fact, the prothrombin time and platelet number are more frequently abnormal than the fibrinogen concentration, which may still be in the normal range. It may have been reduced by the coagulopathy process—but from an initially increased concentration, as is often observed in patients with disseminated cancer, even in the absence of complicating infections. The presence of a high percentage of megathrombocytes is indicative of the peripheral origin of the thromobocytopenia.

Abnormality of all these screening tests suggests the presence of a consumption coagulopathy. Unfortunately, it is not pathognomonic of the syndrome because other pathological processes related to the tumor or its treatment may account for some of these modifications, e.g., liver disease induced by previous chemotherapy, bone marrow depression due to widespread osseous metastasis, or previous extensive radiotherapy or chemotherapy. Therefore, confirmatory tests are needed to support the diagnosis of consumption coagulopathy.

The most frequently used confirmatory tests are based on the presence in the circulating blood of degradation products of the fibrinogen and fibrin molecules (FDP/fdp) (19). Some of these products induce a lengthening of the thrombin time and the reptilase time (40). Both tests can also be abnormal because of an isolated hypofibrinogenemia. In contrast to the thrombin time, the reptilase time is not influenced by heparin and can be used to follow the response of the coagulopathy to an anticoagulant treatment (41). The most useful tests are indeed the ones that directly measure the FDP/fdp blood concentration. Several procedures are available (19). The staphylococcal clumping test provides a measurement of the larger fragments X and Y (14). The tanned red cell hemagglutination inhibition test is sensitive to all degradation products (66), but can give false-negative values in the presence of an anti-D (Rh) antibody (36). The thrombo-Wellcotest based on the agglutination of latex particles coated with antibodies to the smaller fragments D and E is a frequently utilized rapid procedure (24). Although increased FDP/fdp concentration is measured in 95% of consumption coagulopathies, only values higher than 40 μg/ml should be considered characteristic of the syndrome, as moderate elevations are commonly noted in many other clinical conditions (66). On the other hand, the blood euglobulin lysis time is shortened and the circulating plasminogen level decreased in the rare instances when a disseminated intravascular fibrinogenolysis is concomitant to the consumption coagulopathy (47).

Quantification of some of the blood clotting factors is of no great value for the diagnosis of acute coagulopathy. It is a well-known fact that in normal people and those with a large variety of diseases blood clotting factor concentrations may be higher than 100%, and so the lowering by a consumption process may result in a value that is still within the normal range. Possible abnormalities of blood clotting factors V, VII, VIII, and X were investigated in a prospective study of 108 patients with a malignancy (62). The most consistent alteration was a significant depression of blood factor V level, observed in 53% of the cases. Values equal to or higher than 100% were found in 12% of the patients. On the other hand, it has been shown in patients with no clinical signs that a chronic consumption coagulopathy may be suspected when thromboplastin and thrombin generation is accelerated and when blood factor VIII coag and factor VIII ag are increased (43).

As formation of small amounts of thrombin in the circulating blood is considered to be the operating mechanism in the consumption coagulopathies (or at least in some of them), the detection in the patient's plasma of molecules resulting from the action of such a small quantity of thrombin may be another way of confirming the diagnosis. Soluble fibrin monomers may be recognized in the plasma by paracoagulation reactions, e.g., the ethanol gelation test (11) or the protamine sulfate test (33). The latter is not influenced by heparinization. Unfortunately, in 5 to 10% of patients with an acute coagulopathy these reactions may be negative (4). Circulating complexes of fibrinogen or fibrin with a plasma cold-insoluble globulin (CIg) have been reported in cases of consumption coagulopathy (49). This condition is popularly termed "cryofibrinogenemia." More sophisticated methods for detecting fibrin monomers, fibrinogen dimers, and fibrinogen polymers (fibrinogen complexed with various FDP/fdp) have been elaborated (4). They are based on polyacrylamide gel electrophoresis, gel exclusion chromatography, and affinity chromatography on insolubilized fibrinogen. All these techniques are time-consuming and cannot be used at the present time in routine laboratories. Nevertheless, measurement of these compounds will probably play a major role in the future for confirming the diagnosis in some consumption coagulopathies.

Fibrinopeptide A is a low-molecular weight peptide released from the fibrinogen molecule in the presence of a low thrombin concentration (50). It can be measured by a radioimmunoassay method, but its increase in the circulating blood is also observed in several other clinical conditions, e.g., systemic lupus erythematosus and renal transplant rejection.

When thrombin is formed in the systemic circulation, it combines rapidly with a plasma α_2-globulin, antithrombin III (56). This irreversible interaction results in a decreased plasma concentration of the active protein, which may be reduced to 10% of its normal value (5). Here again there are several drawbacks to a more common use of this test. Antithrombin III behaves as an acute phase reactant, and its blood level before the onset of the coagulopathy may be so much elevated that its combination with free thrombin may result in a decreased value that nevertheless remains within the normal range. It is also known that the elevation of the blood antithrombin III level may be due to the presence of a concomitant disease. Moreover, immunologic determination of antithrombin III levels seems to be of no use. Only the biologic antithrombin III levels should be determined. In conjunction with increased factor VIII coag and factor VIII ag levels, its decrease may be considered highly suggestive of a chronic consumption coagulopathy (43).

Estimation of the fibrinogen half-life is a cumbersome method that takes several days to obtain an accurate measurement. Therefore, it is of no use in cases of acute coagulopathy. On the other hand, it may be considered to be another useful method for detecting patients with a well-compensated chronic coagulopathy when the hemostatic tests are normal (32). Consumption of the fibrinogen molecules may occur in extravascular locations (e.g., the tumor itself or ascites), as shown by a very high FDP/fdp concentration in ascites due to peritoneal metastases of a malignant ovarian tumor (63). More recently, techniques based on computerized handling for following the fate of ^{125}I-fibrinogen through various physiological compartments have been elaborated; some of these parameters are useful for indicating nonintravascular fibrin build-up (55).

In patients who are considered candidates for treatment with heparin, plasma reptilase clotting time, protamine sulfate test, and plasma antithrombin III measurement, which are insensitive to heparinization, should be performed before starting the anticoagulant treatment, as they may be used as monitoring tests. Plasma antithrombin III levels are not affected by circulating FDP/fdp. Cases in which an anemia is associated with circulating red blood cell fragments (schistocytes) often present a microangiopathic hemolytic anemia in addition to the coagulopathy.

Differential Diagnosis

Although primary fibrino(geno)lysis seems to be a rare phenomenon, it is considered to be easily distinguished from consumption coagulopathy by its normal platelet count (27). Unfortunately, as stressed previously, thrombocytopenia may occur in cancer patients for several other reasons, and so the platelet count is not a helpful parameter for separating one syndrome from the other. The diagnosis of consumption coagulopathy should be based on more specific tests. A primary fibrino(geno)lysis should be considered when the circulating plasminogen level is low and there are no positive tests indicating the presence of small amounts of circulating thrombin.

Acquired hypofibrinogenemia, acquired dysfibrinogenemia, or both abnormalities may result in major alteration of some of the screening tests, suggestive of a consumption coagulopathy. For instance, plasma fibrinogen levels of less than 100 mg/dl, assessed by the coagulation method, induce marked lengthening of the prothrombin time and the thrombin time (4).

Other less frequent coagulopathies that may occur in patients with cancer are described later in this chapter. Their differentiation from a consumption coagulopathy is much easier.

Initiating Conditions

Malignant tumors as well as some benign tumors may be associated with a consumption coagulopathy. Giant hemangiomas may trigger a consumption coagulopathy, probably by inducing a mechanical injury to the vessel endothelium (19). In some solid malignant tumors and acute leukemias, cellular components able to initiate a consumption coagulopathy are probably released in the circulation. The appearance of an acute coagulopathy or the exacerbation of a pre-existing coagulopathy after the administration of active cytotoxic chemotherapy in some cases of acute leukemia seems to indicate that such a mechanism may be operative (42).

On the other hand, conditions secondary to the existence of a malignant tumor may be the cause of the hemostatic disorder. One of these conditions, systemic infection, is observed in 39% of patients with cancer who develop a consumption coagulopathy (1). Septicemia due to a Gram-negative organism is present in more than 50% of these patients. Mismatched transfusion, a rare event, may also be the trigger mechanism in patients requiring large amounts of blood.

Pathogenesis

It is generally considered that a consumption coagulopathy results from the formation in the systemic circulation of small amounts of thrombin that produce activation and consumption of several blood clotting factors as well as deposition of fibrin thrombi in the microvasculature (47).

In benign hemangiomas, the probable alteration of the vascular endothelial surface results in activation of blood clotting factor XII, which activates the intrinsic pathway of the coagulation cascade. Such a mechanism probably is also operative in the acute coagulopathies observed in systemic infections (47) where septicemia is associated with an activation of factor XII that secondarily activates prekallikrein into kallikrein and transforms plasminogen into active plasmin. Kallikrein formation is followed by a plasma increase in bradykinin that induces generalized vasodilatation and may be related to the hypotension measured in most of the coagulopathies associated with an infection. A decreased blood complement C3 level is also frequently observed.

Consumption coagulopathies occurring in cancer patients without systemic infection are never associated with activation of factor XII. Once considered to result from the release of tissue thromboplastin from the malignant cells into the vascular compartment, recent data do not confirm this hypothesis. Analysis of the procoagulant activity in some normal and malignant human tissues revealed that it is due in normal cells to a thromboplastic factor that is lacking in most malignant cells. On the other hand, the latter cells contain a diisopropylfluorophosphate (DFP)-sensitive serine protease capable of initiating blood coagulation by direct activation of factor X, bypassing the extrinsic pathway of the coagulation cascade, which is mandatory for the action of the thromboplastic factor present in benign cells (26). Direct activation of blood clotting factor X by mucin-rich carcinomatous tissues was described a few years ago (25). As carcinoma of the prostate is a tumor known to be associated with consumption coagulopathies, it is interesting to emphasize that two DFP-sensitive serine proteases capable of limited proteolysis on the fibrinogen and fibrin molecules have been described in the benign hyperplastic tissues as well as in the carcinomatous tissues of this gland (21). Finally, two neutral proteases active against several blood clotting factors, including fibrinogen, are known to be present in granulocytes (23). One may wonder if the enzymes described in the prostate and in the granulocytes may account in some patients for consumption coagulopathies independent from the formation of thrombin as was previously suspected (46).

Coming back to the classic point of view, it is considered, according to experimental data collected in animal studies, that as soon as small quantities of thrombin are formed in the systemic circulation fibrinopeptide A and later fibrinopeptide B are cleaved from the fibrinogen molecules. The large fibrinogen derivatives circulate as soluble fibrin monomers. The fibrinopeptides may cause systemic or pulmonary vasoconstriction. Thrombi of fibrin may be deposited in the microvasculature of several organs (e.g., kidney and brain). Thrombin acts on several other blood clotting factors—V, VIII, XIII—resulting in their activation and ultimate clearing by the reticuloendothelial system (4,19). Such a process leads to a marked decrease in the plasma concentration of these factors. The clearance of the activated forms of some other factors (e.g., IX and X) seems to be rapid in this syndrome. Thrombin also produces platelet aggregation, a phenomenon that contributes to platelet removal from the circulation.

As most consumption coagulopathies are characterized by an increased FDP/fdp concentration, thrombin cannot be considered the only operative enzymatic factor. Concomitant or secondary activation of plasminogen into plasmin by release of tissue plasminogen activator, kallikrein formation, or some other not yet defined process may result in the proteolysis of fibrinogen, fibrin, and some other blood clotting factors (V, VIII, XIII), increasing by this mechanism their rate of disappearance from the circulating blood (4). In most cases this elevated FDP/fdp concentration is not accompanied by signs suggestive of a generalized fibrino(geno)lysis. It must therefore be assumed that the process is a local one, detectable only by the passage in the systemic circulation of the fibrinogen or/and fibrin degradation products. According to the proteolytic enzyme concentration and the duration of the process, the degradation results in FDP/fdp of several molecular weights. Some of the larger fragments are potent inhibitors of fibrin formation, whereas the smaller ones inhibit platelet aggregation (19). The largest fibrinogen derivatives probably form soluble complexes with fibrin monomers. Local fibrino(geno)lysis may be one of the mechanisms that can account for the frequently reported absence at postmortem examination of fibrin thrombi in the microvasculature of patients who died with a consumption coagulopathy.

Treatment

When the presence of a consumption coagulopathy is strongly suggested by the results of the hemostatic tests, the physician in most cases hesitates about the measures to be taken. In spite of the lack of randomized clinical trials in this field, it appears from the available data that the therapeutic attitude depends on the clinical presentation of the coagulopathy.

Acute Coagulopathy

First, a possible initiating condition secondary to the presence of a tumor (e.g., a systemic infection) should be looked for. In patients with septic shock, immediate and aggressive measures to treat the infection and maintain an adequate blood pressure must be taken, although the prognosis is rather poor. Heparin administration does not seem to be beneficial in coagulopathies triggered by an infection (20). However, reappraisal of the therapeutic attitude is mandatory if there is some evidence that another mechanism may be operative. In cancer patients and especially in those with marked immunosuppression, prompt treatment of their infections can avoid the development of the ominous coagulopathy.

In the other cases where the acute coagulopathy is directly related to the presence of a disseminated tumor, only specific and adequate therapy of the neoplasm can result in the disappearance of the hemostatic disorder as is known to happen in patients with a generalized prostate cancer successfully treated with an estrogenic compound (64). If no effective antitumor therapy is available, administration of heparin only induces a short remission of the coagulopathy and is probably not worthwhile. However, there are two situations where anticoagulant therapy may be of some help: in patients with a tumor sensitive to the administered treatment, when some delay must be expected before a sufficient reduction of the tumor masses is achieved, and in patients with a sensitive tumor when administration of an active chemotherapy may induce or exacerbate an acute coagulopathy by rapid destruction of a high number of malignant cells. The latter situation is observed in some cases of acute promyelocytic leukemia, and some authors propose to start heparin therapy together with the administration of chemotherapy in these leukemias (28).

When an anticoagulant treatment with heparin is started in a patient with a malignancy, close medical supervision should be afforded. The contraindications to the administration of heparin are well known (59), but in these patients some of the contraindications may be considered relative because of the life-threatening situation due to the acute coagulopathy. There is still much controversy about the administration regimens of heparin (69). Nevertheless, the following rules may be proposed.

The usual daily dose ranges from 300 to 500 units/kg/24 hr. A study in patients with thromboembolic disorders showed that continuous intravenous infusion of heparin is associated with fewer bleeding complications than the intermittent pulse method and is as efficacious (59), and as a result, the continuous infusion method is becoming more frequently utilized. In some hospitals a first intravenous push dose of 5,000 to 10,000 units of heparin is given, followed by a 24-hr infusion of a 20,000-unit dose. More recently, certain centers have started treatment of acute consumption coagulopathy with a smaller dose (2,500 to 5,000 units) given subcutaneously every 8 to 12 hr (5), but at the present time there is no general agreement about the efficacy of this treatment. In case of failure of this minidose regimen, it seems appropriate to administer the larger doses as indicated above. Adequate monitoring of the anticoagulant treatment with heparin is another field of controversy that cannot be discussed here (69).

The development of an acute coagulopathy by depressing an already decreased blood platelet count may result in values so low that the risk of an intracerebral hemorrhage becomes very high if heparinization is to be started. Therefore, platelets are transfused to restore the platelet count to at least 50,000/mm^3, thereby making the anticoagulant therapy safer.

Response to the heparin treatment is indicated by an increase in the plasma level of blood clotting factor V and fibrinogen, which becomes apparent during the first 48 hr if no concomitant liver disease is present (18). The thrombin and reptilase times, which are an indirect measure of the FDP/fdp level, respond more slowly. Although this level usually starts decreasing after 24 hr of heparin therapy, it may still be elevated after 1 week if its initial value was markedly increased. The blood platelet count is not a reliable parameter for evaluating the response to the treatment because its increase in cases of regression of the coagulopathy is rather slow and frequently incomplete, as several other factors play a role in the thrombocytopenia in cancer patients. The persistence of marked thrombocytopenia when all other hemostatic parameters have reverted to normal raises the strong possibility of a heparin-induced thrombocytopenia (3).

As magnification of the inhibitory properties of plasma antithrombin III is the mechanism of action of heparin, the probability of depletion of this plasma protein, despite adequate heparinization, should be considered in cases that do not respond to heparin treatment. If the dosage reveals a low plasma level of antithrombin III, administration of antithrombin III-containing concentrates may be expected to control the coagulopathy (4). These concentrates have been used on a rather limited scale, but their administration has not been associated with clinical bleeding.

Utilization of oral anticoagulant drugs (e.g., warfarin) has been suggested, but clinical data are scarce and do not suggest that it is of value in the treatment of acute coagulopathies.

Blood clotting factor replacement therapy should never be attempted as an initial treatment, because it may provide additional substrates to the proteolytic factors that started the coagulopathy (7). Moreover, some of the factors are in an activated form, and their administration may lead to vascular thrombosis. When it becomes apparent that the coagulopathy does not respond to the measures detailed previously and that diffuse bleeding is occurring, a detailed analysis of the blood clotting factors of the patient should be performed to indicate the specific replacement therapy needed. Heparin administration should be continued during this additional therapy in order to minimize possible thrombotic manifestations. Blood factors may be given in the form of fresh frozen plasma, cryoprecipitate, prothrombin complex concentrates (II, VII, IX, X), and fibrinogen. The latter factor may be especially valuable in patients whose fibrinogen liver synthesis is decreased by a concomitant liver disease or by administration of L-asparaginase. Whole blood transfusions are required in patients with marked anemia due to major diffuse hemorrhages. The role of platelet transfusion was already discussed.

A possible role for antiaggregating drugs has not been defined. Antifibrinolytic therapy was widely used alone several years ago, but seems to be of value in only a very low percentage of cases (18). It may be tried in patients who do not respond to the measures delineated above and in those with signs of a concomitant disseminated fibrino(geno)lysis. Several proteolytic inhibitors are available: apronitin, epsilon aminocaproic acid, tranexamic acid. Epsilon aminocaproic acid is usually given slowly at an initial intravenous dose of 5 g, followed by 2 g every 1 to 2 hr for 24 hr or until diffuse hemorrhage stops (4). Careful monitoring of the patient is required during this therapy because of the major side effects of the drug: hypotension, ventricular arrhythmias, and hypokalemia. Antifibrinolytic therapy should never be given alone, i.e., without adequate anticoagulant treatment to prevent the appearance of diffuse intravascular thromboses, a life-threatening complication of this therapy (30).

Chronic Coagulopathy

The consensus is that the most important factor for controlling chronic coagulopathy is adequate treatment of the tumor. However, this is not feasible if the chronic coagulopathy is the first sign of the presence of a tumor, if no efficient treatment is available for the type of tumor, or when the tumor becomes resistant to a previously effective therapy. As indicated previously, patients with this form of coagulopathy may develop major and sometimes lethal complications, which may be prevented by adequate anticoagulant therapy. The following therapeutic modalities result from an analysis of cases collected in the literature (58). These recommendations are in fact based on data collected from heterogeneous populations of patients in which some were treated with cytotoxic drugs as well as with anticoagulants.

Therapy with heparin seems to be the most effective anticoagulant treatment in chronic consumption coagulopathies, being active in 78% of the cases reported. These results seem to be much superior to those obtained by the use of oral anticoagulant drugs (e.g., warfarin, which corrects the hemostatic disorder in only 19% of cases). Moreover, a few patients who did not respond to heparin were given warfarin without success, whereas 12 of 26 warfarin failures did respond to subsequent heparin therapy. Another phenomenon showing the role of heparin in controlling the coagulopathy is the recurrence of the clinical signs of the coagulopathy in 19 patients successfully treated with heparin at the time the anticoagulant treatment was interrupted. Many anecdotal cases illustrating this phenomenon are well known to physicians working in this field. Heparin should be started at the same dosage as for acute coagulopathy, and the dosage should be maintained at least during the period in which clinical signs (e.g., thrombophlebitis) are present. Thereafter, provided hemostatic parameters are normalized, heparin may be administered by the subcutaneous route at a dose of 5,000 units every 8 or 12 hr for a long duration, provided the physician performs a careful follow-up of the patient to detect possible complications of this long-term treatment, e.g., thrombocytopenia, alopecia, and bone aseptic necrosis. There are no known criteria for discontinuing the anticoagulant therapy; but in patients who have had episodes of thrombosis, recurrence is very likely if anticoagulation is stopped unless there has been marked shrinking of the tumor mass after antineoplastic therapy.

The danger of antifibrinolytic therapy in the absence of previous control of the coagulation process is the same as in the acute form of the coagulopathy, and there are probably no good reasons to resort to it in the chronic form because of the high rate of vascular thromboses. Likewise, in cases characterized by hypofibrinogenemia, intravenous administration of fibrinogen has been associated with acute thrombotic episodes (58).

PRIMARY FIBRINO(GENO)LYSIS

Tumor-Associated

It was considered several years ago that in some cases of disseminated malignancy, especially of prostatic origin, hypofibrinogenemia resulted from a primary fibrino(geno)lytic process (65). However, at the present time most investigators consider that this phenomenon is in fact concomitant or secondary to a consumption coagulopathy (19). In most cancers associated with such a coagulopathy, the proteolysis probably occurs in localized parts of the body, its presence being demonstrated by a rise in the circulating FDP/fdp concentration. However, in some rare cases, a systemic fibrino(geno)lysis is present, as indicated by a much shortened blood euglobulin lysis time and a low blood plasminogen concentration (37). The differentiation of primary fibrino(geno)lysis from DIC is considered possible, the former being characterized by a normal blood platelet count (27). Unfortunately, as discussed previously, this parameter is rarely helpful because of the various other causes of thrombocytopenia in patients with a disseminated cancer. In some cases considered to be typical primary fibrino(geno)lysis, heparin administration has resulted in a rapid disappearance of the hemostatic disorder; such a response has been interpreted as indicating that a consumption coagulopathy was in fact the primary disorder (47). Nevertheless, as antithrombin III has inhibitory properties against several proteases, including plasmin, this response to heparin cannot be considered satisfactory proof of the presence of a consumption coagulopathy. Malignant tissues contain serine proteases active at least on one blood clotting factor. It is probable that these enzymes do not have such a strict specificity and that they may induce limited proteolysis of other blood proteins. The two proteolytic factors detected in prostatic carcinomatous tissues are active on fibrinogen and fibrin, and one may wonder if the release in the systemic circulation of such enzymes cannot result in a complex situation of concomitant consumption coagulopathy and fibrino(geno)lysis (10).

Primary local fibrino(geno)lysis seems to occur in rare instances. A local hemorrhagic diathesis at the site of a subcutaneous metastatic nodule from a giant cell carcinoma of the lung was observed after a biopsy had been performed, and secretion of a plasminogen activator by the malignant tissue was demonstrated (22). An example of extravascular fibrino(geno)lysis may be the occurrence of high concentrations of FDP/fdp in ascites caused by peritoneal metastases of an ovarian carcinoma (63).

As the operating mechanisms of the consumption coagulopathy and the fibrino(geno)lytic phenomenon associated with a tumor are not well delineated, well-defined therapeutic regimens cannot be recommended even when the clinical picture is highly suggestive of a primary fibrino(geno)lysis. At the present time therapy with fibrinolytic inhibitors alone cannot be considered a safe therapeutic regimen because of the potential risk of inducing massive thromboses. It is therefore suggested that a combination of heparin and a fibrinolytic inhibitor be used, as indicated in the treatment of the acute consumption coagulopathy.

Drug-Associated

Painful subungual hemorrhages have been observed in a few patients treated for a solid tumor with doxorubicin hydrochloride. Complete resolution generally occurred about 6 weeks after cessation of the cytotoxic therapy. Coagulation studies carried out in 10 patients receiving doxorubicin hydrochloride according to a weekly schedule demonstrated an increase in the blood FDP/fdp and plasmin levels in some of them. Complementary investigation suggests that this cytotoxic antibiotic can activate the blood fibrinolytic system (6).

INCREASE IN SOME BLOOD CLOTTING FACTORS

Increased activity of certain blood clotting factors has been reported in patients suffering from a malignant tumor without any complication. An increase in the plasma level of factors II, V, VII, VIII, IX, and X has been reported as well as elevation of the fibrinogen level (43,62). As a matter of fact, hyperfibrinogenemia was measured in 46% of the patients in one study (62), and in many of these cases an increased FDP/fdp level was reported. These coagulation abnormalities are considered as indicating the presence of a hypercoagulable state in these patients, i.e., a low-grade subclinical chronic consumption coagulopathy with a compensatory overproduction of the consumed blood clotting factors. As described previously, accelerated rates of thromboplastin and thrombin generation, as well as the presence of a decreased functional antithrombin III level with a normal immunologic antithrombin III level, are observed in some of these patients (43). No data are available about therapeutic modalities for these subclinical hypercoagulable states, but intermittent heparin administered subcutaneously is suggested, as in the maintenance schedule used in the chronic form of consumption coagulopathy.

OTHER COAGULOPATHIES IN PATIENTS WITH CANCER

Circulating Blood Clotting Inhibitors (Excluding FDP/fdp)

Action on Fibrin Polymerization

Inhibition of the fibrin monomer aggregation process is observed in dysproteinemic syndromes where the pathologic gamma globulin binds, probably through its Fab sites, to fibrin (16). This abnormality results in transparent clots with narrow fibrin strands. According to several studies, the inhibitor is present in 14 to 71% of patients with immunoglobulin (Ig) G myeloma, but may also be present in IgA, IgM, and light-chain dysproteinemias. Its presence is not necessarily associated with a hemorrhagic diathesis, which seems to be more frequent in patients with IgA myeloma and macroglobulinemia. As more than one hemostatic defect may occur in the dysproteinemic syndromes, the bleeding disorders observed in these clinical conditions may be due to multiple factors (38).

Interference with fibrin monomer aggregation results in the prolongation of the thrombin time and the reptilase time. When hemorrhagic manifestations are present, they may improve if cytotoxic chemotherapy is successful and induces a fall in the blood paraprotein level. A much faster fall may be obtained after repeated plasmapheresis (38).

Action on Other Steps of the Blood Coagulation Process

Inhibitors against factor VIII have been described in some patients with a dysproteinemic syndrome or a malignant lymphoma (15,68). In dysproteinemic syndromes also, nonspecific inhibitors of the thromboplastin generation time have been described (38).

REDUCED OR ABNORMAL SYNTHESIS OF BLOOD CLOTTING FACTORS

Dysfibrinogenemia

Synthesis by the liver of a functionally abnormal fibrinogen molecule is observed in only a few clinical conditions. In patients with cancer it may be due to the presence of a concomitant acute or chronic liver disease (39), a hepatoma as primary tumor (29), or administration of L-asparaginase in the chemotherapeutic regimen (12). In the latter case, the intrinsically abnormal fibrinogen molecule that probably results from a reaction between L-asparaginase and the asparagine residues of fibrinogen has a decreased survival unaffected by heparin administration (12).

Acquired dysfibrinogenemia may be clinically inapparent or may be associated with a hemorrhagic diathesis or with a thrombotic diathesis. It is characterized in most cases by prolonged thrombin and reptilase times, and by a normal plasma fibrinogen concentration when measured by an immunological method and a low concentration when measured by a coagulation method. Dysfibrinogenemia may result in defective fibrin polymerization (29). At the end of the treatment with L-asparaginase, the liver progressively resumes the synthesis of normal fibrinogen molecules. In the other cases when hemorrhagic manifestations require treatment, administration of normal fibrinogen may be effective, as has been demonstrated in scarce data from cases of congenital dysfibrinogenemia.

Specific Deficiency in Vitamin K-Dependent Factors

Four blood clotting factors (II, VII, IX, X) require vitamin K for their synthesis. In the absence of this vitamin, the proteins synthesized by the liver are in fact biologically inactive clotting factors.

When the plasma levels of these four factors are much depressed, a hemorrhagic diathesis becomes apparent. The diagnosis is made by finding a prolonged prothrombin time and partial thromboplastin time, which are corrected by adding normal plasma to the patient's plasma, thereby excluding the possibility of a circulating anticoagulant (8).

In patients with a malignancy, depletion of vitamin K may be observed in cases of malabsorption due to prolonged malignant obstructive jaundice, prolonged diarrhea, or intestinal sterilization (8). In the latter condition a preexisting lowered intake of vitamin K is necessary to make development of the coagulopathy possible.

Per os administration of water-soluble analogs of vitamin K (e.g., menadione 50 mg) that are well absorbed from the gastrointestinal tract may be used. Phytonadione may be given by the parenteral route at the same dosage.

Deficiency of Blood Clotting Factors Due to Liver Disease

Concomitant liver cirrhosis, massive metastatic liver involvement, or major liver toxicity due to cytotoxic drugs (e.g., methotrexate, 6-mercaptopurine, cytosine arabinoside, or carmustine) may result in a marked decrease of the synthesis of the vitamin K-dependent blood clotting factors and even of factors V and XI (8). These hemostatic disorders may be associated with a consumption coagulopathy. If the depletion is especially one of the vitamin K-dependent factors, administration of vitamin K or one of its analogs is of no use. In cases of life-threatening bleeding diathesis, administration of prothrombin complex concentrates may be started, but the risk of thrombotic complications seems to be rather high in patients with active liver disease; therefore, one may consider adding 5 units of heparin per milliliter of reconstituted material.

Deficiency of Blood Clotting Factors Due to Cytotoxic Chemotherapy

The abnormal synthesis of fibrinogen induced by L-asparaginase has been reported. Mithramycin is known to be associated in at least 50% of the patients treated with a hemorrhagic diathesis due to depression of factors II, V, VII, and X, probably by an action on their synthesis. In fact, mithramycin seems also to induce an increase in the blood fibrinolytic activity and to alter platelet function (48). Finally, actinomycin D administration is reported to be associated in some cases with a deficiency of the vitamin K-dependent blood clotting factors (52). All these disorders are transient.

Isolated Blood Clotting Factor Deficiency

A reduced plasma concentration or an inactive form of factor XIII (plasma transglutaminase) has been reported in patients with disseminated cancer and in those with acute leukemia (51,53). In one study of patients with acute leukemia, a factor XIII activity of less than 40% of normal was associated with a marked defect of fibrin cross linking as shown by SDS-polyacrylamide gel electrophoresis (53). The deficiency or dysfunction of this factor may play a role in the bleeding diathesis observed in some of these patients. If the plasma level of the factor is very low and the hemorrhage severe, fresh frozen plasma may be administered every 6 to 8 days at a 5 ml/kg dose.

Another deficiency reported in patients with acute leukemia is characterized by decreased plasma levels of factors V and X. As with the former abnormality, its pathogenesis is not elucidated (31).

An isolated factor X deficiency is known to occur as a rare complication of primary amyloidosis, probably induced by a selective absorption of the factor on the amyloid substance (34).

Depression of blood clotting factors apparently not due to circulating inhibitors has been reported in some dysproteinemic syndromes; affected factors are II, V, VII, VIII, and X (38).

THROMBOSIS WITHOUT A CONSUMPTION COAGULOPATHY

Thrombotic manifestations have been described not infrequently in dysproteinemic syndromes, although their cause has not been elucidated (38). Patients treated with estrogenic compounds may also present venous thromboses (13). As a reduced antithrombin III plasma level has been observed in women taking estrogen-containing contraceptives, one may wonder if such a mechanism is also operative in these cancer patients (2).

CONCLUSIONS

This review shows clearly that patients with tumors may present hemostatic disorders ranging from minor or life-threatening bleeding to venous and/or arterial thrombotic manifestations. Although some of these confusing clinical syndromes are probably due to a single well-defined defect, it is now quite evident that many interfering factors play a role in the development of one of the more frequent coagulopathies, disseminated intravascular coagulation. Until now no satisfactory treatment has been elaborated to control these hemostatic disorders, and in most cases reversal to a normal hemostatic situation can be obtained only by a marked reduction of the number of malignant cells. Further progress in the control of the coagulopathies associated with a malignancy will probably result from a better knowledge of (a) the physiological properties and interactions of each of the factors involved in normal hemostasis, including platelet and vessel endothelium (44); (b) the different mechanisms that can activate these factors; (c) the major catabolic pathways and catabolic sites in the organism of the clotting and fibrinolytic factors and inhibitors; and (d) the isolation and identification of the molecules released by the malignant cells capable of activating one or several hemostatic factors. Accumulation of these data may be the first step to devising therapeutic modalities specifically directed at inhibiting activation of the hemostatic factor(s) involved in the more common coagulopathies. Such a therapy would be particularly helpful in patients with a chronic consumption coagulopathy whose life is immediately more jeopardized by the possible thrombotic manifestations of the coagulopathy than by the dissemination of the malignancy.

REFERENCES

1. Al-Mondhiry, H. (1975): Disseminated intravascular coagulation: experience in a major cancer center. *Thromb. Diath. Haemorrh.,* 34:181–193.
2. Ambrus, J. L., Ambrus, C. M., Lillie, M. A., Browne, B. J., Hanson, F. W., Niswander, K., Witul, M., Jung, O. S., and Bartfay-Szabo, A. (1976): Effect of various estrogen treatment schedules on antithrombin III levels. *Res. Commun. Chem. Pathol. Pharmacol.,* 14:543–549.
3. Babcock, R. B., Dumper, C. W., and Scharfman, W. B. (1976): Heparin-induced immune thrombocytopenia. *N. Engl. J. Med.,* 295:237–241.
4. Bick, R. L. (1978): Disseminated intravascular coagulation and related syndromes: etiology, patho-physiology, diagnosis and management. *Am. J. Hematol.,* 5:265–282.
5. Bick, R. L., Dukes, M. L., Wilson, W. L., and Fekete, L. F. (1977): Antithrombin III (AT-III) as a diagnostic aid in disseminated intravascular coagulation. *Thromb. Res.,* 10:721–729.
6. Bick, R. L., Fekete, L. F., and Wilson, W. L. (1976): Adriamycin and fibrinolysis. *Thromb. Res.,* 8:467–475.
7. Bick, R. L., Schmalhorst, W. R., and Fekete, L. (1976): Disseminated intravascular coagulation and blood component therapy. *Transfusion,* 16:361–365.
8. Bowie, E. J. W., and Owen, C. A., Jr. (1977): Hemostatic failure in clinical medicine. *Semin. Hematol.,* 14:341–364.
9. Brain, M. C., Azzopardi, J. G., Baker, L. R., Pineo, G. F., Robert, P. D., and Dacie, J. V. (1970): Microangiopathic haemolytic anemia and mucin-formation adenocarcinoma. *Br. J. Haematol.,* 18:183–193.
10. Brassinne, C., Coune, A., Nijs, M., and Tagnon, H. (1976): Characterization of two direct fibrinogenolytic activities and of one proteolytic inhibitor activity in the human prostate. *Thromb. Res.,* 8:803–818.
11. Breen, F. A., Jr., and Tullis, J. L. (1968): Ethanol gelation: a rapid screening test for intravascular coagulation. *Ann. Intern. Med.,* 69:1197–1206.
12. Brodsky, I., Kahn, S. B., Vash, G., Rosse, M., and Petkov, G. (1971): Fibrinogen survival with (^{75}Se) selenomethionine during L-asparaginase therapy. *Br. J. Haematol.,* 20:477–487.
13. Byar, D. P. (1972): Treatment of prostatic cancer: studies by the Veterans Administration Cooperative Urological Research Group. *Bull. NY Acad. Med.,* 48:751–766.
14. Carvalho, A. C., Ellman, L. L., and Colman, R. W. (1974): A comparison of the staphylococcal-clumping test and an agglutination test for detection of fibrinogen degradation products. *Am. J. Clin. Pathol.,* 62:107–112.
15. Castaldi, P. A., and Penny, R. (1970): A macroglobulin with inhibitor activity against coagulation factor VIII. *Blood,* 35:370–376.
16. Coleman, M., Vigliano, E. M., Weksler, M. E., and Nachman, R. L. (1972): Inhibition of fibrin monomer polymerization by lambda myeloma globulins. *Blood,* 39:210–223.
17. Collins, R. C., Al-Mondhiry, H., Chernik, N. L., and Posner, J. B. (1975): Neurologic manifestations of intravascular coagulation in patients with cancer. *Neurology (Minneap.),* 25:795–806.
18. Colman, R. W., Robboy, S. J., and Minna, J. D. (1972): Disseminated intravascular coagulation (DIC): an approach. *Am. J. Med.,* 52:679–689.
19. Colman, R. W., Robboy, S. J., and Minna, J. D. (1979): Disseminated intravascular coagulation: a reappraisal. *Annu. Rev. Med.,* 30:359–374.
20. Corrigan, J. J., Jr., and Jordan, C. M. (1970): Heparin therapy in septicemia with disseminated intravascular coagulation: effect on mortality and on correction of hemostatic defects. *N. Engl. J. Med.,* 283:778–782.
21. Coune, A., Brassinne, C., and Nijs, M. (1979): Proteolytic and fibrinolytic factors in the human prostate. *Thromb. Haemost.,* 41:628–630.
22. Davidson, J. F., McNicol, G. P., Frank, G. L., Anderson, T. J., and Douglas, A. S. (1969): Plasminogen-activator producing tumor. *Br. Med. J.,* 1:88–91.
23. Egbring, R., Schmidt, W., Fuchs, G., and Havemann, K. (1977): Demonstration of granulocytic proteases in plasma of patients with acute leukemia and septicemia with coagulation defects. *Blood,* 49:219–231.
24. Ellman, L., Carvalho, A., and Colman, R. W. (1973): The Thrombo-Wellcotest as a screening test for disseminated intravascular coagulation. *N. Engl. J. Med.,* 288:633–634.
25. Gordon, S. G., Franks, J. J., and Lewis, B. (1975): Cancer procoagulant A: a factor X activating procoagulant from malignant tissue. *Thromb. Res.,* 6:127–137.

26. Gordon, S. G., Franks, J. J., and Lewis, B. (1979): Comparison of procoagulant activities in extracts of normal and malignant human tissue. *J. Natl. Cancer Inst.*, 62:773–776.
27. Gralnick, H. R. (1971): Intravascular coagulation. I. Differential diagnosis and conditioning mechanisms. *Postgrad. Med.*, 62:68–75.
28. Gralnick, H. R., Bagley, J., and Abrell, E. (1972): Heparin treatment for the hemorrhagic diathesis of acute promyelocytic leukemia. *Am. J. Med.*, 52:167–174.
29. Gralnick, H. R., Givelber, H., and Abrams, E. (1978): Dysfibrinogenemia associated with hepatoma. Increased carbohydrate content of the fibrinogen molecule. *N. Engl. J. Med.*, 299:221–226.
30. Gralnick, H. R., and Greipp, P. (1971): Thrombosis with epsilon aminocaproic acid therapy. *Am. J. Clin. Pathol.*, 56:151–154.
31. Gralnick, H. R., and Henderson, E. (1970): Acquired coagulation factor deficiencies in leukemia. *Cancer*, 26:1097–1101.
32. Gralnick, H. R., Marchesi, S., and Givelber, H. (1972): Intravascular coagulation in acute leukemia. Clinical and subclinical abnormalities. *Blood*, 40:709–718.
33. Gurewich, V., and Hutchinson, B. E. (1971): Detection of intravascular coagulation by a serial-dilution protamine sulfate test. *Ann. Intern. Med.*, 75:895–902.
34. Howell, M. (1963): Acquired factor X deficiency associated with systematized amyloidosis—A report of a case. *Blood*, 21:739–744.
35. Jürgens, R., and Trautwein, H. (1930): Über Fibrinopenie (Fibrinogenopenie) bei Erwachsenen, nebst Bemerkungen über die Herkunft des Fibrinogens. *Dtsch. Ark. Klin. Med.*, 169:28–43.
36. Kickler, T., and Bell, W. R. (1977): False-negative test for fibrinogen-fibrin degradation products. *Am. J. Clin. Pathol.*, 68:78–80.
37. Kwaan, H. C. (1972): Disorders of fibrinolysis. *Med. Clin. North Am.*, 56:163–176.
38. Lackner, H. (1973): Hemostatic abnormalities associated with dysproteinemias. *Semin. Hematol.*, 10:125–133.
39. Lane, D. A., Scully, M. F., Thomas, D. P., Kakkar, V. V., Woolf, I. L., and Williams, R. (1977): Acquired dysfibrinogenemia in acute and chronic liver disease. *Br. J. Haematol.*, 35:301–308.
40. Larrieu, M. J., Rigollot, C., and Marder, V. J. (1972): Comparative effects of fibrinogen degradation fragments D and E on coagulation. *Br. J. Haematol.*, 22:719–733.
41. Latallo, Z. S., and Teisseyre, E. (1971): Evaluation of reptilase-R and thrombin clotting time in the presence of fibrinogen degradation products and heparin. *Scand. J. Haematol.*, 13:261–266.
42. Leavey, R. A., Kahn, S. B., and Brodsky, I. (1970): Disseminated intravascular coagulation—A complication of chemotherapy in acute myelomonocytic leukemia. *Cancer*, 26:142–145.
43. Losito, R., Beaudry, P., Valderrama, J. C., Cousineau, L., and Longpre, B. (1977): Antithrombin III and factor VIII in patients with neoplasms. *Am. J. Clin. Pathol.*, 68:258–262.
44. Majerus, P. W., and Miletich, J. P. (1978): Relationships between platelets and coagulation factors in hemostasis. *Annu. Rev. Med.*, 29:41–49.
45. Mant, M. J., and King, E. G. (1979): Severe acute disseminated intravascular coagulation. A reappraisal of its pathophysiology, clinical significance and therapy based on 47 patients. *Am. J. Med.*, 67:557–563.
46. Merskey, C. (1973): Defibrination syndrome or. . . ? *Blood*, 41:599–603.
47. Minna, J. D., Robboy, S. J., and Colman, R. W. (1974): *Disseminated Intravascular Coagulation in Man.* Charles C Thomas, Springfield, Ill.
48. Monto, R. W., Talley, R. W., Caldwell, M. J., Levin, W. C., and Guest, M. M. (1969): Observations on the mechanism of hemorrhagic toxicity in mithramycin (NSC 24559) therapy. *Cancer Res.*, 29:697–704.
49. Mosseson, M. W. (1977): Cold-insoluble globulin (CIg), a circulating cell surface protein. *Thromb. Haemost.*, 38:742–750.
50. Nossel, H. L., Ti, M., Kaplan, K. L., Spanondis, K., Soland, T., and Butler, V. P., Jr. (1976): The generation of fibrinopeptide A in clinical blood samples: evidence for thrombin activity. *J. Clin. Invest.*, 58:1136–1144.
51. Nussbaum, M., and Morse, B. S. (1964): Plasma fibrin stabilizing factor activity in various diseases. *Blood*, 23:669–678.
52. Olson, R. E. (1964): Vitamin K-induced prothrombin formation: Antagonism by actinomycin D. *Science*, 145:926–928.

53. Rasche, H., Dietrich, M., Gaus, W., and Schleyer, M. (1974): Factor XIII activity and fibrin subunit structure in acute leukemia. *Biomedicine,* 21:61–66.
54. Robboy, S. J., Colman, R. W., and Minna, J. D. (1972): Pathology of disseminated intravascular coagulation (DIC). *Hum. Pathol.,* 3:327–343.
55. Robson, E. B., Murawski, G. F., and Bettigole, R. E. (1977): Use of ^{125}I-fibrinogen kinetic data to detect disseminated intravascular coagulation and deposition of fibrin in patients with metastatic cancer. *Thromb. Haemost.,* 37:484–508.
56. Rosenberg, R. D. (1975): Actions and interactions of antithrombin and heparin. *N. Engl. J. Med.,* 292:146–151.
57. Rosenthal, R. L. (1963): Acute promyelocytic leukemia associated with hypofibrinogenemia. *Blood,* 21:495–508.
58. Sack, G. H., Jr., Levin, J., and Bell, W. R. (1977): Trousseau's syndrome and other manifestations of chronic disseminated coagulopathy in patients with neoplasm: clinical, pathophysiologic, and therapeutic features. *Medicine (Baltimore),* 56:1–37.
59. Salzman, E. W., Deykin, D., Shapiro, R. M., and Rozenberg, R. (1975): Management of heparin therapy-controlled prospective trial. *N. Engl. J. Med.,* 292:1046–1051.
60. Shanberge, J. N., Tanaka, K., and Gruhl, M. C. (1971): Chronic consumption coagulopathy due to hemangiomatous transformation of the spleen. *Am. J. Clin. Pathol.,* 56:723–729.
61. Siegal, T., Seligsohn, V., Aghai, E., and Modan, M. (1978): Clinical and laboratory aspects of disseminated intravascular coagulation (DIC): a study of 118 cases. *Thromb. Haemost.,* 39:122–134.
62. Sun, N. C. J., McAfee, W. M., Hum, G. J., and Weiner, J. M. (1979): Hemostatic abnormalities in malignancy, a prospective study of one hundred eight patients. Part 1. Coagulation studies. *Am. J. Clin. Pathol.,* 71:10–16.
63. Svansberg, L., and Åstedt, B. (1975): Coagulative and fibrinolytic properties of ascitic fluid associated with ovarian tumors. *Cancer,* 35:1382–1387.
64. Tagnon, H. J., Schulman, P., Whitmore, W. F., and Leone, L. A. (1953): Prostatic fibrinolysin. Study of a case illustrating role in hemorrhagic diathesis of cancer of the prostate. *Am. J. Med.,* 15:875–884.
65. Tagnon, H. J., Whitmore, W. F., Jr., and Shulman, N. R. (1952): Fibrinolysis in metastatic cancer of the prostate. *Cancer,* 5:9–12.
66. Thomas, D. P., Niewiarowski, S., Myers, A. R., Block, K. J., and Colman, R. W. (1970): A comparative study of four methods for detecting fibrinogen degradation products in patients with various diseases. *N. Engl. J. Med.,* 283:663–668.
67. Trousseau, A. (1877): *Clinique Médicale de l'Hôtel-Dieu de Paris, Vol. 3,* 5th ed. Baillière, Paris.
68. Wenz, B., and Friedman, G. (1974): Acquired factor VIII inhibitor in a patient with malignant lymphoma. *Am. J. Med. Sci.,* 268:295–299.
69. Wessler, S., and Gitel, S. (1975): Control of heparin therapy. In: *Progress in Hemostasis and Thrombosis,* edited by T. H. Spaet. Grune & Stratton, New York.

Medical Complications in Cancer Patients,
edited by J. Klastersky and M. J. Staquet.
Raven Press, New York © 1981.

Platelet Transfusion for Thrombocytopenic Cancer Patients

Charles A. Schiffer, Joseph Aisner, and *Peter A. Daly

Cell Component Therapy Section, Baltimore Cancer Research Program, National Cancer Institute, University of Maryland Hospital, Baltimore, Maryland 21201

The aggressive multimodality treatment of cancer depends on the ability to support the patient through periods of marrow aplasia and pancytopenia. Although recent attention in the transfusion area has tended to focus on the technical advances allowing infection treatment and prevention with granulocyte transfusion, it is in fact the increased availability and greater understanding of the proper use of platelet transfusion which are primarily responsible for allowing patients with bone marrow failure states to survive long enough to receive effective therapy. Although occasional patients with lymphomas or solid tumors may require extensive transfusion supportive care during the initial treatment of their disease, it is patients with primary bone marrow disorders (e.g., acute leukemia) who most frequently develop prolonged thrombocytopenia and become dependent on the more specialized aspects of platelet transfusion therapy. As a consequence, most published clinical experience deals with leukemia or aplastic anemia patients, and a number of comprehensive reviews are available for reference (1,10,26,34,49,52). In this review we summarize the current thoughts about the proper use of platelet transfusion in cancer patients with an emphasis on the large number of problems still requiring further investigation of which the clinician should be aware.

PLATELET PREPARATION AND STORAGE

Most platelets for tranfusion are prepared as platelet concentrations (PC) as a by-product of whole blood donation, with between 4 and 10 units of pooled PC representing an average transfusion to an adult patient. All platelets are not created equally, however. It has been demonstrated that factors such as the centrifugation forces, temperature during preparation, volume in which the platelets are suspended, necessity for leaving the PC without agitation for 1 to 2 hr after concentration, conditions of transport from the collection center

---

* Present address: Mercers Hospital, Dublin 2, Ireland.

to the blood bank, and perhaps individual donor differences influence the quality of the final product (59). Similarly, although platelets can be stored in research laboratories in the liquid state for 48 to 72 hr without appreciable loss of viability or function, scrupulous attention must be paid to: (a) the platelet concentration and plasma volume (45 to 50 ml); (b) storage at "room temperature" (22 to 24°C); (c) type of agitation (gentle to-and-fro movement in the horizontal plane); and (d) separation of the platelet bags to allow adequate oxygen flow across the bags (34,41,42,56). The controversy between storage at 4 and 22°C which dominated research during the early 1970s has been resolved in favor of the higher temperature in view of the superior platelet recovery, survival, and almost immediate hemostatic effectiveness of the "room temperature" product (19,60).

The techniques of collection and storage vary widely among blood centers and are particularly critical when platelets are stored for more than 24 hr. The quality of platelets provided, therefore, also potentially varies considerably. Quality control regulations in the United States require only occasional measurement of platelet yield and pH and do not include monitoring of the clinical effectiveness of either fresh or stored PC (3). It is important therefore that clinicians provide information to the blood bank about the recovery and function of the stored platelets so that techniques can be modified as necessary. Research aimed at modifying the many storage variables is in progress in many laboratories and includes studies of newer plastics which allow more rapid gas exchange (43), varying ambient oxygen tensions, and different nutrient-enriched suspending media. The effects on platelet storage of the new CPD-adenine anticoagulent recently introduced into the United States is of interest in this regard and is currently under study.

A number of safe and efficient machines are available for the rapid procurement of normally functioning platelets from single donors (2,32,62). It should be noted that centrifugation of multiple units of whole blood drawn and returned from the same donor is also a simple and efficient method of platelet collection that can be done in any blood bank (53). Thus the unavailability of expensive pheresis equipment should not prevent the collection of single donor platelets if clinically indicated. Because most plateletpheresis machines are not "closed" systems, these platelets cannot be stored for more than 24 hr because of concern about bacterial contamination, and most are administered within a few hours of collection. It is likely, however, that closed systems will be developed and therefore the same variables analyzed for single platelet units must be restudied on the plateletpheresis product (37). Furthermore, single-donor HLA-matched platelets are frequently shipped long distances to recipients in other cities or states (24), and currently there are essentially no data on the best container, temperature, etc. for platelet transport. Thus clinicians utilizing such "long distance" donors must keep in mind the problems of transport as well as histocompatibility considerations when interpreting the outcome of transfusion. If necessary, in certain unusual circumstances some donors can be utilized on multiple consecutive days, if their platelet counts are monitored carefully (53).

INDICATIONS FOR PLATELET TRANSFUSION

There is a direct relationship between the circulating platelet count and the incidence of hemorrhage in thrombocytopenic cancer patients, with the incidence of severe spontaneous hemorrhage increasing significantly at counts less than 20,000/μl (5,48). Minor hemorrhagic phenomena such as petechiae in dependent areas, occult blood in the stools, or microscopic hematuria may develop at higher platelet counts and do not necessarily presage the onset of more clinically significant bleeding. Conversely, life-threatening hemorrhage can develop rapidly in the absence of more minor stigmata during episodes of infection, fever, chemotherapy administration with tumor lysis, and disturbances of coagulation, particularly disseminated intravascular coagulation (DIC).

Because of the unpredictability of the onset of hemorrhage and the results of two prospectively randomized trials (33,44), it has become the practice at most cancer centers to administer platelets prophylactically at counts between 10,000 and 20,000/μl to prevent hemorrhage. Many clinical factors may influence the development of hemorrhage at any given count, as noted above, and it is often appropriate to administer platelets at higher counts to seriously ill patients. In addition to patients with serious infection or DIC, patients with rapid tumor lysis, protracted emesis, rapid falls in platelet count, chemotherapy-related mucosal injury, and "precarious" sites of tumor involvement (e.g., intracranial tumors) are at increased risk of bleeding. A recent randomized study by Solomon et al. (61) confirmed other clinical observations that the liberal use of platelets, often at platelet counts greater than 20,000 to 30,000/μl, in patients in high-risk groups can effectively prevent hemorrhage in adult patients with acute nonlymphocytic leukemia. These investigators demonstrated that a rapid fall in platelet count from day to day is a helpful clinical clue suggesting a need for transfusion. Thus for patients with other active clinical problems, it appears that a transfusion policy of this sort is superior to a rigid prophylactic approach based solely on platelet count.

The proper management of clinically stable thrombocytopenic patients is not clear from this or other published studies, however, and it is well known that many patients with platelet counts less than 10,000/μl will remain free of hemorrhage until infection or fever develops. It is difficult to identify such patients prospectively, however. In addition, such patients are usually concurrently granulocytopenic and at risk for the development of infection and accompanying catastrophic bleeding. After balancing all these factors, we recommend prophylactic platelet transfusion at counts less than 15,000 to 20,000/μl, even in stable patients receiving induction chemotherapy and particularly in patients with diseases such as leukemia in whom the frequency of infection and coagulopathy are high and in whom even more profound thrombocytopenia can be expected. Some stable patients with "solid" tumors or patients with leukemia receiving maintenance chemotherapy with shorter periods of severe thrombocytopenia may not require prophylactic platelet transfusion, although there are no good data available concerning this point. If prophylactic transfusions are not given to these patients, they must be followed closely by experienced physicians with ready access to platelet transfusion.

Thrombocytopenic patients frequently require invasive diagnostic or surgical procedures. Although it is well recognized that surgery can be done after provision of platelet transfusions, there is little information available describing the levels of platelet count at which such procedures can be done safely. The only test of *in vivo* platelet function is the bleeding time, which increases in a linear fashion with decreasing platelet counts at counts less than $100,000/\mu l$ (28). Although the bleeding time is considerably prolonged at a count of $50,000/\mu l$ (approximately 15 min, assuming "normal" platelets are circulating), it is this figure which is most frequently mentioned as the "safe" level at which even major surgery can be performed. No recommendations about a safe "bleeding time" level can be made, and clearly a simpler and more reproducible test would be desirable. It should be emphasized, however, that most available data are anecdotal, and there is considerable individual patient variation. In some patients observation for bleeding following other procedures (e.g., bone marrow aspirates or biopsies, cutaneous cutdown sites) can be helpful in predicting the likelihood of hemorrhage following more traumatic procedures. Adequate supplies of fresh platelets should be available for use in these patients should unexpected bleeding occur.

Patients with adult acute leukemia receiving initial induction therapy represent the major users of platelet transfusion, although there is relatively little published information about the transfusion requirements of this group. In a recent study from our institution (11), adults with nonlymphocytic leukemia receiving induction therapy with daunorubicin and a continuous infusion of cytosine arabinoside (Ara-C) were analyzed (51). All patients received prophylactic platelet transfusion at counts less than $20,000/\mu l$. An average of 10.7 transfusions/patient (range 2 to 30) with a total of 67 units/patient (range 9 to 184) were administered. Severe hemorrhage occurred in 11 patients, each of whom was either infected or had active DIC, and it was a major cause of death in only 4 patients (1 with DIC, 3 with severe alloimmunization). These results reflect favorably on the use of prophylactic platelets and are also a reflection of the shorter periods of aplasia when anthracycline–Ara-C combinations are used owing to the high remission rate after a single course of therapy. More rapid remission induction with a consequent lesser duration of supportive care has contributed significantly to the higher remission rates now achievable in "higher risk" and elderly patients.

The major complication noted during this study was the development of hepatitis and alloimmunization with associated transfusion reactions and poor posttransfusion increments. Almost all of the hepatitis was of the "non-A, non-B" variety and produced persistent abnormalities in liver function in some patients. Obviously, serologic testing for this agent (agents?) is urgently needed and is currently under investigation. Other complications, such as overt graft-versus-host disease or bacteremia from inadvertently contaminated platelets (9), were not seen. The most difficult problem encountered in these patients was alloimmunization, the management of which is discussed in detail below.

ALLOIMMUNIZATION

Incidence

Of the 60 patients on this study, 50% developed lymphocytotoxic antibody during the course of induction therapy, and 17 patients (28%) received HLA-matched platelets. This rate of antibody production is similar to our previous experience in patients with acute nonlymphocytic leukemia (ANLL) (54) and is representative of the 50 to 100% range of alloimmunization described by others (25,35,63,67), the incidence depending in part on the patient population being studied and the intensity of cytotoxic and immunosuppressive therapy being administered. Fortunately, because of the perhaps delayed kinetics of antibody formation in these intensively treated patients, alloimmunization frequently did not develop until the patients were about to enter remission and were producing their own platelets. Maintenance and relapse therapy was rendered more difficult in these patients, however.

Diagnosis

Alloimmunization is characterized clinically by the failure to achieve expected platelet count increments after transfusion, often but not invariably accompanied by the presence of transfusion reactions. A number of other factors, however, including severe infection, fever, splenomegaly, hepatomegaly, DIC, brisk hemorrhage, and drug-mediated immune destruction (55), as well as transfusion of platelets with decreased viability due to inappropriate storage techniques, can result in decreased platelet recovery and shortened platelet survivals. The detection of lymphocytotoxic (anti-HLA) antibodies can help confirm the diagnosis, but this test is not readily available in most hospitals. As a rapid and simple alternative, measurement of platelet increments 1 hr posttransfusion can be of help in distinguishing between alloimmunization, which produces very low increments, and most other causes of accelerated platelet destruction, which are characterized by near-normal increments with a subsequent rapid fall in count (14). The major exceptions to these guidelines are septic shock and massive organomegaly, which also tend to produce immediate platelet destruction. Thus measurement of 1-hr posttransfusion increments is indicated as a diagnostic test in patients in whom day-to-day increments following transfusion of *fresh* platelets have been inadequate. If 1-hr increments are low (less than 3,000 per unit in adults), then consideration should be given to the use of HLA-matched platelets.

Management

The recognition that platelets from both family members or nonrelated donors matched at the HLA A and B loci can circulate normally in alloimmunized recipients has markedly improved the prognosis for alloimmunized patients (18,23,27,40,41,64,68). Such preparations are generally available at most major cancer centers, although the large number of HLA antigens (genetic "polymorphism") require that large HLA-typed donor pools be developed for the support of these patients (24). It is extremely expensive to recruit and maintain large HLA donor pools, however, and recent research has focused on donor selection "strategies" designed to increase the number of donors available per patient. A series of investigations by Duquesnoy et al. (4,17,18) suggest that some alloimmunized patients do not require perfectly matched platelets but rather will respond to platelets mismatched for HLA antigens not expressed on platelets (e.g., HLA B12) (4) or for antigens serologically cross-reactive with the recipient's antigens and hence not recognized as "foreign" (17,18). Other, probably more heavily alloimmunized patients, tend not to respond to such "selectively mismatched" platelets (63) and indeed may develop refractoriness to apparently perfectly matched platelets. This latter phenomenon may develop eventually in as many as 25% of alloimmunized patients (57) and is responsible, along with the considerable expense of HLA typing, for the current interest in other cross-matching techniques for donor selection.

It is likely that in most cases antibodies to platelet-specific antigens not detectable on lymphocytes are responsible for refractoriness to perfectly HLA-matched platelets, although the possibility of drug-mediated immune destruction should also be considered in appropriate patients (55). A number of *in vitro* cross-matching techniques with a considerable range of complexity and sensitivity using the platelet as the target cell are available and can be helpful in the selection of donors for individual patients (8,23,66). Most have not been as successful as a means of "mass screening" of donors probably because platelet-specific and anti-HLA antibodies are present in many patients (20). In addition, although HLA typing is a permanent record suitable for computer storage, platelet antibody testing requires that the potential donor make two trips to the blood center—once for cross matching and again for donation. Further advances in platelet cryopreservation may help modify this situation, although the moderate platelet injury produced by current platelet freezing methods may interfere with platelet antibody tests, most of which measure platelet damage as an endpoint. Cross matching by lymphocytotoxicity testing, which can utilize a frozen cell panel, is plagued by a high rate of "false negative" results and therefore is also unreliable for donor screening (20,31). Thus HLA typing remains the most reliable method for selecting matched platelet donors for the majority of alloimmunized patients. If HLA typing is not available, empiric use of family members is recommended with follow-up counts at 1-hr intervals as a test of compatibility.

The management of alloimmunized patients for whom no HLA-matched donors can be found is difficult. Prophylactic transfusions should not be given to such patients because the risks of hepatitis and transfusion reactions seem to outweigh any potential benefits. In addition, there is some evidence that the transfusion reactions associated with mismatched platelet transfusions can produce a decrease in circulating granulocyte count and hence an increased risk of infection (30). When such patients bleed, however, infusions of massive doses (greater than 20 to 30 units) of platelets are occasionally of clinical benefit, sometimes in the absence of sustained platelet count increments. Possible mechanisms for this salutary effect include the "accidental" administration of a fortuitously matched platelet unit as well as temporary binding of circulating platelet antibody, allowing subsequently transfused platelets to survive and exert hemostatic effectiveness (45). Pharmacologic doses of corticosteroids have also been utilized as a means of achieving short-term hemostasis, possibly by the mechanism of improving blood vessel wall endothelial "integrity" (6,39). Most of the anecdotal observations utilizing corticosteroids seem to have been in patients with immune-mediated thrombocytopenia or in animals (6,39), and good studies in humans are lacking. As with all thrombocytopenic patients, infections should be treated promptly, drugs which affect platelet function should be avoided, severe coughing and emesis should be eliminated as best as possible, and menses should be suppressed in premenopausal females.

Prevention

It is of note that a significant number of patients never become sensitized despite repeated exposure to platelet and leukocyte antigens behaving as if they were "immune tolerant." Preliminary analyses have failed to distinguish differences in immunoglobulin levels, sex, type of therapy, HLA type, skin test reactivity, or the interval between the cytotoxic therapy and antigenic exposure between antibody responders and nonresponders (54). More detailed studies of this type are indicated in the hope of discovering clinical manipulations capable of reducing the immune response to histocompatibility antigens.

Recently it was suggested that removal of mononuclear cells, which are present in units of PC in concentrations up to 10^8 cells per unit of PC, may decrease the rate of alloimmunization following platelet transfusion (7). In this study, PC with a lymphocyte contamination of less than 10^7 per unit were utilized. Other data suggest that if indeed the observation by Brand et al. (7) is correct, the dose of contaminating lymphocytes may be of importance because reducing the lymphocyte count from 1.4×10^8 to 0.4×10^8 per unit of PC failed to alter the rate of alloimmunization (46). Both available studies were retrospective and nonrandomized, and no attempt was made to control the type of red blood cells administered in the later report (46). Randomized studies, one of which is in progress at our institution, are necessary before the use of "leukocyte-poor" PC can be recommended. Although centrifugation to remove the leukocytes is a relatively simple step, the platelet loss can be considerable and averages 15 to 30% depending on the force used. In addition, leukocyte-poor or frozen red blood cells would have to be used exclusively to reduce antigenic exposure from this source, thereby drastically increasing the overall blood costs. The mechanism by which this putative prevention or delay of immunization takes place is not clear. Although leukocytes may well be more antigenic than platelets, HLA antigens are well expressed on platelets (13) and can be recognized and processed *in vivo* as indicated by transfusion experience in immunized patients. The observation by Herzig et al. (29) that removal of leukocytes from platelet preparations may enhance the response to partially matched platelets in occasional alloimmunized patients may provide some supportive background for this approach, but clearly further clinical and laboratory investigation is needed.

PLATELET CRYOPRESERVATION

Methodology allowing long-term platelet storage can be of considerable assistance in the management of alloimmunized patients. Autologous and HLA-typed platelets have been frozen, thereby maintaining a ready supply for alloimmunized patients and decreasing the crisis atmosphere which frequently occurs when an HLA-matched donor is required at short notice (50,52). In the autologous setting, platelets are obtained from patients between courses of chemotherapy during remission of their leukemia, are frozen and stored, and are then transfused during subsequent periods of thrombocytopenia (52). In our institution, approximately 40% of the transfusion needs of leukemic patients receiving maintenance chemotherapy are met by the use of autologous frozen platelets (Fig. 1). In addition, patients with chronic myelogenous leukemia have been supported through the blast crisis phase of their disease using autologous platelets harvested during the chronic phase. An analogous approach should be feasible in the many ongoing studies of patients receiving intensive chemotherapy with autologous marrow reconstitution.

Cryopreservation techniques using both dimethylsulfoxide (DMSO) and glycerol (16) have been described, but to date only the DMSO methodology has been sufficiently reproducible for general usage. Using 5% DMSO, polyolefin freezing bags, and a variety of freezing rates and conditions, recoveries varying between 60 and 70% of fresh platelets with satisfactory hemostatic results have been noted in a number of laboratories (38,50,52,65). Because the DMSO is largely removed after thawing, there are no side effects following these transfusions; moreover, the technology is simple enough for use outside of research laboratories. Successful transfusion of platelets frozen at liquid nitrogen temperatures ($-120°C$) for 3 years or more has been described and should therefore permit long-term storage of HLA-matched platelets as well as random-donor platelets for emergency use (15).

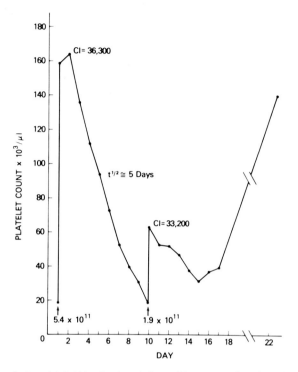

FIG. 1. Posttransfusion platelet kinetics in a patient with acute nonlymphocytic leukemia (ANLL) receiving autologous frozen platelets obtained and frozen 2 to 3 months previously. In this splenectomized patient the $t_{1/2}$ and corrected increment (CI)

$$CI = \frac{\text{absolute increment} \times \text{body surface area (M}^2)}{\text{no. of platelets transfused} \times 10^{11}}$$

were equivalent to results expected with transfusion of fresh platelets. Marrow recovery occurred on days 17 and 18.

SINGLE-DONOR PLATELET TRANSFUSION

Single-donor platelets have been used predominantly in the setting of alloimmunization, which developed following transfusion of more readily available and less costly random donor platelets. With the development of efficient plateletpheresis machines, there has been an increased interest in the use of single-donor platelets from the initiation of transfusion with the goals of decreasing hepatitis acquisition and possibly modifying the pattern of recipient alloimmunization. Although long-term support is possible using family members (22), there are almost no contemporary data available concerning the rate of alloimmunization in patients receiving platelets with higher degrees of leukocyte contamination prepared using pheresis machines. In addition to the increased expense, other as yet theoretical problems may result from the provision of single-donor platelets. If an attempt is made to use closely HLA-matched platelets from nonrelated donors, one may select for the development of antibodies against non-HLA platelet antigens which are not easily detectable and which could make further donor selection difficult if not impossible. Similarly, providing partially matched platelets in order to produce a restricted pattern of sensitization only against the mismatched antigens may not be successful because of the considerable serologic cross reactivity in the HLA system. Thus antibody formed by exposure to a limited number of HLA antigens may have activity against a broad range of HLA antigens, resulting in a situation analogous to that which occurs following random donor transfusion. Indeed, in a canine model it was shown that the incidence of alloimmunization is similar in dogs supported by a single random donor as compared to a pool of multiple random donors (47). Of note, however, was that alloimmunization actually developed earlier in the dogs receiving single-donor platelets. Certainly further careful research is necessary before single-donor platelet transfusion is utilized as "standard" supportive care with the exception of the requirements of the alloimmunized patient. This is particularly true because, although the available collection machines have an enviable safety record to date, the possibility of donor side effects and morbidity is always present. Furthermore, it is possible that the risk of graft-versus-host disease (GVHD) in severely immunosuppressed patients may be increased because of the larger doses of lymphocytes administered with single-donor platelets, particularly those prepared by the Haemonetics Model 30 blood separator (2,12,21). Because GVHD is extremely rare in nonmarrow transplant recipients, it is premature to recommend routine irradiation of either random-donor or single-donor platelets administered to other patients with cancer. Nonetheless, more descriptions of GVHD in leukemic patients have been published recently, and clinicians should be aware of the protean manifestations of this unusual complication of blood component transfusion (12,21).

CONCLUSIONS

The increased availability of platelets and the remarkable successes achieved with their proper use have made many physicians consider platelet transfusion and collection as "routine" and not requiring further intensive investigation. In the preceding sections we described a number of problems as well as serious side effects which still remain in the area of platelet transfusion support. Close collaboration between clinicians and blood bank personnel is required to address these issues and to continue to provide the most suitable platelet product for the prophylaxis and treatment of hemorrhage.

REFERENCES

1. Aisner, J. (1977): Platelet transfusion therapy. *Med. Clin. North Am.,* 61:1133–1145.
2. Aisner, J., Schiffer, C. A., Wolfe, J. H., and Wiernik, P. H. (1976): A standardized technique

for efficient platelet and leukocyte collection using the model 30 blood processor. *Transfusion,* 16:437–445.

3. American Association of Blood Banks (1978): *Standards for Blood Banks and Transfusion Services,* pp. 10–11. Washington, D.C.
4. Aster, R. H., Szatkowski, N., Liebert, M., and Duquesnoy, R. J. (1977): Expression of HLA-B12, HLA-B8, w4, and w6 on platelets. *Transplant. Proc.,* 9:1695–1696.
5. Belt, R. J., Leite, C., Haas, C. D., and Stephens, R. L. (1978): Incidence of hemorrhagic complications in patients with cancer. *JAMA,* 239:2571–2574.
6. Blajchman, M. A., Senyi, A. F., Hirsh, J., Surya, Y., Buchanan, M., and Mustard, J. F. (1979): Shortening of the bleeding time in rabbits by hydrocortisone caused by inhibition of prostacyclin generation by the vessel wall. *J. Clin. Invest.,* 63:1026–1035.
7. Brand, A., Van Leeuwen, A., Eernisse, J. G., and Van Rood, J. J. (1976): Platelet immunology with special regard to platelet transfusion therapy. In: *Proceedings of the 16th International Congress of Hematology,* Kyoto, September 5–11.
8. Brand, A., Van Leeuwen, A., Eernisse, J. G., and Van Rood, J. J. (1978): Platelet transfusion therapy. Optimal donor selection with a combination of lymphocytotoxicity and platelet fluorescence tests. *Blood,* 51:781–788.
9. Buchholz, D. H., Young, V. M., Friedman, N. R., Reilly, J. A., and Mardiney, M. R., Jr. (1971): Bacterial proliferation in platelet products stored at room temperature. *N. Engl. J. Med.,* 285:429–433.
10. Cash, J. D. (1972): Platelet transfusion therapy. *Clin. Haematol.,* 1:395–411.
11. Chang, P., Wiernik, P. H., Lichtenfeld, J. L., and Schiffer, C. A. (1978): Levamisole (L), cytosine arabinoside (Ara-C), and daunorubicin (DNR) induction therapy of adult acute nonlymphocytic leukemia (ANLL). *Proc. Am. Assoc. Cancer Res. Am. Soc. Clin. Oncol.,* 19:370.
12. Cohen, D., Weinstein, H., Mihm, M., and Yankee, R. (1979): Nonfatal graft-versus-host disease occurring after transfusion with leukocytes and platelets obtained from normal donors. *Blood,* 53:1053–1057.
13. Cook, K. M. (1974): Distribution of HL-A antigens on blood cells. *Tissue Antigens,* 4:202–209.
14. Daly, P. A., Schiffer, C. A., Aisner, J., and Wiernik, P. H. (1980): Platelet transfusion therapy—One hour post-transfusion increments are valuable in predicting the need for HLA-matched preparations. *JAMA,* 243:435–438.
15. Daly, P. A., Schiffer, C. A., Aisner, J., and Wiernik, P. H. (1979): Successful transfusion of platelets cryopreserved for more than 3 years. *Blood,* 54:1023–1027.
16. Dayian, G., and Rowe, A. W. (1976): Cryopreservation of human platelets for transfusion. *Cryobiology,* 13:1–8.
17. Duquesnoy, R. J., Filip, D. J., and Aster, R. H. (1977): Influence of HLA-A2 on the effectiveness of platelet transfusions in alloimmunized thrombocytopenic patients. *Blood,* 50:407–412.
18. Duquesnoy, R. J., Filip, D. J., Rodey, G. E., Rimm, A. A., and Aster, R. H. (1977): Successful transfusion of platelets "mismatched" for HLA antigens to alloimmunized thrombocytopenic patients. *Am. J. Hematol.,* 2:219–226.
19. Filip, D. J., and Aster, R. H. (1978): Relative hemostatic effectiveness of human platelets stored at 4° and 22°C. *J. Lab. Clin. Med.,* 91:618–624.
20. Filip, D. J., Duquesnoy, R. J., and Aster, R. H. (1976): Predictive value of cross-matching for transfusion of platelet concentrates to alloimmunized recipients. *Am. J. Hematol.,* 1:471–479.
21. Ford, J. M., Lucey, J. J., Cullen, M. H., Tobias, J. S., and Lister, T. A. (1976): Fatal graft-versus-host disease following transfusion of granulocytes from normal donors. *Lancet,* 2:1167–1171.
22. Freireich, E. J., Kliman, A., Gaydos, L. A., Mantel, N., and Frei, E., III (1963): Response to repeated platelet transfusion from the same donor. *Ann. Intern. Med.,* 59:277–287.
23. Gmur, J., von Felten, A., and Frick, P. (1978): Platelet support in polysensitized patients: Role of HLA specificities and crossmatch testing for donor selection. *Blood,* 51:903–909.
24. Graw, R. G., Jr., Herzig, R. H., Langston, M. G., Perdue, S. T., and Terasaki, P. I. (1977): National donor registry and computer transfusion programs for platelet transfusions. *Transplant. Proc.,* 9:225–227.
25. Green, D., Tiro, A., Basiliere, J., and Mittal, K. K. (1976): Cytotoxic antibody complicating platelet support in acute leukemia. *JAMA,* 236:1044–1046.

26. Greenwalt, T. J., and Jamieson, G. A., editors (1978): *The Blood Platelet in Transfusion Therapy.* Alan R. Liss, New York.
27. Grumet, F. C., and Yankee, R. A. (1970): Long-term platelet support of patients with aplastic anemia. *Ann. Intern. Med.,* 73:1–7.
28. Harker, L. A., and Slichter, S. J. (1972): The bleeding time as a screening test for evaluation of platelet function. *N. Engl. J. Med.,* 287:155–159.
29. Herzig, R. H., Herzig, G. P., Bull, M. I., Decter, J. A., Lohrmann, H.-P., Stout, F. G., Yankee, R. A., and Graw, R. G., Jr. (1975): Correction of poor platelet transfusion responses with leukocyte-poor HL-A-matched platelet concentrates. *Blood,* 46:743–750.
30. Herzig, R. H., Poplack, D. G., and Yankee, R. A. (1974): Prolonged granulocytopenia from incompatible platelet transfusions. *N. Engl. J. Med.,* 290:1220–1223.
31. Herzig, R. H., Terasaki, P. I., Trapani, R. J., Herzig, G. P., and Graw, R. G., Jr. (1977): The relationship between donor-recipient lymphocytotoxicity and the transfusion response using HLA-matched platelet concentrates. *Transfusion,* 17:657–661.
32. Hester, J. P., Kellogg, R. M., Mulzet, A. P., Kruger, V. R., McCredie, K. B., and Freireich, E. J. (1979): Principles of blood separation and component extraction in a disposable continuous-flow single-stage channel. *Blood,* 54:254–268.
33. Higby, D. J., Cohen, E., Holland, J. F., and Sinks, L. (1974): The prophylactic treatment of thrombocytopenic leukemic patients with platelets: A double blind study. *Transfusion,* 14:440–446.
34. Hoak, J. C., and Koepke, J. A. (1976): Platelet transfusion. *Clin. Haematol.,* 5:69–79.
35. Holme, S., Vaidja, K., and Murphy, S. (1978): Platelet storage at 22°C: Effect of type of agitation on morphology, viability, and function in vitro. *Blood,* 52:425–435.
36. Howard, J. E., and Perkins, H. A. (1978): The natural history of alloimmunization to platelets. *Transfusion,* 18:496–503.
37. Katz, A., Houx, J., and Ewald, L. (1978): Storage of platelets prepared by discontinuous flow centrifugation. *Transfusion,* 18:220–221.
38. Kim, B. K., and Baldini, M. G. (1974): Biochemistry, function, and hemostatic effectiveness of frozen human platelets. *Proc. Soc. Exp. Biol. Med.,* 145:830–835.
39. Kitchens, C. S. (1977): Amelioration of endothelial abnormalities by prednisone in experimental thrombocytopenia in the rabbit. *J. Clin. Invest.,* 60:1129–1134.
40. Lohrmann, H.-P., Bull, M. I., Decter, J. A., Yankee, R. A., and Graw, R. G., Jr. (1974): Platelet transfusions from HL-A compatible unrelated donors to alloimmunized patients. *Ann. Intern. Med.,* 80:9–14.
41. Mittal, K. K., Ruder, E. A., and Green, D. (1976): Matching of histocompatibility (HL-A) antigens for platelet transfusion. *Blood,* 47:31–41.
42. Murphy, S., and Gardner, F. H. (1971): Platelet storage at 22°C; metabolic, morphologic, and functional studies. *J. Clin. Invest.,* 50:370–377.
43. Murphy, S., and Gardner, F. H. (1975): Platelet storage at 22°C: Role of gas transport across plastic containers in maintenance of viability. *Blood,* 46:209–218.
44. Murphy, S., Koch, P. A., and Evans, A. E. (1976): Randomized trial of prophylactic vs. therapeutic platelet transfusion in childhood acute leukemia. *Clin. Res.,* 24:379A.
45. Nagasawa, T., Kim, B. K., and Baldini, M. G. (1978): Temporary suppression of circulating antiplatelet alloantibodies by the massive infusion of fresh, stored, or lyophilized platelets. *Transfusion,* 18:429–435.
46. Ness, P. M., and Perkins, H. A. (1978): Cytotoxic antibody formation from platelets with different degrees of WBC contamination. *Transfusion,* 18:388.
47. O'Donnell, M. R., and Slichter, S. J. (1979): Platelet (PLT) alloimmunization—Correlation with donor source. *Clin. Res.,* 27:390A.
48. Roy, A. J., Jaffe, N., and Djerassi, I. (1973): Prophylactic platelet transfusions in children with acute leukemia: A dose response study. *Transfusion,* 13:283–290.
49. Schiffer, C. A. (1978): Some aspects of recent advances in the use of blood cell components. *Br. J. Haematol.,* 39:289–294.
50. Schiffer, C. A., Aisner, J., and Wiernik, P. H. (1976): Clinical experience with transfusion of cryopreserved platelets. *Br. J. Haematol.,* 34:377–385.
51. Schiffer, C. A., Aisner, J., and Wiernik, P. H. (1978): Platelet transfusion therapy for patients with leukemia. In: *The Blood Platelet in Transfusion Therapy,* edited by T. A. Greenwalt and G. A. Jamieson, pp. 267–279. Alan R. Liss, New York.

52. Schiffer, C. A., Aisner, J., and Wiernik, P. H. (1978): Frozen autologous platelet transfusion for patients with leukemia. *N. Engl. J. Med., 299*:7–12.
53. Schiffer, C. A., Buchholz, D. H., and Wiernik, P. H. (1974): Intensive multiunit plateletpheresis of normal donors. *Transfusion,* 14:388–394.
54. Schiffer, C. A., Lichtenfeld, J. L., Wiernik, P. H., Mardiney, M. R., Jr., and Joseph, J. M. (1976): Antibody response in patients with acute nonlymphocytic leukemia. *Cancer,* 37:2177–2182.
55. Schiffer, C. A., Weinstein, H. J., and Wiernik, P. H. (1976): Methicillin-associated thrombocytopenia. *Ann. Intern. Med.,* 85(3):338–339.
56. Shulman, N. R. (1966): Immunological considerations attending platelet transfusion. *Transfusion,* 6:39–49.
57. Slichter, S. J. (1978): Efficacy of platelets collected by semi-continuous flow centrifugation (Haemonetics model 30). *Br. J. Haematol.,* 38:131–140.
58. Slichter, S. J. (1978): Selection of compatible platelet donors. In: *Platelet Physiology and Transfusion,* edited by C. A. Schiffer, pp. 83–92. American Association of Blood Banks, Washington, D.C.
59. Slichter, S. J., and Harker, L. A. (1976): Preparation and storage of platelet concentrates. I. Factors influencing the harvest of viable platelets from whole blood. *Br. J. Haematol.,* 34:395–402.
60. Slichter, S. J., and Harker, L. A. (1976): Preparation and storage of platelet concentrates. II. Storage variables influencing platelet viability and function. *Br. J. Haematol.,* 34:403–419.
61. Solomon, J., Bofenkamp, T., Fahey, J. L., Chillar, R. K., and Beutler, E. (1978): Platelet prophylaxis in acute non-lymphoblastic leukaemia. *Lancet,* 1:267.
62. Szymanski, I. O., Patti, K., and Kliman, A. (1973): Efficacy of the Latham blood processor to perform plateletpheresis. *Transfusion,* 13:405–411.
63. Tejada, F., Bias, W. B., Santos, G. W., and Zieve, P. D. (1973): Immunologic response of patients with acute leukemia to platelet transfusions. *Blood,* 42:405–412.
64. Tosato, G., Applebaum, F. R., and Deisseroth, A. B. (1978): HLA-matched platelet transfusion therapy of severe aplastic anemia. *Blood,* 52:846–854.
65. Valeri, C. R., Feingold, H., and Marchionni, L. D. (1974): A simple method for freezing human platelets using 6% dimethylsulfoxide and storage at −80°C. *Blood,* 43:131–136.
66. Wu, K. K., Hoak, J. C., Thompson, J. S., and Koepke, J. A. (1975): Use of platelet aggregometry in selection of compatible platelet donors. *N. Engl. J. Med.,* 292:130–133.
67. Wu, K. K., Thompson, J. S., Koepke, J. A., Hoak, J. C., and Flink, R. (1976): Heterogeneity of antibody response to human platelet transfusion. *J. Clin. Invest.,* 58:432–438.
68. Yankee, R. A., Grumet, F. C., and Rogentine, G. N. (1969): Platelet transfusion therapy. The selection of compatible platelet donors for refractory patients by lymphocyte HL-A typing. *N. Engl. J. Med.,* 282:1208–1212.

Medical Complications in Cancer Patients,
edited by J. Klastersky and M. J. Staquet.
Raven Press, New York © 1981.

Neurological Disorders in Cancer Patients and Their Treatment

J. Hildebrand

Medical Service and Henri Tagnon Laboratory of Clinical Investigation, Tumor Center, Free University of Brussels, Institut Jules Bordet, 1000 Brussels, Belgium

Prolongation of life in cancer patients because of recent advances in the treatment of malignant disease creates new problems in supportive care due to allowing the appearance or increasing the incidence of certain manifestations of the neoplasms. Lesions of the nervous system are among the most serious complications of malignant tumors because they pose an immediate threat to the duration and quality of the survival. These complications are fairly common as one patient in five with generalized cancer develops major signs of nervous system dysfunction.

A recent attempt was made to provide a classification and description of the clinical features of nervous system lesions in cancer patients (24). The purpose of the present chapter is to emphasize their treatment. Because early recognition improves the therapeutic results, the first and most prominent clinical features of the various lesions of the nervous system are briefly summarized.

The neurological disorders seen in patients with cancer can be classified into four categories according to their pathogenesis: (a) lesions caused by metastases and local extension of the tumor; (b) lesions produced by antineoplastic treatments; (c) lesions attributed to the remote effect of cancer on the nervous system; and (d) neurological diseases concomitant but unrelated to the malignancy. The vast majority of treatments reviewed here concern the first category.

BRAIN METASTASES

Clinical Features

In our experience, brain metastases are the most common neurological lesions seen in cancer patients, accounting for over 30% of all neurological disorders. Lung cancer is by far the most common primary tumor. In addition, most of the brain metastases of undetermined origin are likely to originate from occult bronchogenic carcinomas. Thus in patients with lung carcinoma, brain metastases may be the first and even the only clinical manifestation of the disease.

In other malignant diseases, brain metastases usually occur when the neoplastic spread is evident elsewhere, particularly in the lungs. Among those neoplasms, breast carcinoma and melanoma figure prominently. Melanoma is a relatively rare neoplasm; however, when it becomes generalized there is about a 50% chance of developing brain metastases. Early symptoms and signs of brain metastases are extremely polymorphic. In an unselected population of patients with cancer, signs of diffuse brain lesions (e.g., changes in alertness, intellectual impairment, or gait abnormalities) are seen as the first manifestations of brain metastases in 50% of the patients (23). In patients with focal neurological deficits, a single neurological sign or a combination of signs may be expected since brain metastases are distributed at random in proportion to the mass of the brain area. Moreover, because in most cases brain metastases are multiple, the onset of the focal neurological signs may be acute, mimicking stroke. The differential diagnosis may be made even more difficult by spontaneous temporary remission (48). Finally, about 25% of brain metastases are asymptomatic and discovered at autopsy.

The electroencephalogram (EEG) and isotope brain scan are good complementary screening examinations, and computerized tomographic (CT) brain scan is currently the most accurate method for detecting and localizing brain neoplasms and for assessing their growth in response to treatment.

Treatment

Prophylactic Treatment

In patients with solid tumors, prophylactic treatment of brain metastases has been advocated and is still used in patients with small cell anaplastic carcinoma (oat cell carcinoma). The reasons for this prophylaxis are: (a) the high incidence of brain metastases in oat cell carcinoma (43); (b) the fairly good sensitivity of this tumor to irradiation; and (c) the prolongation of life of these patients by applying a combination of drugs that do not easily cross the blood–brain barrier and so leave the brain unprotected for the development of secondary tumors. Thus theoretically brain metastases appear as a major factor limiting further therapeutic progress in this disease.

The prophylactic treatment of brain metastases in patients with oat cell carcinoma of the lung consists in irradiation of the whole brain, the most current dose being 3,000 rads given in 10 to 14 fractions. During the first trials using prophylactic brain irradiation, the effect of this treatment on the incidence of brain metastases was not quantitatively evaluated nor did these studies contain nonirradiated controls (31,36). The first two controlled studies (29,30,64) demonstrated a significant decrease in the incidence of brain metastases in patients treated by cranial irradiation (Table 1) but no significant increase in the survival. In the larger of the two studies (64), the benefit of prophylactic brain irradiation was found only in patients who did not achieve a complete remission (Table

TABLE 1. *Trials testing prophylactic brain irradiation in small cell lung carcinoma*[a]

Ref.	Stage of disease	No. of cases	Prophylactic treatment	Frequency of metastases	p	Mean survival	p
30	Not specified	29	14 received 3,000 rads in 10 fractions	0 (0%)	0.05	9.8 months	ns
			15 Controls	4 (27%)		7.2 months	
64	Limited and extensive	151/171	69 received 3,000 rads in 10 fractions	2 (3%)	0.01	8.7 months	ns
			82 Controls	15 (17%)		8.5 months	
	Only patients with complete remission	48/151	22 received 3,000 rads in 10 fractions	2 (9%)	ns	Not specified	
			26 Controls	4 (15%)		Not specified	
35	Limited	15	All received 3,000 rads in 12 days	CR 0/8 PR 3/7	—	35 weeks	
	Extensive	14	Same treatment	CR 0/1 PR 2/8 NR 0/5	—	23 weeks	
11	Limited but unresectable	24	2,000 rads in 10 fractions and 2 weeks	4 (17%)	ns	Not specified for patients with oat cell carcinoma	
		21	Controls	5 (24%)			
27	Limited	111	55 received 4,000 rads in 4 weeks	5 (9%)	ns	310 days	ns
			56 Controls	7 (13%)		281 days	

[a]ns: not significant. CR, complete remission; PR, partial remission; NR, no remission.

1). This observation conflicts somewhat with the data published by Levitt et al. (35) where, despite cranial irradiation, brain metastases were found only in patients with partial remission (Table 1).

The decrease in cerebral metastases by prophylactic irradiation with 2,000 rads was not demonstrated by Cox et al. (11) in patients with oat cell carcinoma. However, the irradiation was sufficient to reduce or delay the appearance of brain metastases in patients with squamous large cell carcinoma and adenocarcinoma of the lung.

Finally, a recent study by Hirsch et al. (27) does not confirm earlier results which indicated that cranial irradiation decreases the incidence of brain metastases in patients with small cell anaplastic carcinoma of the lung (Table 1).

In conclusion, prophylactic cranial irradiation does not seem to prolong the life of patients with oat cell carcinoma. It possibly decreases the incidence of brain metastases, but this has not been unequivocally established. One study (11) suggests that in other types of lung cancer the prophylactic irradiation of the cranium may increase the delay in the development of brain metastases.

Treatment of Symptomatic Brain Metastases

Choice of treatment in the various clinical situations where brain metastases are seen remains difficult despite the large number of studies devoted to the subject. This is due mainly to the lack of adequately controlled trials. In addition, the duration and quality of the survival, often chosen as criteria for evaluating treatment of brain metastases, are not related to brain metastases alone in patients with disseminated disease. Another frequently used criterion for treatment evaluation is objective remission. This parameter is of course directly related to the effect of a given therapy on brain metastases, but it is difficult to measure with accuracy.

Clinical improvement of patients with brain metastases is often due to corticosteroids, which act primarily on brain edema surrounding the tumor. In a vast majority of the studies, this effect is not clearly dissociated from those of specifically antineoplastic treatments. Brain CT scan possibly allows such a distinction, but only a few recent studies include this examination.

Neurosurgery

Several reports indicate that surgical removal of brain metastases is superior to no treatment at all. However, these retrospective and nonrandomized studies are probably biased by the selection for neurosurgery of the patients with the best prognosis. Probably the strongest argument in favor of surgical removal of brain metastases is the rate of long survivals observed in series of operated patients. Störtebecker (62) operated on 125 patients and reported that 21.6% were alive 1 year after operation; 1 patient with hypernephroma survived 17 years. In a small series of 16 patients operated by Perese (49), 3 (18.8%) were alive after 2.5 years. Even more encouraging results were obtained by Furlow (17): 16.2% of 37 patients were alive at 6 years. Lang and Slater (34) operated on 208 patients with brain metastases. Excluding those with positive chest X-rays, they observed a 35% survival at 1 year, 15% at 3 years, and 10% at 5 years. Out of 155 cases operated by Vieth and Odom (65), 21 (13.5%) survived the operation by 1 year and 6 were still alive more than 3.5 to 10 years later. More recently, Raskind et al. (53) reported that among 51 operated patients there was a 30% survival 1 year after neurosurgery and 8% were still alive after 3 years. Adequate (i.e., randomized) controls were not used in any of these studies, and it is likely that the patients chosen for neurosurgery were those with the best prognosis. Nevertheless, it is reasonable to assume that exceptionally long survivals are due to the surgical removal of the secondary tumor. However, the benefit provided by neurosurgery to a restricted number of patients is balanced by the high rate of early mortality, which was higher than 25% and even higher than 50% in several studies (49,56,60,62). Therefore, the question is not so much to know whether one should or should not operate on patients with cerebral metastases but rather how to select the cases for neurosurgery. Obviously, postoperative mortality may be reduced to acceptable figures (e.g., 5.4%) by adequate patient selection (17). Although it is not possible to establish rigid eligibility rules for neurosurgery in patients with brain metastases, several criteria emerge from most studies:

1. Patients must be in good general condition and have a minimal extraneural neoplastic burden.
2. In the case of a favorable neurosurgical outcome, the expected survival should be greater than 6 months.
3. Brain metastases must appear unique after a careful investigation and should appear totally removable, as biopsies and partial resections are accompanied by an increased rate of early death.
4. Slowly growing tumors—those which have a long interval between the diagnosis of the primary neoplasm and the control metastases—probably have a better postneurosurgical prognosis. These tumors, however, include hypernephroma, thyroid carcinomas, or testicular tumors which account, unfortunately, for a small percentage of primaries in brain metastases.

Substantial prolongation of life and improvement of its quality is the main goal of neurosurgery in the treatment of brain metastases. Another aim of surgery is the relief of intracranial hypertension. This can be achieved either by decompression and removal of large tumor masses or by the derivation of the cerebrospinal fluid (CSF). The last procedure may be particularly useful in tumors of the posterior fossa.

Finally, the decision to operate on cerebral metastases should be tempered in the future by the progress made in treatment by radiotherapy and chemotherapy.

Radiotherapy

Radiotherapy appears today to be essentially a prophylactic treatment; its goal is to prolong and improve the quality of the survival. The improvement of life quality may be achieved through partial or total regression of the neurological symptoms and signs. Such remissions have been observed in 37 to 80% of patients treated mainly, but not exclusively, with radiotherapy (9,16,41,43,44, 47,58).

These rates of objective remissions, although very high, are not superior to those obtained with corticosteroids, which were given to most of the patients studied in these trials. In addition, a similar rate of objective remissions was found by Horton et al. (28) in a randomized and prospective study where patients were treated either with prednisone (40 mg/day for 4 weeks) or a combination of radiotherapy and prednisone. However, the duration of the remission tended to be longer in the irradiated patients. The fact that the initial improvement in patients irradiated for brain metastases may be due primarily to the administration of steroids—which act on the peritumoral brain edema and which activity is not related to tumor pathology—is further consistent with the rather surprising observation (9,44) that the rate of objective remissions after irradiation is not related to the nature of the primary tumor. In another study (16), patients with squamous cell bronchogenic carcinoma did even better than those with a much more radiosensitive oat cell tumor. Thus it is reasonable to assume that the initial improvement of the neurological status in patients with brain metastases treated by radiotherapy and corticosteroids is due to regression of the peritumor brain edema. Radiotherapy produces, in patients who respond to treatment, more sustained remissions. This would explain why, in the study by Nisce et al. (44), the average duration of the remission was longer in patients with breast carcinoma (6 months) than in those with malignant melanoma (3 months). The lack of melanoma brain metastases to respond favorably to irradiation was observed in other studies.

Therefore, the duration of the neurological palliation seems to be a much better criterion than the rate of objective remission for the evaluation of radiotherapy in patients with brain metastases. The survival time is not a very good criterion to appreciate the efficacy of a treatment on brain metastases because death may be related to other, usually neoplastic, lesions. There is evidence, however, from successive and uncontrolled studies that radiotherapy is prolonging the survival of those patients.

What is the best radiotherapy schedule? There is a large consensus that the whole cranium should be irradiated because in the majority of cases the metastases are multiple and disseminated. The doses and the time of irradiation are not standardized, however. By comparing the results from different medical centers, it appears that, in terms of rates of objective remission and duration of survival time, similar results are obtained by different treatments ranging from 1,000 rads given in one dose to 4,500 rads delivered over 4 weeks. As indicated above, however, those evaluation criteria are open to criticism when steroids are used. A single dose of 1,000 rads increases the rate of complications, at least in patients with intracranial hypertension (51). From large prospective studies now in progress, it will probably emerge that the administration of 3,000 rads over a 12-day period combines safety and best efficacy.

Corticosteroids and Chemotherapy

Corticosteroids reduce the peritumoral cerebral edema with regularity and thereby improve the neurological functions, usually within 24 to 48 hr, in the majority of patients with brain metastases. The total daily doses vary from 10 to 16 mg, but in some cases higher doses improve the therapeutic results. The clinical effects of corticosteroids are sustained as long as their administration is maintained. However, because of some serious side effects (e.g., proximal myopathy or depression in the immune mechanisms), unnecessarily high doses of corticosteroids must be avoided during the maintenance phase.

Glycerol, given at daily doses of 1.5 g/kg p.o. in four fractions, is also effective in reducing brain edema in patients with brain metastases (4). In cases of emergency, a perfusion with 20% mannitol reduces rapidly but temporarily the edema.

Today the role of chemotherapy in the treatment of brain metastases appears modest and requires further evaluation. Chemotherapeutic agents are usually combined with radiotherapy and corticosteroids, so that studies testing their efficacy alone are scarce. Often preference is given to studying lipid-soluble drugs crossing the blood–brain barrier. However, since brain metastases do not usually infiltrate the normal brain to an extent comparable to primary tumors, and since the barrier is not preserved in the metastatic nodules, this limitation may not be justified. In our experience (25) breast carcinoma brain metastases respond better to the combination of CCNU, vincristine, and methotrexate than do bronchogenic secondaries. A similar difference between the response of breast and lung cerebral metastases was reported by Pouillart et al. (52) using the combination VM-26 and CCNU. Cunningham and Baxter (12) suggested that the addition of CCNU to radiation and corticosteroids may prolong the survival in patients with intracerebral metastases from lung cancer.

Finally, individual examples of successful treatment of brain metastases of relatively rare origin [e.g., Wilm's tumor (63) and testicular teratoma (33)] have been reported.

EXTRADURAL SPACE METASTASES

Clinical Features

Spinal cord compression due to epidural metastases occurs, according to tumor pathology, in 1 to 4% of cancer patients. In most cases the involvement of the epidural space by the neoplastic tissue originates from vertebral metastases.

Hence this complication is seen most commonly in such tumors as breast, lung, kidney, prostate, or thyroid carcinomas, which readily metastasize to bone, as well as lymphomas and myelomas.

Clinical symptoms and signs of epidural metastases are remarkably stereotyped, but their progression is related to the growth rate and location of the tumor and therefore varies considerably from one patient to another. The most common initial presentation is back pain, which has a radicular distribution and is usually increased by straining, coughing, or sneezing. Weakness and muscle atrophy may develop if the delay between root involvement and compression of the spinal cord lasts long enough. Signs of spinal cord compression may develop suddenly, within a few hours, or progressively. It is believed that impairment of the spinal blood flow is an important factor in the pathogenesis in patients with acute dysfunction of the spinal cord. Complementary examinations consist essentially of: (a) plain X-rays, which demonstrate vertebral metastases in at least 80% of the patients; (b) analysis of the CSF, which usually shows a blockage of CSF and consistently high protein levels; and (c) myelography, which reveals partial or complete block of the dye product.

Treatment of Epidural Space Metastases

Various treatments of epidural metastases aim at relieving pain and producing functional neurological improvement. The latter goal, however, is achieved less frequently than the former. Several prognostic factors must be considered in relation to the response to treatment:

(a) Nature of the primary tumor. Patients with lymphomas have a much better prognosis than those with other solid tumors. Patients with lung carcinoma are poor responders.

(b) Neurological status. Sudden onset of signs of spinal cord compression, severe paraplegia, and the presence of major sensory loss or of sphincter dysfunction are unfavorable prognostic factors.

(c) Effect of the duration of the neurological signs before laminectomy and the outcome of the operation are controverted (3,7,61).

Prophylactic Treatment

Prophylaxis of spinal cord compression by epidural metastases per se is not a standard procedure. However, treatment of patients with Hodgkin's disease includes (in stages I, II, and IIIa) irradiation of cervical, mediastinal, and lumbo-aortic areas. Patients with non-Hodgkin's lymphomas in stages I and II are similarly treated. Thus in all these patients, the epidural space is irradiated totally or partially with approximately 3,000 to 4,500 rads. Because lymphomas do not usually relapse in irradiated areas, one may consider these irradiations as prophylactic treatment of epidural space metastases. We do not have figures proving the efficacy of this prophylaxis, but it is reasonable to assume that the extremely low percentage (0.1%) of spinal cord compressions observed [e.g., by the Southwest Oncology Group in 1,039 cases of non-Hodgkin's lymphoma registered between 1972 and 1977 (22)] is related to irradiation of the spinal cord area.

Among patients with other solid tumors, those with vertebral metastases appear to be at high risk with respect to epidural spinal compression. Myelography performed in such patients reveals a high percentage of partial or even complete blocks (37). We suggest that this examination be performed in every patient with vertebral metastases, even in the absence of signs of spinal cord compression, especially if pain is present. Lipid-soluble dye is used for the procedure, as it allows subsequent objective evaluation of the effects of radiotherapy, which is used as a prophylactic treatment of spinal compression in patients with abnormal myelography.

Treatment of Spinal Cord Compression

A question often asked and not yet definitively answered is whether laminectomy is useful. There is a wide agreement that in lymphomas, including Hodgkin's disease, spinal cord compression should be treated by radiotherapy and chemotherapy (NH_2 mustard, vincristine, procarbazine, and prednisone) without laminectomy (42,59). These patients, however, should be kept under supervision, and laminectomy may be useful if the neurological signs fail to improve or become more conspicuous.

With other solid tumors, laminectomy has been recommended as the first treatment despite a high percentage of disappointing results (restoration of gait and sphincter functions has been achieved in only 10 to 35%) and a high rate of morbidity (3,7,61,66,69). Recently Gilbert et al. (18) analyzed 130 consecutive cases of spinal cord compression by extradural metastases treated by radiotherapy and 105 previously reported cases treated for the same complication at the Memorial Sloan-Kettering Cancer Center. Of the 235 patients, 65 underwent surgical decompression followed by radiotherapy and 170 were treated by irradiation alone. There was no significant difference between the two groups, even when patients with various grades of weakness at the onset of treatment were considered separately. Although this study is retrospective and nonrandomized, it strongly suggests that the role of laminectomy is limited even in patients with tumors poorly sensitive to irradiation.

Chemotherapy may be added to radiotherapy. The choice of drugs is related to the nature of the primary tumor. It should be pointed out that metastases of the epidural space are in no way protected by the blood–brain barrier.

Administration of corticosteroids at doses similar to those used in patients with brain metastases is a current practice in some centers. It aims to reduce the possible spinal cord edema which may have been increased by irradiation.

Summary

1. Early detection of metastases of the epidural space by myelography is recommended in order to start their treatment before the appearance of signs of spinal cord compression.

2. In patients with clinical signs of spinal cord compression, radiotherapy, chemotherapy, and administration of corticosteroids should be started as soon as possible. The place of neurosurgery in the management of epidural metastases remains controversial. We feel that laminectomy should be performed when: (a) the diagnosis is uncertain; or (b) the combination of radiotherapy and chemotherapy cannot be given or fails to improve the neurological status rapidly.

If laminectomy is to be performed as the first treatment, the cases in which success is most often achieved appear to be those with slowly progressing neurological signs of spinal cord compression by epidural metastases originating from tumors relatively resistant to irradiation.

MENINGEAL CARCINOMATOSIS

Clinical Features

Meningeal carcinomatosis (MC) is a widespread infiltration of the leptomeninges by neoplastic cells. Its incidence is related to the primary neoplasm. During recent years the rate of MC has rapidly changed in a number of neoplasms: It increases with the prolongation of the survival time and then decreases with the use of prophylactic treatment. The best example is children with acute lymphoblastic leukemia (ALL) where the rate of meningeal leukemia (ML) first increased from 5% to more than 50%, then fell from 5 to 10% with the systemic use of central nervous system (CNS) leukemia prophylaxis. An increased rate of ML is also observed in adult acute leukemia (AL). For instance, only 2 of 230 adults with AL followed by Dawson et al. (15) before 1970 had clinical signs of ML; whereas from 1970 to 1972, 7 of 41 patients with acute granulocytic leukemia (AGL) and 7 of 12 with ALL developed ML. A similar rate (22%) of ML was reported by Renoux et al. (55) among 68 adults with AGL, its frequency being higher in young patients. Among 101 patients with chronic granulocytic leukemia (CGL) reported by Schwartz et al. (57), 7 developed ML during the blastic phase of the disease. Meningeal involvement has even been described in chronic lymphocytic leukemia (CLL) but is exceptional (1).

In solid tumors ML is becoming particularly frequent in lymphomas. Of 50 patients with ML seen by Olson et al. (46) between 1967 and 1971, 14 had lymphomas. In contrast, in a recent series of 1,039 non-Hodgkin's lymphoma patients, the rate of clinically apparent leptomeningeal involvement was 3.7% (22). A diffuse histiocytic subtype was by far the most frequent histology associated with CNS involvement. In a smaller series of 52 patients with diffuse histiocytic and undifferentiated lymphomas reported by Bunn et al. (8), 15 (29%) had leptomeningeal involvement. Finally, in 140 complete autopsies of patients with lymphoma, 15 had MC; also in this study the histiocytic subtype was most commonly associated with meningeal metastases (19).

In earlier series, however, lymphomas were a rare source of MC, the most common primary tumors being gastric, breast, and lung carcinomas. In nonlymphoma solid tumors, where therapeutic advances are less spectacular, the changes in the rates of MC are less conspicuous. However, in a recent report by Brereton et al. (6), the incidence of MC in 58 consecutive patients treated for oat cell carcinoma of the lung was 9%.

The clinical picture of MC is characterized by a widespread, multifocal, usually asymmetrical involvement of the nervous system consisting essentially of: (a) encephalopathy and intracranial hypertension; (b) meningeal syndrome; and (c) cranial nerve and spinal root lesions. Mental changes, confusion, irritability, headaches, and vomiting are the most prominent first manifestations of MC, especially in leukemic children. Cranial nerves and spinal roots are more frequently involved in adults with primary solid tumors than in leukemic children. CSF is characterized by the presence of neoplastic cells. In patients with leukemia, the finding of two blasts in the CSF is sufficient to establish the diagnosis of ML. However, among patients with solid primary tumors, neoplastic cells may also be found (although less frequently and in smaller numbers) in the CSF of patients with cerebral metastases. Therefore, the diagnosis of ML requires other CSF changes (e.g., higher protein concentrations or low glucose levels) associated with the clinical signs described above.

Prophylactic Treatment

The benefit of the prophylactic treatment of CNS leukemia has been clearly demonstrated only in ALL, where its use greatly contributed to the dramatic improvements achieved in the treatment of the disease. What this prophylaxis should be, however, remains to be established. Cranial irradiation plus five intrathecal injections of 12 to 15 mg methotrexate (MTX) over 2.5 weeks is the most common procedure, although frequent CT brain scan abnormalities and persistent changes in intellectual performances were recently reported after this treatment (50). On the other hand, equally good prophylaxis of ML in ALL patients was obtained by Haghbin and Galicich (21) using intraventricular injections of MTX through an Ommaya reservoir without cranial irradiation. In Haghbin's treatment, MTX is also given during the maintenance treatment and systemic chemotherapy includes BCNU. It is likely, therefore, that in the future cranial irradiation could be omitted or at least reduced during prophylaxis in children with ALL.

In view of the increasing incidence of meningeal involvement, the use of a prophylactic treatment has also been advocated in other diseases, but its efficacy and modalities of treatment remain to be established by adequately controlled trials.

Dahl et al. (13) showed that in patients with AGL, 2,400 rads of craniospinal irradiation can reduce the incidence of CNS relapse, but the treatment has little impact until marrow remissions can be significantly prolonged. Therefore recent progress achieved in the management of AGL provides a solid rationale for CNS prophylaxis in this disease. Also, patients with diffuse non-Hodgkin's lymphoma who have bone marrow or bone involvement initially and in whom a complete clinical remission is achieved could be considered for CNS prophylaxis (71).

Treatment of Overt Meningeal Carcinomatosis

Overt meningeal carcinomatosis is a very serious complication because eradication of neoplastic cells invading the leptomeninges is exceptional. In patients with AL, satisfactory results were reported by Bleyer et al. (5) with MTX given via Ommaya reservoir. Two regimens were used (either 12 mg/m² or 1 mg q 12 hr × 6), each being repeated every 4 to 8 days for 8 weeks, and then monthly. The two regimens gave a mean remission of more than 300 days, and only 1 of 19 patients failed to achieve remission. Neurotoxicity was markedly lower with the low-dose schedule. In patients with overt ML, irradiation does not appear to be useful if chemotherapy is maintained.

Cytosine arabinoside (Ara-C) may be administered intrathecally at doses as high as 70 mg/m² (2,67). Intrathecal thio-tepa has also been used in the treatment of ML in doses ranging from 1 to 10 mg/m² body surface area (20). Studies comparing the efficacy of these three drugs in the treatment of ML are lacking, and the experience with thio-tepa is limited. It seems reasonable to use Ara-C when cells become resistant to MTX.

Although drugs given systematically cannot be considered the treatment of choice for MC, those crossing the blood–meningeal barrier (e.g., nitrosoureas or pyrimethamine) have some effects. Corticosteroids relieve signs of ML and should be used as emergency therapy when other treatment must be delayed for a short time.

The therapy of MC with solid tumors has not been investigated in any systematic way. Retrospective studies indicate that the majority of lymphoma patients treated by a combination of craniospinal irradiation (most frequently 3,000 to 3,500 rads) and intrathecal chemotherapy (usually MTX 10 to 15 mg twice a week) responded to treatment (8,19,71). With solid tumors other than lymphomas the results are less encouraging: however, prolonged clinical functional improvements and clearing of CSF abnormalities have been observed in women with breast carcinoma after craniospinal irradiation and intrathecal chemotherapy (26,46,70). In MC secondary to lung and gastric carcinoma or melanoma, the effects of even an aggressive therapy combining craniospinal irradiation and intrathecal and systemic chemotherapy have been disappointing in our experience. In all cases where favorable results were achieved, it was necessary to maintain intrathecal chemotherapy.

MISCELLANEOUS LESIONS

This section deals with treatment of various neurological lesions which are not exclusively associated with malignancies, but the incidence of which is increased in neoplastic diseases.

Lesions Caused by Antineoplastic Treatment

Chemotherapy and radiation therapy cause a variety of dysfunctions of the cerebral and peripheral nervous systems. Unfortunately, none can be treated with efficacy.

The neurotoxicity due to chemotherapy is dose-related in most cases, appears during drug administration, and usually regresses when the adminstration is discontinued. Therefore, persistent neurotoxicity due to chemotherapeutic agents is easier to avoid than severe lesions caused by radiation therapy, which occur after a delay of several months or years.

Infections of the Nervous System

Infections of the nervous system in patients with malignant tumors are rare. They account, in our experience, for about 1% of all neurological lesions seen in cancer patients. However, it is important to recognize these complications because some may be successfully treated. These infections are seen primarily in patients with lymphoma or leukemia, and after neurosurgery. The distribution of agents causing the CNS infections differs considerably from that found in the general population, but is similar to what is observed in conditions where the immune defenses are impaired, suggesting that immunodepression is important in the pathogenesis of CNS infection with neoplastic disease. Granulopenia (particularly that with a count under 500 cells/mm^3) and head and spine surgery are other major predisposing factors.

Herpes zoster is the most frequent nervous system infection in cancer patients. It occurs primarily in patients with lymphomas, CLL, or myeloma; radiotherapy and intensive use of chemotherapy and corticosteroids are the main predisposing factors. The greatest problems of this infection are residual pain and dissemination with visceral involvement (54). Passive immunization with herpes zoster immunoglobulin or plasma, if given early, may decrease the percentage of dissemination in immunodepressed patients. This treatment together with discontinuation of chemotherapy and corticosteroids is recommended in cancer patients who develop herpes zoster infections. The administration of adenine arabinoside 10 mg/kg/day, when given during the first 6 days of the disease, helps to eliminate pain, clear the virus from vesicles, and prevent the formation of new vesicles and pustulation in immunodepressed patients (68). High doses of interferon appear to decrease acute pain, diminish the severity of postherpetic neuralgia, limit cutaneous dissemination, and produce a sixfold reduction of visceral complications (39).

Bacterial meningitis is likely to develop in the presence of severe neutropenia, impaired immunity, and neurosurgery. The distribution of germs causing those infections is characterized by a high incidence of *Listeria monocytogenes,* Gram-negative bacilli, *Staphylococcus,* and various types of *Streptococcus.* Meningitis due to *Pneumococcus* has been associated with splenectomy (10). *Listeria monocytogenes* is susceptible to many antibiotics, but intravenous ampicillin appears as the most effective and safest treatment. In the treatment of Gram-negative meningitis, a combination of potentially synergistic antibiotics such as carbenicillin and gentamicin is preferred to chloramphenicol. Intraventricular injections of gentamicin (10 mg every 24 hr) or tobramicin may be necessary to eradicate the infection, especially when ventriculitis develops. Staphylococcal meningitis requires the administration of antistaphylococcal penicillin or vancomyin.

Fungal meningitis caused primarily by *Cryptococcus neoformans* is seen mainly in patients with depressed immunological defenses: those with lymphomas and CLL. Favorable results have been observed in the treatment of this meningitis with the combination of 5-fluorocytosine and amphotericin B. However, the presence of the underlying malignancy, corticosteroid administration, low CSF glucose, a CSF leukocyte count of less than 20/mm^3, the presence of *Cryptococcus* or CSF smear isolation of *Cryptococcus* from extraneural sites, and high titers of cryptococcal antigens in CSF and in serum are unfavorable factors for cure.

Abscesses caused by a variety of organisms including *Staphylococcus aureus, Streptococcus, Escherichia coli, Pseudomonas, Bacteroides,* and *Aspergillus* are not common in patients with cancer. Their treatment is primarily neurosurgical, but requires the addition of antibiotics at full therapeutic doses.

Encephalitis is the least common form of CNS infection. Progressive multifocal leukoencephalopathy occurs predominantly but not exclusively in immunodepressed cancer patients (mainly lymphoma and CLL). It is caused by a papovavirus. Individual cases have been treated by 5-iodo-2'-deoxyuridine or cytosine arabinoside, but the efficacy of those treatments is not unequivocally established.

Herpes simplex virus (HSV) is the most common cause of encephalitis in Western countries. The increase of its incidence in cancer patients has not been clearly demonstrated. The benefit of adenine arabinoside, which reduces the mortality of patients with HSV encephalitis in the general population, should also be given to patients with cancer.

Acquired forms of CNS toxoplasmosis are seen almost exclusively in states of impaired immunity such as lymphoma patients. Despite the activity of sulfonamides combined with pyrimethamine on *Toxoplasma gondii,* death is the usual outcome in patients with *Toxoplasma* encephalitis and an underlying cancer.

Carcinomatous Neuropathies

The so-called carcinomatous neuropathies are a group of relatively rare diseases attributed to a remote effect of cancer on the nervous system. In most of these diseases, the pathogenesis remains obscure and there is no treatment. In particular, there is no correlation between the response to treatment of the neuropathy and that of the underlying malignancy. There are, however, two possible exceptions: the Eaton-Lambert syndrome (ELS) and the myeloma peripheral neuropathies.

ELS has been reported in patients without malignant disease, but it is primarily associated with oat cell lung carcinoma. ELS is characterized by a proximal weakness which predominates in the lower limbs. The strength may be increased by repetition of movements, and a marked facilitation of muscle potentials is seen after repetitive stimulation of the nerve at 10 to 50 cycles/sec. The syndrome is due to a reduction in acetylcholine (ACh) vesicles released at the motor nerve endings. Therefore, drugs which specifically increase the number of ACh packets, e.g., guanidine (32) or 4-aminopyridine, which increases neurally evoked transmitter release from the motor nerve (40), are effective in the treatment of ELS (38). In addition, in some cases ELS improves after treatment of the underlying tumor (45).

Peripheral neuropathies of myeloma patients are of two types: one with and one without amyloidosis. The latter variety represents a form of carcinomatous polyneuritis. It is associated primarily with osteosclerotic forms of myeloma and may improve after various treatments of the neoplasm, especially radiotherapy (14), but the response is not guaranteed.

ACKNOWLEDGMENT

This work was supported in part by contract N01-CM-53840 of the National Cancer Institute, Bethesda, Maryland.

REFERENCES

1. Amiel, J. L., and Droz, J. P. (1976): Lymphocytose rachidienne au cours de la leucémie lymphocitaire chronique. *Nouv. Presse Med.,* 5:94.
2. Band, P. R., Holland, J. F., Bernard, J., Weil, M., Walker, M., and Rall, D. (1973): Treatment of central nervous system leukemia with intrathecal cytosine arabinoside. *Cancer,* 32:744–748.
3. Bansal, S., Brady, L. W., Olsen, A. O., Faust, D. S., Osterholm, J., and Kazem, I. (1967): The treatment of metastatic spinal cord tumors. *JAMA,* 202:686–688.
4. Bedikian, A. Y., Valdivieso, M., and Withers, H. R. (1977): Glycerol, a new alternative to dexamethasone in patients receiving brain irradiation. *Abstr. AACR,* p. 50.
5. Bleyer, W. A., Poplack, D. G., Ziegler, J. L., Leventhal, B. G., Ommaya, A. K., and Chabner, B. A. (1976): "Concentration time" methotrexate therapy of meningeal leukemia via a subcutaneous reservoir: A controlled clinical trial. *ASCO Abstr.,* p. 253.
6. Brereton, H. D., O'Donnell, J. F., Kent, C. H., Matthews, M., Dunnick, R. N., and Johnson, R. E. (1978): Spinal meningeal carcinomatosis in small-cell carcinoma of the lung. *Ann. Intern. Med.,* 88:517–519.

7. Brice, J., and McKissock, W. (1965): Surgical treatment of malignant extradural spinal tumours. *Br. Med. J.,* 1:1341–1344.
8. Bunn, P. A., Schein, P. S., Banks, P. M., and De Vita, V. T. (1976): CNS complications in patients with diffuse histiocytic and undifferentiated lymphoma: Leukemia revisited. *Blood,* 47:3–10.
9. Chao, J. H., Phillips, R., and Nickerson, J. J. (1954): Roentgen-ray therapy of cerebral metastases. *Cancer,* 7:682–689.
10. Chilcote, R. R., Bachner, R. L., and Hammond, D. (1976): Septicemia and meningitis in children splenectomized for Hodgkin's disease. *N. Engl. J. Med.,* 295:798–800.
11. Cox, J. D., Petrovich, Z., Paig, C., and Stanley, K. (1978): Prophylactic cranial irradiation in patients with inoperable carcinoma of the lung. Preliminary report of a cooperative trial. *Cancer,* 42:1135–1140.
12. Cunningham, T., and Baxter, D. (1974): Effect of CCNU on survival of patients with intracerebral metastasis treated with radiation and corticosteroids. *Abstr. AACR,* p. 87.
13. Dahl, G., Simone, J., Hustu, H. O., and Mason, E. W. (1976): Preventive CNS irradiation in acute myelogenous leukemia. *Blood,* 48:961.
14. Davis, L. E., and Drachman, D. B. (1972): Myeloma neuropathy. *Arch. Neurol.,* 27:507–511.
15. Dawson, D. M., Rosenthal, D. S., and Moloney, W. C. (1973): Neurological complications of acute leukemia in adults: Changing rate. *Ann. Intern. Med.,* 79:541–544.
16. Deeley, T. J., and Edwards, J. M. R. (1968): Radiotherapy in the management of cerebral secondaries from bronchial carcinoma. *Lancet,* 1:1209–1212.
17. Furlow, L. T. (1963): Metastatic tumors of the brain. *Clin. Neurosurg.,* 7:63–78.
18. Gilbert, R. W., Kim, J. H., and Posner, J. B. (1978): Epidural spinal cord compression from metastatic tumor: Diagnosis and treatment. *Ann. Neurol.,* 3:40–51.
19. Griffin, J., Thompson, R. W., Mitchinson, M. J., Kiewiet, J. C., and Welland, F. H. (1971): Lymphomatous leptomeningitis. *Ann. J. Med.,* 51:200–208.
20. Gutin, P. H., Weiss, H. D., Weirnik, P. H., and Walker, M. D. (1976): Intrathecal N,N',N''-triethylenethiophosphoramine (thio-tepa) (NSC-6396) in the treatment of malignant meningeal disease. Phase I–II study. *Cancer,* 38:1471–1475.
21. Haghbin, M., and Galicich (1977): A long-term follow-up of Ommaya reservoir for prophylaxis and treatment of central nervous leukemia. *Abstr. ASCO,* p. 342.
22. Herman, T. S., Hammond, N., Jones, S. E., Butler, J. J., Byrne, G. E., and McKelvey, E. M. (1979): Involvement of the central nervous sytem by non-Hodgkin's lymphoma. *Cancer,* 43:390–397.
23. Hildebrand, J. (1973): Early diagnosis of brain metastases in an unselected population of cancerous patients. *Eur. J. Cancer,* 9:621–626.
24. Hildebrand, J. (1978): *Lesions of the Nervous System in Cancer Patients, (EORTC, Vol. 5).* Raven Press, New York.
25. Hildebrand, J., Brihaye, J., Wagenknecht, L., Michel, J., and Kenis, Y. (1973): Combination chemotherapy with 1-(2-chloro-ethyl-3-cyclohexyl-1-nitrosourea) (CCNU), vincristine, and methotrexate in primary and metastatic brain tumors. A preliminary report. *Eur. J. Cancer,* 9:627–634.
26. Hildebrand, J., and Debusscher, L. (1977): Meningeal carcinomatosis. In: *Recent Advances in Cancer Treatment,* edited by H. J. Tagnon and M. J. Staquet, pp. 241–253. Raven Press, New York.
27. Hirsch, F., Hansen, H. H., Paulson, A. B., and Vraa-Jensen, J. (1979): Development of brain metastases in small cell anaplastic carcinoma of the lung. In: *CNS Complications of Malignant Disease,* edited by M. M. B. Kay and G. Whitehouse, pp. 175–184. Macmillan, New York.
28. Horton, J., Baxter, D. H., Olson, K. B., and The Eastern Cooperative Oncology group (1971): The management of metastases to the brain by irradiation and corticosteroids. *Am. J. Roentgenol. Radium Ther. Nucl. Med.,* 111:334–336.
29. Jackson, D. V., Richards, R., Cooper, R., Feree, C., Muss, H. B., White, D. R., and Spurr, C. L. (1977): Prophylactic cranial irradiation in small cell carcinoma of the lung. A randomized study. *JAMA,* 237:2730–2733.
30. Jackson, D. V., Cooper, M. R., Richards, F., II, Ferree, C., Muss, H. B., White, D. R., and Spurr, C. L. (1977): The value of prophylactic cranial irradiation in small cell carcinoma of the lung: A randomized study. *Abstr. ASCO,* p. 319.
31. Johnson, R. E., Brereton, H. D., and Kent, C. H. (1976): Small-cell carcinoma of the lung: attempts to remedy causes of post-therapeutic failure. *Lancet,* 2:289–291.

32. Kameskaya, M., Elmavist, D., and Thesleff, S. (1975): Guanidine and neuromuscular transmission. *Arch. Neurol.,* 32:505–518.
33. Kaye, S. B., Begent, R. H. J., Newlands, E. S., and Bagshawe (1979): Successful treatment of malignant testicular teratoma with brain metastases. *Br. Med. J.,* 1:233–234.
34. Lang, E., and Slater, J. (1964): Metastatic brain tumors. Results of surgical and neurological treatment. *Surg. Clin. North Am.,* 44:865–872.
35. Levitt, M., Meikle, A., Murray, N., and Weinerman, B. (1978): Oat cell carcinoma of the lung: CNS metastases in spite of prophylactic brain irradiation. *Cancer Treat. Rep.,* 62:131–133.
36. Livingston, R. B., and Moore, T. N. (1976): Combined modality treatment of oat cell carcinoma of the lung. *Proc. Am. Assoc. Cancer Res.,* 17:152.
37. Longeval, E., Hildebrand, J., and Vollont, G. H. (1975): Early diagnosis of metastases in the epidural space. *Acta Neurochir. (Wien),* 31:177–184.
38. Lundh, H., Nilsson, O., and Rosen, I. (1977): 4-Aminopyridine—A new drug tested in the treatment of Eaton-Lambert syndrome. *J. Neurol. Neurosurg. Psychiatry,* 44:1109–1112.
39. Merigan, C. T., Rand, K. H., Pollard, R. B., Abdallah, P. S., Jordan, G. W., and Fried, R. P. (1978): Human leucocyte interferon for the treatment of herpes zoster in patients with cancer. *N. Engl. J. Med.,* 298:981–987.
40. Molgo, M. J., Lemeignon, M., and Lechet, P. (1975): Modification de la libération du transmetteur à la jonction neuromusculaire de la grenouille sous l'action de l'amino-4 pyridine. *C. R. Acad. Sci. (Paris),* 281:1637–1639.
41. Montana, G. S., Meacham, W. F., and Caldwell, W. L. (1972): Brain irradiation for metastatic disease of lung origin. *Cancer,* 29:1477–1480.
42. Mullins, G. M., Flynn, J. P. G., El-Madhi, A. M., McOreen, D., and Owens, A. H., Jr. (1971): Malignant lymphoma of the spinal epidural space. *Ann. Intern. Med.,* 74:416–423.
43. Newman, S. J., and Hansen, H. H. (1974): Frequency, diagnosis and treatment of brain metastases in 247 consecutive patients with bronchogenic carcinoma. *Cancer,* 33:492–496.
44. Nisce, L. Z., Hilaris, B. S., and Chu, F. C. H. (1971): A review of experience with irradiation of brain metastasis. *Am. J. Roentgenol. Radium Ther. Nucl. Med.,* 111:329–333.
45. Norris, F. H., Izzo, A. J., and Garvey, P. H. (1965): Brief report: tumor size and Lambert-Eaton syndrome. In: *The Remote Effect of Cancer on the Nervous System,* edited by L. Brain and F. H. Norris, pp. 81–82. Grune & Stratton, New York.
46. Olson, M. E., Chernik, N. L., and Posner, J. B. (1974): Infiltration of the leptomeninges in systemic cancer. *Arch. Neurol.,* 30:122–137.
47. Order, S. E., Hellman, S., Vonessen, C. F., and Kligerman, M. M. (1968): Improvement in quality of survival following whole-brain irradiation for brain metastasis. *Radiology,* 91:149–153.
48. Paillas, J. E., Soulayrol, R., Combalbert, A., Vigouroux, M., Salomon, G., and Lavielle, J. (1966): Etude sur les métastases cérébrale solitaires des cancers viscéraux. *Neurochirurgie,* 12:337–360.
49. Perese, D. M. (1959): Prognosis in metastatic tumors of the brain and the skull: An analysis of 16 operative and 162 autopsied cases. *Cancer,* 12:609–613.
50. Poplack, D. G., Peylan-Ramu, N., Oliff, A., Bode, U., Moss, H., Nannes, E., and Levine, A. S. (1978): Sequellae of central nervous system prophylaxis in patients with acute lymphoblastic leukemia. *Abstr. SIOP Meeting, Brussels,* p. 97.
51. Posner, J. B., Chu, F. C. H., and Nisce, L. Z. (1974): Rapid course radiation therapy of brain metastases. *Abstr. ASCO,* No. 752, p. 172.
52. Pouillart, P., Mathe, G., Poisson, M., Buge, A., Huguenin, P., Gautier, H., Morin, P., Hoang Thy, H. T., Lheritier, J., and Parrot, R. (1976): Essai de traitement de glioblastomes de l'adulte et des métastases cérébrales par l'association d'adriamycine, de VM 26 et de CCNU. *Nouv. Presse Med.,* 5:1571–1576.
53. Raskind, R., Weiss, S. R., Manning, O., and Wermuth, R. A. (1971): Survival after surgical incision of single metastatic tumors. *Am. J. Roentgenol. Radium Ther. Nucl. Med.,* 3:323–328.
54. Reboul, F., Donaldson, S. S., and Kaplan, H. S. (1978): Herpes zoster and varicella injection in children with Hodgkin's disease. *Cancer,* 41:95–99.
55. Renoux, M., Dhermy, D., Bernard, J. F., Brousse, N., Hening, D., Amar, M., and Boivin, P. (1977): Localisations cérébro-méningées des leucémies aigües myéloblastiques de l'adulte. Etude clinique et anatomo-pathologique de 15 cas. *Nouv. Rev. Fr. Hematol.,* 18:23–34.

56. Richards, P., and McKissock, W. (1963): Intracranial metastases. *Br. Med. J.,* 1:15–18.
57. Schwartz, J. H., Canellos, G. P., Young, R. C., and DeVita, V. T. (1975): Meningeal leukemia in the blastic phase of chronic granulocytic leukemia. Am. J. Med., 59:819–828.
58. Sherata, W. M., Hendrickson, F. R., and Hindo, W. A. (1974): Rapid fractionation technique and re-treatment of cerebral metastases by irradiation. *Cancer,* 34:257–261.
59. Silverberg, I. J., and Jacobs, E. M. (1971): Treatment of spinal cord compression in Hodgkin's disease. *Cancer,* 27:308–313.
60. Simionescu, M. E. (1960): Metastatic tumors of the brain. A follow-up study of 195 patients with neurosurgical considerations. *J. Neurosurg.,* 17:361–373.
61. Smith, R. A. (1965): An evaluation of surgical treatment for spinal cord compression due to metastatic carcinoma. *J. Neurol. Neurosurg. Psychiatry,* 28:152–158.
62. Störtebecker, T. P. (1954): Metastatic tumors of the brain from a neurosurgical point of view (a follow-up study of 158 cases). *J. Neurosurg.,* 11:84–111.
63. Traggis, D., Jaffe, N., Tefft, M., and Vawter, G. (1974): Successful treatment of Wilm's tumor with intracranial metastases. *Pediatrics,* 56:472–473.
64. Tulloh, M. E., Maurer, L. H., and Foncier, R. J. (1977): A randomized trial of prophylactic whole brain irradiation in small cell carcinoma of the lung. *Proc. Am. Soc. Clin. Oncol.,* 18:268.
65. Vieth, R. G., and Odom, G. L. (1965): Intracranial metastases and their neurosurgical treatment. *J. Neurosurg.,* 23:375–383.
66. Vieth, R. G., and Odom, G. L. (1965): Extradural spinal metastases and their neurosurgical treatment. *J. Neurosurg.,* 23:501–508.
67. Wang, J. J., and Pratt, C. B. (1970): Intrathecal arabinosyl-cytosine in meningeal leukemia. *Cancer,* 25:531–534.
68. Whitley, R. J., Ch'ien, L. T., Dolin, R., Galasso, G. J., Alford, C. A., Jr., and The Collaborative Study Group (1976): Adenine arabinoside therapy of herpes zoster in immunosuppressed NIAID collaborative antiviral study. *N. Engl. J. Med.,* 294:1193–1199.
69. Wright, R. L. (1963): Malignant tumors of the spinal extradural space. Results of surgical treatment. *Ann. Surg.,* 157:227.
70. Yap, B. S., Yap, H. Y., Benjamin, R. S., Blumenchein, G. R., Hart, J. S., and Bodey, G. P. (1977): Treatment of meningeal carcinomatosis. *Abstr. ASCO,* p. 287.
71. Young, R. C., Howser, D. M., Anderson, T., Fisher, R. I., Jaffe, E., DeVita, V. T. (1979): Central nervous system complications of non-Hodgkin's lymphoma. The potential role of prophylactic therapy. *Am. J. Med.,* 66:435–443.

Medical Complications in Cancer Patients,
edited by J. Klastersky and M. J. Staquet.
Raven Press, New York © 1981.

Psychological Aspects of Cancer Diagnosis

Melvin J. Krant

Department of Medicine, University of Massachusetts Medical Center,
Worcester, Massachusetts 01605

In 1970 Bard (1) described the patient with cancer as "a person under a special and severe form of stress." He concluded that all too many individuals were technically cured of their disease, but were left with an incapacitating psychological injury. Just how many of today's patients with cancer adapt reasonably well to their lives, for as long as they live those lives, and how many suffer emotional complications related to the cancer experience cannot be stated, for no statistics of this nature exist. What does exist is a breadth of publications that testify to the psychological consequences following in the wake of a cancer diagnosis. Few of these publications present carefully evaluated and researched data for which appropriate control populations are employed. Although most writings are anecdotal, with a few controlled studies verifying the more descriptive reports, there is little need to argue academically whether cancer patients suffer more emotional complications than do patients with other major medical dislocations in their lives. The nature of the suffering cannot be called "psychiatric," and I doubt if the psychiatrist is the person who can serve as the primary therapist or be visualized as a preventing agent. An appreciation of the psychological dimensions is an inherent role in the cancer physician's ministrations to patients. Therefore, I write this chapter as an internist concerned with understanding, as well as minimizing, the suffering of the cancer patient.

The nature of the "cancer" stress appears to be, as Bard indicated, an especially stressful phenomenon, yet basically similar to many other of life's assaults. There are a number of studies of individuals who experienced significant trauma, such as approaching death, loss of a cherished other, or loss of a limb, or who were caught in an environmental disaster (2). All such events appear to inaugurate a set of emotional responses—shock, denial, anxiety, anger, guilt, frustration, and depression—in somewhat sequential manner over time (3). The latter, depression, appears to result from continued frustration to restore the state of the individual to the way things were, resulting in a growing awareness that the former valued steady state is irrevocably lost (4). The event itself (e.g., the diagnosis of cancer) is the stress, the inciting circumstance. The individual to whom the stressful event is occurring may react in a number of possible modes, depending on age, life circumstance, ego strength, perceived support, and the specific conscious or unconscious meaning that the stress may have for him. For many people in the general Western culture, stress is relative to a number of inferences regarding the human condition, such as a sense of personal power, a sense of control of one's destiny, a sense of "belongedness," and a belief in a limitless future. These human inferential configurations constitute a belief system for "safety" or "security" in a difficult world.

The fundamental impact of cancer, then, relates to how it strikes to the core of beliefs regarding one's personal security in the world. I examine four elements in the human belief system that are part of this personal security sense: (a) the physical body and its valued parts; (b) the sense of personal invulnerability—perhaps better defined as a sense of control and power to effect wanted events in life; (c) the sense of aloneness, portrayed as the despairing conviction that no one can "understand me and my plight"; and (d) a forced confrontation with "futurelessness," with death at the end of a limited road. These four states constitute an existential (philosophical) strain associated with a set of painful emotions. How an individual handles such aroused, internal strains, attempting to prevent total disorganization of his/her personality, can be defined as coping. The stresses and an individual's responses may be said to constitute a "morale" system. The charge to the physician caring for the cancer patient is to work toward keeping up the morale of the patient. The failure of the individual morale system to be sustained results in a personal set of perceptions that can be called suffering, a word which implies a broad sense of human despair. Keeping up morale is best accomplished by being aware of the nature of the strains that are apt to reduce it.

Since human beings differ in so many ways, it would be unwise to speak categorically of suffering without understanding how elements such as age, sex, social position, and finances impinge on a person's perceptions of himself. Cancer impacts on an individual who is somewhere in the arc of a life career in which ambitions, responsibilities, life tasks, and postponed gratifications exact a strong influence in determining an individual's outlook toward his disease as well as his/her life (5). Bearing cancer means something different to differing people (6). Nevertheless, we can search for predictors of breakdown in the morale system, examine possible ways of preventing breakdown, and structure relevant investigational questions.

According to Morris (7), personal adaptation in the cancer patient appears to be similar to a general pattern of adapting to other life stresses. In a lengthy review of the psychological responses to mastectomy, Morris alludes to the work of Cobb (8), who opined that the impact of any given stress is mediated by factors such as antecedent personal coping style, established psychological needs, genetic predispositions, past experience, and current life situation (including work load, responsibility, roles). The concept of social support appears especially pertinent to adaptability. Cobb defined social support as meaning the sense of being loved and cared for, esteemed, and valued, and part of a network of mutual obligations. Brown et al. (9) defined an "intimate confiding tie" as a major bulwark against depressive breakdown following a major life stress. Interwoven are two other paradigms that pose unique stress–reaction potentials on cancer patients, i.e., the long-term threat that cancer poses and the intimate body problems that are inherent to the diagnosis and treatment. The cancer patient does not face a one-time event which then can be integrated as a once-and-for-all phenomenon, painful as the event might be. The cancer patient faces chronic threat of recurrence despite all that may have been done and the sacrifices made. Furthermore, the patient must deal with the chronic, long-term loss of the safe reliability of the body.

The anxiety in the cancer experience may be said to begin when a person is signaled by a body symptom, the personal uncovering of a sign, or a physical examination, and the possibility of cancer is thrust into consciousness. The prediagnostic period is important to understand as a time of panic.

PREDIAGNOSTIC PERIOD

Patients come into a cancer-care system after a sign or symptom is unraveled or becomes severe enough for a patient to seek remedial action. The handling of the threat of possible cancer seems dependent on an individual's personality make-up, as well as on the cognitive grasp of the situation. Cancer of the breast has been most studied in regard to specific patient behaviors. Thomas (10) reported a multistaged paradigm for understanding the breast cancer patient's actions from the prediagnostic period to death. He found that after discovery certain patients may react by minimizing or completely denying the message, resulting in delay in seeking medical attention. Greer (11) clarified the nature of such delays when he reported that 60% of the patients whom he observed to have delayed for longer than 3 months were habitual deniers in the face of life stresses. Fear and anxiety about the diagnosis were paramount in the minds of those who delayed as reported in another study, but elements such as guilt, depression, and states of indecision played a role as well (12). Another study, based on psychological tests administered to 41 women referred because of breast symptoms, concluded that the very "independent" woman delayed because she felt threatened by the idea of dependency on her doctor, hospital, staff, or family (13). Worden and Weisman (14), on the basis of interviews with 125 patients with various cancers, concluded that women with breast cancer who delayed seeking medical attention were older, lived alone with no one to depend on, and were fearful of an extended illness. Delayers (all cancers) were seen as having: more denial as to the serious nature of their illness, a stronger belief that the condition was not serious, more marital problems, more reports of isolation, and a greater sense of powerlessness. Other reports emphasize social class, reporting that women from higher socioeconomic classes seem to delay significantly less in seeking diagnosis (15).

Whether delaying or rushing into medical care, the diagnostic period is one of acute anxiety. Forty-two percent of patients in one study (16) characterized this period as the most emotionally stressful in their course with cancer. The same study indicated that many patients could not, or did not, share these tense feelings with spouses or with medical staff. Maguire (17) commented that these anxiety signals were seldom picked up by surgeons in an outpatient clinic, and that the patients did not openly communicate their feelings to the staff on admission. This anxiety as to the possibility of cancer and the lack of open communication may result in painful phenomena following hospital admission, e.g., nightmares, insomnia, restlessness, crying spells, etc. This initial anxiety is greatly augmented during the waiting times between diagnostic tests and definitive medical reports and procedures.

The physician or his/her surrogate, aware of this anxiety state, might well understand that at least two interventions are needed for the patient living with the possibility of cancer: (a) shortening the work-up period as much as possible and coming up with a definitive diagnosis and treatment plan in rapid order; and (b) exhibiting a sensitivity to a patient's anxieties and fears and encouraging open communication about these feelings. The physician who can empathize with his patient's anxiety at this time and encourage communication initiates a secure feeling in these threatened individuals.

PROBLEMS IN THE BODY

People vary in their investments in their bodies. The investment is not always the same degree for each bodily zone. The head and neck, breast, rectum, and extremities have been most explored as highly valued parts of the self, especially the breast and bowel. The problems of body mutilation and cancer impact as such are difficult to separate, but many anecdotal reports emphasize the mutilation aspects, apart from the cancer, as being central to some person's adaptation. In 1955 Bard and Sutherland (18) noted that for some women losing a breast was interpreted as a worse assault on their integrity than was the fear of death associated with cancer. Many patients, they argued, were convinced that they could expect only pity, revulsion, intolerance, or some other equally disturbing reaction from the community, especially from other women. Bard and Sutherland did not do systematic studies, and factors such as age, culture, social relationships, etc. were not delineated. Neither did they carefully distinguish whether these patients were struggling only with the issue of breast loss and not the impact implicit in the amputation, i.e., that cancer had been diagnosed. Sutherland (19) concluded that "serious change in body form and function creates stress determined by the specific conscious or unconscious meaning of the sacrificed organ and its function." He concluded that mastectomy became an intolerable insult to women whose expectation of esteem in the eyes of others was to a large extent based on their beauty and shapeliness.

Further specific organ-oriented behaviors have been recorded. Mourning for the lost breast has been noted (20). Phantom breast sensations are not at all infrequent (21,22). Even suicide has been reported as a consequence of mastectomy and subsequent abandonment by the husband (23). Suicide ideation may not be at all uncommon during the postoperative period, and in one reported study 25% of 41 middle-class, middle-aged women were reported seriously to have considered killing themselves. These women had considerable anxiety about resuming sexual relationships with their partners (16).

In 1964 Quint reported on a small cohort (21 patients) of middle-aged, middle-class women who had undergone radical mastectomy for cure (24). She followed these patients at home during their first postoperative year and found that with the ups and downs present in their lives during this interval sensations of defeminization, mutilation, and de-enervation were frequent, interlocked with a sense of doom that, despite the lack of recurrence, death was impending. Delayed wound healing greatly intensified these feelings. These women exhibited impairment in work function, be it looking after their homes or reporting to an out-of-home job. Just how these women were selected for the study was not made clear, and the reader is left with an uncertainty as to whether all women are expected to respond to mastectomy in similar manner.

Jamison et al. studied 41 postmastectomy women approximately 10 months after surgery (radical or modified radical procedures) and reported that 36% of these women significantly increased their chronic use of tranquilizers, some 16% noted increased alcohol intake, and 25% reported deteriorated sex lives (16). In this study women over the age of 45 with long and stable marriages fared better in emotional, social, and sexual adaptation than did younger and currently unmarried women. The reactions of the patient's consort, husband or lover, was seen as critical to the patient's adaptation, but specific data were not alluded to.

In an accompanying report (25), the same authors studied the effects of mastectomy on the patient's male partners and concluded that mastectomy has a "ripple effect" from patient to spouse, and that the ensuing crisis could be profound. The sample of men they studied by mail questionnaire was small and appeared highly selective inasmuch as only 15% of the sample contacted responded. One of the important findings was that the patient's psychological functioning was correlated with the man's visiting pattern in the hospital, his involvement with the surgical planning decision, and his involvement in postoperative care. The greater the male involvement, the more complete was the return to a normal life style. Even in this selected sample, a number of men indicated a reluctance to look at their partner's scar or to be involved with the painful hospitalization. Although many authors who have worked with breast cancer patients emphasize the importance of the consort to a woman's psychological recovery, virtually no other empirical studies exist that help identify the supportive from the nonsupportive mate.

Polivy (26) reinforced the "breast loss" as key to emotional suffering and found that mastectomized women had lower body-image scores 3 months after surgery than patients undergoing a breast biopsy or those classified as noncancer, noncosmetic surgical controls.

Weisman and Wordan (27), however, believe that the postoperative period is characterized by a predominance of concern with life and death and not specifically with the breast. Maguire et al. (28), in a recent study, reported that 55% of patients studied were primarily concerned with the diagnosis of cancer, whereas only 18% were concerned primarily with breast loss. These studies indicated that mastectomy patients experience a peak in distress 1 to 2 months post-operation, after the patient has been at home for a while. Anger against the surgeon for the loss of the breast has been noted; this anger may spill over to the husband, and, in turn, the husband may well respond with anger to the surgeon, creating a cycle of unresolving anger.

Further adjustment problems have been the basis of several recent studies. Maguire's report details the results of a study conducted in a breast clinic in which 196 mastectomy patients were followed for at least 1 year after surgery and compared to an age-matched sample of benign breast lesion patients whose breasts were not resected. Fifty-six percent of the cancer patients were judged to have experienced considerable short-term emotional difficulties in relation to problems identified as: adjusting to a breast prosthesis, concern about attitudes of their sex partners, concern about their shapes and their scars, and concern about their ability to face other people when at home. Longer-lasting effects (1 year) included a disabling depression that was present in 20% of the cancer patients (versus 5% for a benign control group), ongoing difficulty in coping with work in 44% (versus 3% for the benign group), and continued sexual difficulties in 28% (versus 3% for the benign group). Maguire emphasized that upward of 30% of patients in this sample claimed that they had inadequate information about their diagnosis from their surgeons, and that this lack of information and a general sense of noncommunication played a major role in their long-term emotional upset (28).

Morris et al. (29) found that 23% of patients were apt to have depressive symptoms (measured by the Hamilton Rating Scale for Depression) 1 year following surgery, even when simple mastectomy had been performed. At 2 years, 22% of the patients continued to be depressed. Patients who were perimenopausal at the time of surgery were especially apt to have long-term sexual problems, as were patients judged, by psychological testing presurgically, to have depressive symptoms. Approximately 30% of the patient sample continued to dwell on the loss of the breast 2 years after surgery, clearly indicating the specific mutilating perception.

Certain psychological tests have been employed as "predictors" of later adjustment to mastectomy. Schonfield (30) examined a group of patients undergoing radiotherapy with a relatively good prognosis. He observed that those patients who returned to work posttherapy, as opposed to those who did not, scored significantly lower on a pretreatment Morale Loss Scale of the Minnesota Multiphasic Personality Inventory (MMPI) and significantly higher on the Sense of Well-Being Scale. Women who contemplated suicide in Jamison's study (16) were distinguished by a highly significant difference in the Eysenck Personality

Inventory (EPI) Neuroticism Scale. Morris' study supported the latter finding by demonstrating that patients who adjusted poorly over a long follow-up had significantly higher preoperative scores on the Neuroticism Scale of the administered EPI.

How much weight the breast itself, as opposed to cancer per se, carries for the emotional adaptation of breast cancer patients may not be totally clear, but procedures have been developed and are being further refined to either preserve as much breast tissue and surrounding musculature as is possible or to create via reconstructive mammoplasty a simulated normal breast. Lumpectomy (tumor removal, preserving surrounding breast tissue) with radiotherapy and/or chemotherapy (31), primary interstitial radiation implantation with external beam radiation amplification, and simple (total) mastectomy with node sampling are all being tested. Reconstructive mammoplasty, either at the time of the original breast cancer surgery or some months later, is gaining adherents (32). There is little reason to doubt that for some women maximum tissue preservation or the availability of reconstructive mammoplasty eliminates much suffering. It is critical that physicians do not minimize the importance of breast tissue preservation or reconstruction. Age is not a critical determinant, for as Asken (33) pointed out, a mastectomy may connote the debilitating prospects of aging for an older person, carrying significant emotional pain. If women are helped to understand the alternatives available in breast cancer surgery, encouraged to consider the possibilities of reconstructive surgery, and supported in their deliberations and choices, the issue of the breast as such may well be minimized. To berate, chide, or mock an older postmenopausal woman for wondering about the possibility of reconstruction may well be to destroy her feelings of trust and self-esteem. Not to raise alternatives is to rob a patient of feelings of "being understood," for many patients will not raise such issues with their busy doctors, either because of personal shame, reticence, or guilt. It is the physician's or his surrogate's obligation to explore these alternatives with each patient.

Curable carcinoma of the rectum and lower sigmoid colon, with resultant abdominoperineal resection and permanent colostomy, can also result in serious long-term adjustment problems, depending on colostomy function, personality organization, and perceived significant-other support. Indices and predictors for colostomy adaptation in the literature are far fewer than with breast cancer, but there is no *a priori* reason to doubt that the same stress and strain concepts apply. Rowbotham (34) pointed out that colostomies frequently impose long-term problems despite a "myth" that time alone results in resolution. Dysfunctions such as intermittent discharge of feces fluid and gas need continual reassessment and professional guidance. Underlying chronic depression is not uncommon and can interfere with social adjustment. Bronner-Huszar (35) observed that in the compulsively clean personality colostomy can engender feelings of self-hate and self-disgust, as well as phobic responses to cleansing that can keep a person tied to a toilet for hours at a time. Marital problems are not rare. Sexual impotence may be aggravated in the male (neurological damage, interfering with erection capacity); figures quoted for loss of potency range from 20 to 90% of cases studied. For women the sense of being sexually acceptable may be injured. Concerns of being rejected by one's partner may cause retreat from attempting contact. The partner may well have problems with body image and wounds and may so signal the patient.

Druss et al. (36) observed that depression, accompanied by libidinal reduction, was common after colostomy. A year or longer of adaptive time has been reported in long-term colostomy survivors. In one study approximately 60% of 110 rectal cancer patients followed for longer than 1 year said they experienced depression, feelings of invalidism, feelings of limited acceptance by spouses, friends, and fellow workers, and a reduction in work capacity (37). Olin and Fischer (37) commented that where family or social relationships were characterized by tension, hostility, or lack of care preoperatively, a delay in self-image recovery could be expected.

There is a dearth of reports on preoperative evaluation counseling, patient and family preparation, and postoperative psychosocial assistance plans. Yet it is hard not to believe that preparing the patient and family, as well as attempting to recognize preoperatively those patients at high risk for emotional suffering, would not be of enormous value.

VULNERABILITY

Cancer is a disease that evokes helplessness, and feeling helpless to exert influence on one's destiny may well be one of the most unbearable aspects of the human condition. Much of our life efforts, singularly and in the collective, are organized to give us a sense of feeling able, or sufficiently powerful, to influence our life space and to feel safe from chaotic invasion, be it by nature, enemies, government, or disease. To feel that one can bring effective influence to bear on one's present and future appears to be the essence of coping. Whereas patients with such conditions as heart disease, diabetes, and asthma can be taught to have control over the expressions of illness through exercise, diet, abstention from incident-arousing stimuli, etc., the cancer patient has traditionally felt helpless to influence the outcome of his illness. His source of power rests in the physician or in God. Without a confirmatory attitude in the latter, a feeling of utter vulnerability to all life's vicissitudes may be aroused. Such feelings can breed such emotional responses as guilt, anger, and resentment.

Abrams and Finesinger (38) explored guilt feelings in cancer patients and hypothesized that human beings need to believe in an "orderly" world in which chaos cannot be ascribed to randomness. Therefore, self-blame for disease or blame of another's actions is frequently resorted to in order to "feel" an explanation. Shands (39) pointed out that placing blame outside the self as the cause for disaster is not uncommon. Shame frequently accompanies guilt and appears to be a publicly oriented emotion for having been singled out for an uninvited and undesired disaster, or for letting others down in a manner which threatens role-relationship and one's definition of self-worth. "Feeling like a burden" is a common expression of cancer patients.

Personalized guilt, especially in areas of perceived past actions that might have been immoral or sinful, may be lessening as certain of our value systems change and as the external world comes to bear the brunt of etiology. Radiation exposure, industrial carcinogenesis, and home-food carcinogens (e.g., saccharin) are now seen as causative, and personal self-examination may be less necessary for explanation. Nevertheless, the physician should be aware that patients may harbor guilt sensations that aggravate their suffering. "If only" comments are important to unearth and explore. "If only . . . I had come to see you sooner, doctor" may be personally heard; and "If only . . . I had made him come to you sooner, doctor" is important to listen to in order to identify the spouse's anguish and guilt. The idea of punishment for immoral themes still abounds and requires voicing and gentle unwrapping.

A recent autobiographic publication by a young psychologist with testicular cancer addressed a number of critical existential issues (40). "Patient's mind and body are powerful factors in the fight against cancer," he wrote, and "failure to use these factors may result in patient resistance to treatments, depression, and loss of the will to live." Fiore (40) observed that "the vast technical expertise available tends to take all decisions out of the patient's hands," with resultant emotional distress for the patient. Feeling a sense of control over one's destiny is the antidote to despairing helplessness. When patients feel helpless in controlling medical events in their life, one form of control may be to resist treatment. When patients are given a sense of choice and responsibility rather than a sense of having to do something for somebody else, they can then accept a prolonged, painful therapy.

Prolonged and painful therapies are more and more commonplace in cancer treatment. Adjuvant therapies in breast cancer may be administered for 6 months to 2 years, as may multimodality (e.g., radiation plus chemotherapy) treatment in leukemia, Hodgkin's disease, osteogenic sarcoma, etc. Patients have varied and sometimes debilitating reactions to such lengthy treatments. Meyerowitz et al. (41) studied 50 women undergoing lengthy adjuvant postmastectomy chemotherapy and found that all these women experienced negative changes in their lives during the treatment. These changes, including repetitive nausea, vomiting, and anorexia, a general sense of lethargy and heavy fatigue, lack of ambition, and a sense of emotional inhibition, were distressing and upsetting. Thirty-eight percent gave up activities in which they had previously engaged, and 32% were unable to continue work-related activities they had performed in the past. Many found themselves irritable, nervous, tearful, and agitated. Only 12% of these 50 women reported a complete return to their normal level of behaviors and feelings. Nevertheless, nearly all commented that they would recommend such treatment to a friend should the occasion arise. It is hard to judge the latter response. Perhaps the women were persuaded that their futures looked particularly bleak owing to the possibility of recurrent cancer and that the long-term adjuvant therapy was a bulwark against that grim perspective. If so, it is possible that their symptoms were a reflection of their "entrapment" into treatment; or perhaps the upset was endurable and preferable to living with the "helplessness" of an uncontrollable future in which cancer could return.

An alliance with the physician and a positive commitment to treatment is obviously a comforting coping strategy. As Fiore pointed out (40), this cannot be a totally passive and dependent action. Some patients need to feel some sense of control. In addition to an open communication style and an attitude of the physician to share responsibility with the patient (recognizing that some patients cannot take on any responsibility), other methods of producing some positive sense of personal control and battle have been developed. In some centers the patient may be encouraged to take on responsibility for his cancer and his life, and through psychotherapeutic techniques explore personality problems that may have contributed to the evolution of the malignancy (42,43). A technique for battling the cancer by image-focusing and the mobilizing of immune, natural defenses has become popular (43). Meditation and relaxation techniques have also been suggested (44). Such procedures are reported to help patients feel that they are exerting some influence on the course of the illness and allow for an improved confederacy with an understanding physician and medical treatments. Special dieting and exercise promote the same general feeling of exerting a positive influence on the cancer. The goal in these efforts is to self-heal, which can be equated with undoing helplessness to influence events in one's life and to foster powerful feelings in order to deflect unwanted events. Alliance with the physician and the treatments promotes the sense of power; self-directed behavior augments this alliance. Active and open communication, and an overt invitation to shared responsibility in decision-making, move in the same direction. A good deal of skepticism exists in traditional medical settings for such techniques, but exploration of their potential in a creditable investigational manner should be furthered.

ISOLATION

A companion to helplessness is isolation. When a person feels that he/she has no influence on life events, he/she is also apt to feel alone and bewildered. Part of the physician's responsibility is to foster a sense of community and relationship. The manner of a physician's bearing toward the patient has received frequent comment. Brewin (45) recently advised that "a few words at the right time can make a big difference to the morale of a frightened, depressed patient." Always have a plan, he advises, and tell it to the patient: "Lack of information can greatly increase anxiety and stress, but so can too much of it. . . . Always have something to be positive and optimistic about." The defeated, depressed physician produces a defeated, depressed patient. The attitude in the relationship is critical. Part of that attitude should include an awareness that patients frequently do not communicate their feelings to medical staff people easily, and that physicians often do not listen to, or pick up on, a patient's attempts to communicate. In studies already alluded to, mastectomized women with suicidal ideation felt that they had a poor relationship with their surgeons (16). Maguire (17) pointed out the frequency with which patients noted that they were neither listened to nor helped to express their feelings. Physicians tend to detect very little of the distress their patients experience, perhaps as a device to protect their own equilibrium, which comes under challenge when the physician feels helpless to do anything about his patient's upset. Weisman and Worden (27) also pointed out that the patient's distress is frequently overlooked, and that specific interviewing techniques are required to uncover the problems patients feel. Quint (24) observed that her patients felt that interaction with the study interviewers was one of the few outlets they had for expressing their most painful fears and feelings. Quint's team was impressed by the amount of loneliness experienced by these patients.

The latter observations point out that isolation is a product of patient withdrawal, staff unavailability, and family withdrawal. That husband and wife mutually support isolation should not come as a surprise. Grandstaff (46) depicted a postmastectomy process, similarly described by Jamison et al. (16), in which the wife has trouble showing the scar to her husband but finally does so; the husband refuses to look at the scar, and the patient then does not allow herself to show her chest again (46). Inevitably, the husband perceives her withdrawal as rejection and responds by further withdrawal. The cycle of mutual withdrawal, once initiated, continues. As withdrawal develops, social and leisure activities may decline, enhancing the isolation. Certain patients may withdraw from work, again furthering their sense of isolation.

As already mentioned, emotional vulnerability seems well correlated with social circumstances and the perceived presence of strong and intimate ties. In Cobliner's study (47) of 300 women with early gynecological and breast malignancies, 10 factors were structured that influenced emotional adjustment. Four of these were regarded as social support factors; and of the others, involvement in satisfying activity seemed important. As already indicated, Brown et al. (9) postulated that women are more liable to depressive breakdown following stressful events when "not being in employment," in contrast to those who are.

Weisman (48) reported that newly diagnosed cancer patients who exhibit emotional vulnerability during the 3-month postdiagnosis period tend to come from multiproblem families, have current marital problems, and looked forward to little family support in their struggles. Other characteristics were that they had hesitated for some time in seeking medical treatment after suspecting cancer, were generally pessimistic about their status and their future, had regrets about the past, had a history of depression, and expressed a tendency to feel worthless and destructive. These patients tended to cope with their problems by suppressing emotion, acting out their tensions, withdrawing into isolation, and expressing feelings of being victimized. They differed significantly from the "good" copers, who adapted readily, had good resolution of their problems, were able to confront the facts, redefined problems to look more favorable, and accepted the support of significant others. As opposed to the poor copers, the good copers were able to forge a strong alliance with the physician. It should be noted that even the good copers had short-lived episodes of experiencing helplessness, anxiety, loneliness, and even anguish.

Several strategies have been suggested as interventions to deal with patient isolation. One is patient education; another is patient and family counseling; and a third is self-help groups. These strategies are frequently linked. Patient education has always been understood to be a major medical role. "Knowledge is the antidote to fear," wrote Emerson (49), and giving patients knowledge as to what to do to combat the effects of illness is certainly a physician's role. Collective patient education, however, has emerged as a new tactic. Patients are brought together for a collective educational endeavor whose purpose is to enhance cognitive grasp and coping. In the process, more than cancer and associated treatments may be on the agenda. In a program reported from Minneapolis, 52 newly diagnosed cancer patients participated in an 8-week education program that presented such topics as learning to cope with daily health problems, learning to communicate with others, learning to like yourself, and learning to live with limits, in addition to more standard topics such as learning about cancer and about available resources. The 52 patients were examined on three variables before and after the course: anxiety, meaningfulness in life, and knowledge of cancer. A control group of patients from the same institution receiving all modalities of medical care except for the course were also tested. The "educated patient" group experienced a significant reduction in anxiety compared to controls and to their own pretest scores, and also reported a heightened meaningfulness of life score (50). In general, patient education efforts appear to enhance adaptation and rehabilitation, as patients come to have a better grasp of their illness as well as an appreciation that they are not alone in their affliction or in their responses to it.

Self-help groups for patients and families also serve to bring people together for shared support. The Reach-to-Recovery postmastectomy program employs breast cancer patients as visitors to newly mastectomized patients. Usually the visits are limited to one or two while the patient is in the hospital, and in most state-wide programs the physician must ask for the volunteer visit. Group-oriented activities have been established in many communities organized under the banner "no one understands what it is like to have cancer except another cancer patient." Pursell and Tagliareni report on issues raised in a particular group (51). "Helplessness" was a common issue explored, as were questions about the value of treatment and side effects. Patients sometimes shared their feelings and often compared secrets for keeping up their spirits. The group might praise a member for his/her courage or strength. Difficulties in sharing feelings in the family were discussed. Such problems ensue when a patient is not sure that the family member(s) "could take it," with resultant conflicts between wishing to "spare" or "protect" their families and yet needing their knowledgeable support.

Dumont (52) explored the value of self-help groups in general psychiatric treatment and quotes a phrase attributable to Sir Geoffrey Vickers: "The major threat at every level [of human harmony] is the lack of what I have called an appreciation system sufficiently widely shared to mediate communication, sufficiently apt to guide action, and sufficiently acceptable to make personal experience bearable." Not all patients desire groups, and lengths of involvement are quite varied for those who participate. That they serve a purpose in alleviating isolation is undeniable. Their availability may, for the right patient, make an enormous difference in the sense of morale.

Lewis and Bloom (53) point out that, although there is a general awareness among health-care professionals that "significant others" are important to a patient as the primary source of social interaction and support, designed intervention for these people is seldom enacted. For example, there are few reports of integrated husband-wife support programs for breast cancer, although a number of rehabilitation and counseling hospital-based programs for the patient have been described (54,55).

Professional support programs for individual patients appear organized to aid the patient's coping through encouraged emotional release, anticipatory problem-solving, and information exchange. Just who the supportive individual should be and what long-term effects can be accomplished is far from resolved. Intervening with the needy patient presents some problem, since patients and physicians seem to be able to disguise the visibility of emotional unrest. Ervin (23) emphasized that it is a significant other (e.g., a spouse) who is the pivotal figure in psychological adjustment, and that the physician should acknowledge a role in teaching the spouse ways to be supportive. The physician must be exquisitely sensitive to this possibility, however, and an available and willing spouse must exist.

FUTURELESSNESS

Shands (39) described a loss of orientation for the future as one of the major psychological reactions to the diagnosis of cancer. He described patients reporting that they felt as if they had experienced "a sudden amputation of the future," and that this realization came as "a blow on the head" with devastatingly shocking impact. In somewhat overblown rhetoric, Brennan (56) took this case deeper in commenting that "in an industrial, technological society which perforce expends most of its efforts in the construction of future benefits and accomplishments, and characteristically places its hopes of achievements, order, and happiness in the future to provide escape from the present, not to have a potentially triumphant future which one can share with others for all practical purposes, is not to exist in the present either." Cancer, in this sense, is a sudden confrontation with life's limits, and for many individuals who prefer not to stare at death during their healthy lives such sudden confrontation is deeply upsetting. Futurelessness may become the dominant perspective for the patient, and such a perspective may be shared by family and by society at large. Such a perspective disenfranchises the cancer patient, as he sees himself and as others view him. Thus, continues Brennan, the cancer patient can best be understood as a victim of deprivation and isolation. These feelings of being deprived of a fit place in society, and the sense of being unwelcomed in the sharing of life pursuits may be at the root of the despair, depression, and resentment so often expressed by patients.

An "amputation of the future" can well be visualized as age-related, although there are few studies that have examined this issue. The young patient with a yet "unlived" life may harbor resentful thoughts about life curtailed, thoughts rather different than those of an elderly patient who might feel that life has been lived and most acts already completed. Such implications should not be accepted too glibly, for elderliness is a state of mind (not of chronology exclusively), and many years, no matter how many they may be, do not free people of resentments for "wasted" and "unfinished" years nor convert them into peaceful, accepting patients.

Much has been written about "hope" as an ingredient in patient care. Hope is future-oriented, a sentiment expressed for a potential change, an improvement of the present state. Physicians are often implored never to take hope away from patients, for a hopeless state is utterly despairing. This requisite seems to have been the root of noncommunicating the diagnosis in the past (57), especially when the medical potential and atmosphere was that "nothing more could be done." Present dictum is that much can be done and that there is always another "something" that can be offered, even when the management plan is requisitely shifting to a palliative, from a curative, mode as conditions worsen.

A considerable effort has been expended during the past decade to restore a confidence in the world for the cancer patient. Efforts are medical and social. All are founded on the notion of a future and are basically comprised of trying to turn a negative, disenfranchised attitude into a positive, forward-looking stance. Cancer societies emphasize the increasing curability of the disease and openly employ the word cancer in order to mitigate against its secretive and unmentionable death image. Therapeutic patient-oriented groups have been organized with "attitude" implications, e.g., Reach-to-Recovery for mastectomy patients, CanSurmount (Colorado) for all patients, and Make-Every-Day-Count. These patient-to-patient self-help groups emphasize a future, an attitude toward hope.

Once the shock is allowed to settle, patients often integrate the experience of diagnosis and move on into treatments and rehabilitation with a positive belief for the future. A hopeless physician attitude is utterly destructive to this integration. As already pointed out, patients will bear extraordinary physical and even psychological disability for a length of time in the protection of a future.

Nevertheless, long-term treatments (e.g., radiotherapy and the adjuvant programs) do tax people and continue to serve as reminders that the disease state exists. This state of "illness-being" can dominate a person's life. Lyon (58) reported that as many as 50% of patients receiving radiation therapy experience a severe depression, and that thoughts of suicide occurred to approximately 13% of the patients studied during the course of treatment. Concluding treatment is frequently a moment of celebration and a gateway to return to "normal" life without constant reminders of disease. Some patients need help, however, giving up treatment. They may visualize that their source of "power and support" is being cut off, throwing them back onto their own resources for getting on with life. Illness, of course, has secondary gains for many, and certain patients have great difficulty in "letting go" of either the illness state or its extension, the treatment state. Physicians should be aware that "terminating" long-term treatment may be difficult for some patients, and in fact offering counseling for return to normalcy may be highly beneficial for those individuals expressing concern about a future without illness and without the healer's immediate proximity.

RECURRENCE

Should disease recur after initial treatment, the patient's sense of helplessness and emotional vulnerability may become explosively visible again. A shaky adaptation may fall apart, and concentrated effort to re-establish a set of "safety" conditions may be necessary. Deep dependency may recur, but confidence in the medical system and in the physician and his or her recommended treatment may be difficult to maintain. Nevertheless, many patients get on with subsequent treatments and begin to alter their focus from a long-term cure to a few weeks, or months, ahead. It is at this point that the search for possible "miracle" cures may begin, in fantasy if not in reality. The pathway with chronic, active disease is strewn with adaptational difficulties, and a myriad of publications have appeared about the management of the late-stage, dying patient. It is well to remember that certain patients (e.g., those with breast cancer metastatic to bone) may live for years, undergoing various manifestations of illness. The physician's task is to keep the quality of life of such patients as high as possible as long as they are alive. The hospice movement, with its emphasis on psychosocial issues, symptom control, and family involvement, has much to teach in this regard.

SUMMARY

Understanding the nature of the psychological wounds that accompany the cancer diagnosis can help the physician formulate plans to promote morale upkeep of his patient. Recognizing that his attitude and availability are critical components of total caring, the physician can facilitate assessment of potential emotional vulnerability and potential for therapeutic interventions. Much is yet to be learned about assessments and long-term therapeutic strategies and outcomes for patients and families. Nevertheless, enough is known to suggest that cancer patients need available, concerned support from significant others, as well as professional staff. Such effort appears to be growing in many communities.

REFERENCES

1. Bard, M. (1970): The price of survival for cancer victims. In: *Where Medicine Fails,* edited by A. Strauss, pp. 99–110. Aldine, Chicago.
2. Lazarus, R. S. (1966): *Psychological Stress and the Coping Process.* McGraw-Hill, New York.
3. Falek, A., and Britton, S. (1974): Phases in coping: The hypothesis and its implications. *Soc. Biol.,* 21:1.
4. Bard, M. (1952): The sequence of emotional reactions in radical mastectomy patients. *Public Health Rep.,* 64:1144.
5. Krant, M. J., (1978): Cancer: Action for improving socialization and family support, and reducing stigma and negative attitudes. In: *The Role of Vocational Rehabilitation,* edited by L. Pearlman. National Rehabilitation Association, Washington, D.C.
6. Hinton, J. (1973): Bearing cancer. *Bri. J. Med. Psychol.,* 46:105–113.
7. Morris, T. (1979): Psychological adjustment to mastectomy. *Cancer Treat. Rev.,* 6:41–61.
8. Cobb, S. (1974): A model for life events and their consequences. In: *Stressful Life Events: Their Nature and Effects,* edited by N. S. Dohrenwend and B. P. Dohrenwend, pp. 151–156. Wiley, New York.
9. Brown, G. W., Bhrolchain, M. N., and Harris, T. (1975): Social class and psychiatric disturbance among women in an urban population. *Sociology,* 9:225.
10. Thomas, S. G. (1978): Breast cancer: The psychosocial issues. *Cancer Nurs.,* 1:53.
11. Greer, S. (1974): Psychological aspects: Delay in the diagnosis of breast cancer. *Proc. R. Soc. Med.,* 67:470–473.
12. Gold, M. A. (1964): Causes of patient delay in diseases of the breast. *Cancer,* 17:564–577.
13. Hammerschlag, C. A., Fisher, S., DeCosser, J., and Kaplan, E. (1964): Breast symptoms and patient delay: Psychological variables involved. *Cancer,* 17:1480–1485.
14. Worden, W. J., and Weisman, A. D. (1975): Psychosocial components of lag-time in cancer diagnosis. *J. Psychosom. Res.,* 19:69–79.
15. Hackett, T. P., Cassem, N. H., and Raker, J. W. (1973): Patient delay in cancer. *N. Engl. J. Med.,* 289:14–20.
16. Jamison, K. R., Wellisch, D. K., and Pasnau, R. P. (1978): Psychological aspects of mastectomy. 1. The woman's perspective. *Am. J. Psychiatry,* 135:432–436.
17. Maguire, P. (1976): The psychological and social sequellae of mastectomy. In: *Modern Perspectives in Psychiatric Aspects of Surgery,* edited by J. G. Howells, pp. 390–421. Brunner/Mazel, New York.
18. Bard, M., and Sutherland, A. M. (1955): Psychological impact of cancer and its treatment. Adaptation to radical mastectomy. *Cancer,* 8:656–72.
19. Sutherland, A. M. (1967): Psychological observations in cancer patients. *Int. Psychiatr. Clin.,* 4:75–92.
20. Rosen, V. H. (1950): The role of denial in acute post-operative affective reactions following removal of body parts. *Psychosom. Med.,* 12:356–361.
21. Roberts, M. M., Furnival, S. G., and Forrest, A. (1972): The morbidity of mastectomy. *Br. J. Surg.,* 59:301–302.
22. Bressler, B., Cohen, S. I., and Magnussen, F. (1956): The problem of phantom breast and phantom pain. *J. Nerv. Ment. Dis.,* 123:181.
23. Ervin, C. J. (1973): Psychological adjustment to mastectomy. *Med. Aspects Hum. Sexuality,* 7:42–65.

24. Quint, J. (1964): Mastectomy—Symbol of cure or warning sign. *GP,* 29:119–124.
25. Wellisch, D. K., Jamison, K. R., and Pasnau, R. O. (1978): Psychological aspects of mastectomy. II. The man's perspective. *Am. J. Psychiatry,* 135:543–546.
26. Polivy, J. (1977): Psychological effects of mastectomy on a woman's feminine self-concept. *J. Nerv. Ment. Dis.,* 164:77–87.
27. Weisman, A. D., and Worden, W. (1976): The existential plight in cancer: Significance of the first hundred days. *Int. J. Psychiatry Med.,* 7:1–15.
28. Maguire, G. P., Lee, E. G., Bevington, D. J., Kuchemann, C., Crabtree, R. J., and Cornell, C. E. (1978): Psychiatric problems in the first year after mastectomy. *Br. Med. J.,* 1:963.
29. Morris, T., Greer, J. S., and Pettingale, K. W. (1977): Psychological and social adjustment to mastectomy: A two-year follow-up study. *Cancer,* 40:2381–2387.
30. Schonfield, J. (1972): Psychological factors related to delayed return to an earlier life style in successfully treated cancer patients. *J. Psychosom. Res.,* 16:41–46.
31. Levene, M. B., Harris, T. R., and Hellman, S. (1977): Treatment of carcinoma of the breast by radiation therapy. *Cancer,* 39:2840–2845.
32. Snyderman, R. K. (1976): On breast reconstruction after mastectomy for cancer. *Plast. Reconstr. Surg.,* 57:224–226.
33. Asken, M. J. (1978): Psychoemotional aspects of mastectomy: a review of recent literature. *Am. J. Psychiatry,* 132:56–59.
34. Rowbotham, J. L. (1971): Colostomy problems—Dietary and colostomy management. *Cancer,* 28:219–238.
35. Bronner-Huszar, J. (1971): The psychological aspects of cancer in man. *Psychosomatics,* 12:133–138.
36. Druss, R. G., O'Conner, T. F., and Stern, L. O. (1969): Psychological response to colectomy. II. Adjustment to permanent colostomy. *Arch Gen. Psychiatry,* 20:419–427.
37. Olin, B., and Fischer, H. K. (1976): Psychiatric aspects of colostomy and ileostomy. In: *Modern Perspectives in Psychiatric Aspects of Surgery,* edited by J. G. Howells. Brunner/Mazel, New York.
38. Abrams, R., and Finesinger, J. F. (1963): Guilt reactions in patients with cancer. *Cancer,* 6:474–482.
39. Shands, H. C. (1966): The informational impact of cancer in the structure of the human personality. *Ann. NY Acad Sci.,* 159:883–889.
40. Fiore, N. (1979): Fighting cancer—One patient's perspective. *N. Engl. Med. J.,* 300:284–289.
41. Meyerowitz, B. E., Sparks, F. C., and Spears, I. K. (1979): Adjuvant chemotherapy for breast cancer: Psychosocial implications. *Cancer,* 43:1613–1618.
42. LeShan, L. (1977): *You Can Fight For Your Life. Emotional Factors in the Confrontation of Cancer.* M. Evans, New York.
43. Simonton, J., and Simonton, S. (1975): Belief symptoms and management of the emotional aspects of malignancy. *J. Transplant. Psychiatry,* 7:29–47.
44. Pelletier, K. (1977): *Mind As Healer, Mind As Slayer,* pp. 134–149. Delta Books, New York.
45. Brewin, T. B. (1977): The cancer patient: Communication and morale. *Br. Med. J.,* 2:1623–1627.
46. Grandstaff, N. W. (1975): The impact of mastectomy on the family. Paper presented at Medical Social Consultants Meeting, San Francisco.
47. Cobliner, W. G. (1977): Psychosocial factors in gynecological or breast malignancies. *Hosp. Physicians,* 10:38.
48. Weisman, A. D. (1976): Early diagnosis of vulnerability in cancer patients. *Am. J. Med. Sci.,* 27:187–196.
49. Emerson, R. W. (1877): Quoted in ref. 45.
50. Johnson, J. (1978): The effects of a patient-centered educational program on a person's adaptability to living with a chronic disease. In: *Abstracts: American Society of Clinical Oncology Meeting.*
51. Pursell, S., and Tagliareni, E. M. (1974): Cancer patients help each other. *Am. J. Nurs.,* 74:650–651.
52. Dumont, M. P. (1974): Self-help treatment groups. *Am. J. Psychiatry,* 131:631–635.
53. Lewis, F. M., and Bloom, T. R. (1978): Psychosocial adjustment to breast cancer: A review of selected literature. *Int. J. Psych. Med.,* 9:1–17.
54. Schmidt, W. L., Kiss, M., and Bibert, L. (1971): The team approach to rehabilitation after mastectomy. *AORN J.,* 19:821–836.

55. Winick, L., and Robbins, G. F. (1977): Physical and psychological readjustment after mastectomy: An evaluation of Memorial Hospital's PMRG program. *Cancer,* 39:478–486.
56. Brennan, M. J. (1970): The cancer gestalt. *Geriatrics,* pp. 96–101.
57. Holland, J. (1973): Psychological aspects of cancer. In: *Cancer Medicine,* edited by J. F. Holland and E. Frei, pp. 991–1021. Lea & Febiger, Philadelphia.
58. Lyon, J. S. (1977): Management of psychological problems in breast cancer. In: *Breast Cancer Management—Early and Late,* edited by B. A. Stoll, pp. 225–235. Heinemann, London.

Medical Complications in Cancer Patients,
edited by J. Klastersky and M. J. Staquet.
Raven Press, New York © 1981.

Cancer Pain

John J. Bonica

*Department of Anesthesiology, University of Washington School of Medicine,
Seattle, Washington 98195*

Cancer pain has long been, and continues to be, one of the most important and pressing issues of the American (and the world) health care system. This importance stems from several factors: (a) cancer pain afflicts 750,000 Americans annually; (b) although when properly used the drugs and other therapeutic modalities currently available are effective in relieving the pain of most cancer patients, they are often inadequately applied; consequently, (c) most patients spend their last weeks and months of life in great discomfort, suffering, and disability which preclude a "quality of life" that is vital to them (16,17).

The purpose of this presentation is to give a very brief overview of several aspects of this problem including: (a) the incidence and magnitude of cancer pain; (b) the physiologic and psychologic effects of cancer pain; (c) the current status of its control and the reasons for deficiencies; (d) the etiology and possible mechanisms of cancer pain; and (e) a very brief evaluation of various modalities currently available for its management. Following long tradition, I use the term "cancer pain" generically to include pain caused by any malignant neoplasm, pain that is a consequence of therapeutic intervention for the disease, or both.

MAGNITUDE OF THE PROBLEM

Incidence

In the United States there are about 700,000 new cases of cancer diagnosed and nearly 400,000 deaths from cancer annually (4) (Table 1). Although cancer is not usually painful at its onset and during its early phases, and a significant percent of patients are cured (4,12), a large number of patients with recurrent or metastatic cancer eventually develop pain which becomes progressively more severe and finally develops into a relentless suffering that greatly aggravates the physiologic and psychologic deterioration of the patient caused by the disease itself (12,22). Moreover, a significant number of patients develop pain as a result of the therapy (31). Although precise data from large-scale epidemiologic

TABLE 1. *Cancer statistics*

Parameter	No.	%
Incidence in USA (1978 ACS estimates)		
New cases diagnosed	700,000	
Cancer deaths	390,000	
Cancer: leading causes of death		
Lung	92,400	23
Colon-rectum	52,000	13
Breast	34,000	8.5
Uterus and ovary	21,500	5.5
Lymphomas	21,500	5.5
Prostate	20,600	5.1
Pancreas	20,000	5
Leukemia	15,000	3.8
Stomach	14,500	3.7
Central nervous system	9,000	2.3

studies on the incidence of cancer pain are not available, a number of surveys suggest that moderate to severe pain is experienced by about 40% of patients with intermediate stages of the disease and by 60 to 80% of the patients with advanced cancer.

TABLE 2. *Incidence of advanced cancer pain*

Study	%[a]	Ref. no.
Average data		
Cartwright et al. (England)—terminal cancer	87	25
Foley (NYC)—33% of 397 pts., in terminal pts.	60	31
Pannuti et al. (Italy)—advanced cancer	65	60
Parkes (London)—advanced cancer	65–70	62
Twycross (St. Christopher's)—500 admissions	80	83
Wilkes (Sheffield)—300 admissions	60	87
Specific lesions[b]		
Bone	85	
Cervix	85	
Stomach	65–75	
Lung	50–70	
Female genitourinary	70	
Pancreas	70	
Male genitourinary	60–75	
Breast	55–70	
Intestine	60	
Kidney	55	
Colon-rectum	50–60	
Leukemia	5	

[a] Percents are rounded to the nearest multiple of five.
[b] Single percent represents data from one report or averages; the ranges are from Foley, Pannuti et al., Wilkes, and other literature (22).

Table 2 summarizes the results of some of these surveys. Wilkes (87) studied nearly 300 patients admitted to a 25-bed unit for the care of dying patients in an English provincial city and found that pain was the major symptom in 58% on admission and occurred more frequently later. Twycross (83) reviewed the records of the patients admitted consecutively to St. Christopher's Hospice, where about 500 patients are admitted each year, and found that over 80% required diamorphine (heroin) for severe pain sometime during their hospital stay. In another survey Parkes (62) interviewed the surviving spouses of 276 patients who had died of cancer, and who had been managed in hospitals in South London or in the home. The survey revealed the following: Among patients managed in the hospital, 40% had mild or no pain, 38% had moderate pain, and 22% had severe or very severe pain; among the patients cared for in the home, 31% had mild or no pain, 21% had moderate pain, and 48% had severe or very severe pain. In still another British study, Cartwright and associates (25) found that 87% of patients who died from cancer had pain prior to death. Foley (31), Houde, and their co-workers found that among 397 patients with cancer in the Memorial Sloan Kettering Cancer Center 38% had pain related to cancer, but the figure rose to 60% among the terminally ill patients in the hospital. The survey reported by Pannuti and associates (60) involved 290 patients with advanced specific tumors admitted to the cancer service of the Malphigi Hospital, Bologna, Italy. Extrapolation of these data suggests that yearly about 250,000 Americans have severe or very severe cancer pain, and another 500,000 have moderate pain related to their cancer or as a result of cancer therapy.

Physiologic and Psychologic Effects of Cancer Pain

Relatively recent studies emphasize that chronic pain induces physiologic and psychologic effects which are similar regardless of etiology (20,75). Persistent pain and suffering produces a progressive physical deterioration due to disturbances in sleep and appetite and often excessive medication. All of these factors contribute to the general fatigue and debility. Moreover, in many patients with chronic pain, the pain perception threshold and pain tolerance thresholds are decreased, possibly owing in part to depletion of endorphins which have been shown to be lower in the cerebrospinal fluid of these patient than in normal patients (2,3). Many patients with chronic pain also undergo serious emotional, affective, and behavioral changes (75). They develop anxiety, depression, hypochondriasis, somatic preoccupation with disease conviction, somatic focusing, and a tendency to deny life problems unrelated to their physical problems. This cluster of psychologic changes, which Pilowsky et al. (63) labeled "abnormal illness behavior," is characteristic of chronic pain whether due to somatogenic or psychogenic etiology. Chronic pain increases levels of neuroticism (10,75). Moreover, as a consequence of debility, there is a progressive reduction in physical and social activities. Because of the prolonged disability, chronic pain is now generally considered a serious national health and economic problem (15,19).

Usually, the physiologic and psychologic impact of cancer pain on the patient is greater than that of nonmalignant chronic pain (12,16,17). The physical deterioration is more severe because these patients have greater problems with sleep disturbance and with lack of appetite, nausea, and vomiting. Cancer patients also develop greater emotional reactions of anxiety, depression, hypochondriasis, somatic focusing, and neuroticism to the pain when it develops than is found in patients with nonmalignant chronic pain (9–11,89). Woodforde and Fielding (89) examined cancer patients with and without pain using the Cornell Medical Index and demonstrated that the former group was significantly more emotionally disturbed than the latter group and that they responded less well to treatment of their cancer and died sooner. The main cause of emotional morbidity was found to be depression, although hypochondriasis and psychosomatic symptoms were also recorded. They commented that the combination of intractable pain and depression represent symptoms that indicate a state of helplessness or inability to cope with disease, damage to the body, and the threat to life, and that this is a response to having a progressive and potentially fatal illness. Bond (10,11) found that cancer patients with pain had raised levels of hypochondriasis and neuroticism whereas pain-free cancer patients had low levels. He further noted that the scores of patients with high-level emotionality fell after the pain was relieved by percutaneous cordotomy. This led Bond to conclude that personality factors are distorted by severe pain and that its relief results in restoration in the direction of normality.

The social effects of the uncontrolled cancer pain are equally devastating. Many patients develop interpersonal problems with members of their family, friends, and the community. The fact that most patients with advanced cancer have to stop working poses not only an economic but also an emotional stress as well as a feeling of dependency and uselessness. The physical appearance and behavior produced by the patient's pain and suffering stresses the family emotionally, which is in turn perceived by the patient and consequently aggravates the pain and suffering. Some patients with severe intractable pain become so discouraged and desperate as to contemplate suicide.

Figure 1, developed by Chapman (26), presents a model of the pain associated with recurrent or metastatic cancer. The basic building block of this pain experience is the barrage of noxious sensory impulses that arise in diseased or damaged tissue caused by the cancer or by complications of cancer therapy. It is to be noted that various factors contribute to the anxiety, depression, and anger experienced by the patient. Moreover, the bidirectionality of the arrows going from one of these to the other and from these to the noxious sensory input emphasizes that each of these factors enhances the activity of the others and thus aggravates the pain, which in turn increases the emotional responses. The clinical implication is that unless the pain is interrupted, the vicious circle continues and the pain and associated responses become greater.

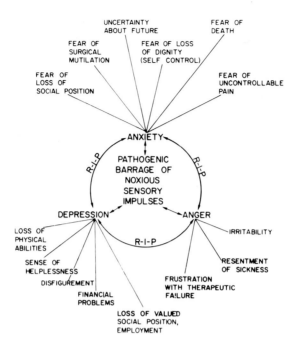

FIG. 1. Psychologic dimensions of the pain experience in the patient with advanced cancer. Anxiety, depression, and anger are presented for visualization purposes as three independent components of the patient's experience, but it should be recognized that these three problems mutually support and feed one another. The relationship among the three dimensions is defined as the rational–imaginative process (R-I-P). (From ref. 26.)

Current Status of Cancer Pain Control

Various sources of information suggest that, like chronic pain in general, cancer pain is improperly managed. A study carried out by Marks and Sochar (53) of Montefiore Hospital in New York revealed that many physicians prescribed inadequate amounts of analgesics for patients with cancer pain (and other medical disorders) and that most patients actually received only about 20 to 25% of the (inadequate) amount prescribed. Consequently, in most patients moderate to severe pain persisted after the narcotic therapy. The reason for the inadequate therapy is discussed in the next section.

In his survey of 276 cancer patients, Parkes (62) found that, of the hospital patients who had severe or very severe pain, the pain *remained unrelieved* even during the terminal stage of the disease. Moreover, among the patients managed in their homes, the incidence of unrelieved severe to very severe pain during the terminal phase increased nearly sixfold of that experienced during the period prior to the terminal phase of the disease. These figures suggest that pain control was inadequate in the hospital and even worse in the home. Parkes noted this was in contrast to what happened to patients managed in St. Christopher Hospice, where pain control is effectively carried out: The incidence of severe and unrelieved pain was 36% during the preterminal period, but this dropped to 8% during the terminal phase of the disease. Cartwright and associates (25) found that 87% of the patients who died from cancer had pain just prior to death that apparently remained unrelieved. Similar reports were made by many participants of the International Symposium on Pain of Advanced Cancer which was held in Venice in May 1978 (22).

In 1974 the problem of inadequate relief of severe pain of advanced cancer in America was brought to national attention by Stewart Alsop, the late highly respected newspaperman and writer who died of cancer. Speaking on national television, Alsop described observing the agony and suffering manifested by a fellow patient at the Clinical Center of the National Institutes of Health, whose severe pain was inadequately relieved by morphine and other potent analgesics. His vivid, heart-rending report prompted the eventual organization of the National Committee on the Treatment of Intractable Pain, a nonprofit organization with the primary goal of effecting better pain control in patients with advanced cancer (64). Since it was founded in September 1977 it has received thousands of letters from family, friends, and physicians describing one or more patients who spent their last few months with severe, excruciating cancer pain that remained unrelieved until death (64). Although admittedly these are anecdotal reports, the fact that the Committee received several thousand such letters within a 12-month period suggests that a not insignificant number of patients who die from cancer spend the terminal part of their lives with unrelieved severe pain. Colin MacInnes (51), the famous British novelist and social commentator, in an article he wrote just before he died of stomach cancer, reported similar personal experiences and referred to the inadequate pain control as "the great defect in English public hospital treatment which to my mind, is a cruel and callous disgrace."

Reasons of Therapeutic Deficiencies

In view of the great advances in biomedical scientific knowledge and technology, and especially the great amount of interest in cancer research and therapy, why is cancer pain so poorly managed? Serious consideration of this important question during the course of the past quarter-century has suggested to me that it is due to neglect of the problem of pain (in contrast to the cancer) by oncologists, educators, investigators, research institutions, and national and international cancer agencies (12,16,17). Consequently, like chronic pain in general, there are voids in our knowledge of cancer pain, and whatever knowledge is currently available is improperly applied.

Improper Application of Current Knowledge

The most important reason for inadequate cancer pain control is improper application of what we do know. This in turn is due to a number of interrelated factors: (a) lack of organized teaching of medical students and physicians and other health professionals in the management of cancer pain; (b) the meager amount of published information about the proper treatment of cancer pain; (c) lack of data based on comprehensive controlled evaluation of the various modalities currently available for this purpose; (d) insufficient knowledge or lack of consideration by the managing physician of the various mechanisms and types of cancer pain and the associated physiologic, emotional, affective, and behavioral responses which must be considered if the pain and suffering are to be effectively treated; (e) lack of appreciation of the greater efficacy of therapeutic modalities other than drugs in certain patients combined with the lack of personnel with the interest and expertise in the proper application of these modalities; and (f) the fact that cancer pain is a complex array of sensory, perceptual, and emotional events which often require the concerted and well-coordinated efforts of specialists from different disciplines working as a team, combined with the fact that traditional medical practice is not conducive to the team approach.

Review of curricula of the medical schools in the United States reveals that few, if any, teach students basic principles of the use of narcotics and other therapeutic modalities that effectively relieve cancer pain (16). Moreover, many physicians in residency training for specialization in surgical, medical, and radiation oncology receive little or no teaching about the proper management of cancer pain. Usually the senior house officer, who has vague and scanty information about cancer pain and its proper control, teaches the junior house officer how to deal with the problem in a rather empirical way and passes on some of the misconceptions that are mentioned below (16).

Inadequate or total lack of interest or concern about the problem of pain by oncologists is further attested to by the fact that very little if any information about the proper management of the pain problem is found in the oncology literature, voluminous as it is. Of the many textbooks on various aspects of cancer, only a few deal with the problem of pain management and then do so in a totally inadequate manner. For example, review of 11 of the most important textbooks and monographs on cancer published in English—including two on surgical oncology (56,65), four educational monographs published by three of the most influential cancer groups (5,27), and four comprehensive books on clinical oncology (1,41,42)—reveals the startling facts summarized in Table 3. Thus it is noted that these seven volumes, totaling nearly 9,500 pages, devote fewer than 18 pages to the treatment of cancer pain. Moreover, review of the current literature reveals only a small number of papers on pain, which is miniscule compared to the hundreds of articles written on other aspects of cancer each year. The only conclusion that can be drawn from these data is that pain has not been considered important by oncologic scientists and clinicians.

As a result of this lack of education of students, graduate physicians, and other health professionals, the pain of cancer is treated in an empirical manner. Insufficient knowledge or lack of consideration of the various mechanisms and types of cancer pain, the associated physiologic and psychologic responses, and the failure to appreciate the role of all the therapeutic modalities currently

TABLE 3. *Discussion of pain in oncology textbooks*

Title of book	Authors	Year of publ.	Total pages	Pages devoted to pain therapy
Cancer Medicine	Holland & Frei	1974	2,018	13
Clinical Oncology	Horton & Hill	1977	819	2.5
Cancer Diagnosis, Treatment and Prognosis	Ackerman & Del Regato	1970	783	None[a]
Cancer: Manual for Practitioners	Massachusetts Division, American Cancer Society	1968	408	None
Clinical Oncology: Manual for Students and Doctors	Comm. Prof. Education U.I.C.C.	1973	322	1.25
Advances in Cancer Surgery	Najerian & Delaney	1976	608	None
Principles of Surgical Oncology	R. W. Raven (ed.)	1976	510	None
Clinical Oncology	U.I.C.C.	1978	304	None
Clinical Oncology for Medical Students and Physicians (3rd ed.)	Rubin & Bakemeier, American Cancer Society	1971	429	None
Cancer, Vols. 1–6	Becker	1975–1977	3,082	None

[a] This volume contains a brief description of pain associated with different types of cancer, but does not discuss pain therapy.

available are partly responsible for mismanagement of the pain. Consequently, most practitioners rely on narcotic analgesics, which, although very useful and with a definite role in the control of pain in cancer, for a variety of reasons are often misused. In a small percentage of patients, potent narcotics are used initially for mild pain which could be relieved by nonnarcotic analgesics alone or combined with psychotropic drugs. The practice of some physicians to "snow the patient under" because the patient has recurrent or metastic cancer denotes a lack of understanding of the problem (12,13). Because it is difficult to estimate the length of life in individual cases, such false humanitarianism may potentiate the depressant effects of the disease and cause the patient to have narcotic-induced anorexia, nausea, and vomiting and thus aggravate the physiologic effects of the cancer.

At the other end of the spectrum of the problem, many, if not most, patients with moderate to severe pain of advanced cancer are given inadequate amounts of narcotics. The very high incidence of undertreatment of cancer pain with narcotics is due to inadequate knowledge of the pharmacology of these drugs and, particularly, serious misconceptions among physicians and nurses about "the risk of addiction." As part of the study previously mentioned, Marks and Sochar (53) surveyed 102 physicians in training in two major hospitals and found that because of inadequate knowledge most physicians underestimated the effective dose range of narcotics, overestimated their duration of action, and had an exaggerated opinion of the dangers of addiction.

Apparently, this problem of inadequate knowledge and misconception about addiction is widespread, because many others have reported similar findings. The English reports of Parkes (62), MacInnes (51), and Cartwright et al. (25) have been cited. Ford (33), of the British National Health Services, emphasized similar findings, as did Saunders (73), Director of St. Christopher's Hospice. From the hundreds of reports received by the National Committee on the Treatment of Intractable Pain, it is obvious that all of the patients with advanced cancer pain who were managed with drugs either received insufficient amounts of potent narcotics or were managed with ineffective drugs.

In some patients, even properly administered systemic drugs are not sufficiently effective and other modalities must be used alone or in combination with drugs. These include nerve blocks and neurosurgical interruption of pain pathways as well as some of the old and newer psychologic techniques which have been shown to be effective in helping or totally relieving cancer pain. Unfortunately, for the aforementioned reasons the roles of these other therapeutic modalities are not known by most practitioners and even many oncologists. Consequently, in most patients who could be more effectively relieved by one of these procedures or a combination of therapies, they are not considered, or if they are considered it is done too late. Related to this is the lack of personnel with interest and expertise in the proper application of these other therapeutic modalities.

It is obvious that more effective management of patients with cancer pain requires an intensive educational campaign for medical students and other health professionals, as well as physicians in practice, including: (a) knowledge about the causes and mechanisms of pain; (b) the efficacy, indications, limitations, and complications of current methods of pain relief; and (c) specific guidelines about proper management of these patients. In addition to courses in the curriculum and postgraduate programs, it is essential to provide better sources of information through the oncologic literature, including books and special articles as well as brochures on cancer pain and its management. Moreover, because cancer pain problems are often too complex for one person to manage, it is highly desirable to have multidisciplinary cancer pain diagnostic and therapy teams, especially in the larger comprehensive cancer centers (14,16,18). Such teams should be composed of basic scientists and clinicians with special interest and expertise in chronic pain in general and cancer pain in particular who would devote the time and effort to carefully evaluate each patient with severe cancer pain and determine the best method or methods of relieving the pain. The team should include medical, surgical, and radiation oncologists, clinical pharmacologists, anesthesiologists, neurosurgeons, psychologists, social workers, nurses with special knowledge and expertise in pain, theologians, and others with special expertise and skills that might be needed in the diagnostic work-up and in the development of the most appropriate therapeutic strategy.

Lack of Knowledge

A void in our knowledge of the basic mechanisms and physiopathology of cancer pain constitutes a second reason for its inadequate control. This can be at least partly attributed to the lack of sufficiently scientifically trained persons working on the problem. Related to this has been the meager amount or total lack of funds for research or research training in this field.

In the United States over $1 billion was spent in 1978 for cancer research by the National Cancer Institute (NCI) and other federal, state, and municipal agencies and by voluntary agencies, private institutions, and the pharmaceutical industry. These funds support the research of hundreds of thousands of scientists, technicians, physicians, and other health professionals who are investigating the cause, prevention, and treatment modalities of every form of cancer. However, until recently, research on cancer pain per se, which from the viewpoint of the patient and his family is one of the most important aspects of this dreadful disease, was virtually nonexistent. Analysis of a computer printout for the period 1971 to 1975 revealed that NCI spent a total of nearly $2.5 billion to support its program and of this amount $560,000 was spent for cancer pain and its research. This averages about $112,000 annually, which represents 0.022% of the annual budget for those years of the major federal agency which supports cancer research. As a member of the committee that reviewed applications for cancer pain research and therapy, I was greatly disappointed by the totally inadequate number of meritorious proposals submitted to the Institute. This re-emphasizes the point made that there is an obvious lack of scientific manpower interested in carrying out pain research.

Another impressive and distressing aspect of this whole problem is the fact that there are no accurate data from large epidemiologic studies on the incidence and magnitude of cancer pain. Again using NCI as an example, we note that it has a biometry branch and an epidemiologic branch which carry out very detailed epidemiologic studies on the incidence of every kind of cancer, and which have the most sophisticated computer system for the storage and easy retrieval of data. The efforts of these two branches have produced accurate information on every aspect of cancer including detailed data on the most infrequent types of cancer. However, at the time of this writing, the Institute has no data on the incidence, magnitude, and cost of the pain associated with malignant disease. This neglect of epidemiologic studies pervades the entire network for cancer hospitals, cancer centers, and agencies (16).

Fortunately, things have begun to improve. Three years ago NCI initiated a pain control program which is beginning to bear fruit. In 1976 the Institute spent $330,000 (more than double the amount spent in 1975), and in 1977 it spent $661,000. In addition, the Institute supported hospice projects and rehabilitation programs which included pain therapy (30). Very recently it initiated two major programs: epidemiologic studies of the most frequent types of cancer and evaluation of the multidisciplinary approach to cancer pain therapy. Although these should help rectify some of the deficiencies, there remains the urgent need for much greater research efforts.

Future research should provide much new information on the exact biochemical, neurophysiologic, and psychologic substrates of chronic pain in general and cancer pain in particular. Once such information is available, we can use the vast amount of knowledge and technology now available in chemistry, pharmacology, and biochemistry to develop agents that can act in an exquisitely specific way to prevent or promptly terminate the various biochemical and neurologic factors that act at molecular and cellular levels to produce pain. Such new agents would produce complete relief without any side effects. Moreover, future studies should permit more specific definition of the impact of various emotional, psychologic, sociologic, and environmental factors on cancer pain and how this information could be applied more effectively in its relief.

Until we acquire new information, we should be able to effectively use the knowledge currently available to do a much better job in relieving the suffering and pain of cancer. To achieve this goal, it is necessary to consider the causes and possible mechanisms of cancer pain and what role psychologic, emotional, environmental, and sociologic factors play in causing suffering and pain in cancer patients. Once these are defined, it is essential to evaluate the efficacy, indications, advantages, limitations, disadvantages, and complications of the various therapeutic modalities available at the present time and select the most effective therapy.

ETIOLOGY OF CANCER PAIN

The etiology of cancer pain may be classified into one of the three major categories: (a) pain caused by the oncologic process; (b) pain that develops as a result of therapy; and (c) pain that develops coincidental with, but unrelated to, the cancer. In the average cancer hospital population, pain is caused by the oncologic process in 75%, posttherapy pain is present in 20%, and about 5% have coincidental pain (31).

Pain Caused by the Oncologic Process

The following classification of cancer-induced pain is a modification of the one first proposed by Bonica (12,13) a quarter-century ago and taking into consideration recently acquired information (18,31).

Bone Tumor Invasion

Tumor invasion of bone by either primary or metastatic lesion is the most common cause of pain in patients with cancer (31). Pain may be the presenting complaint as, for example, in patients with multiple myeloma or it may represent the first sign of metastatic disease as occurs in patients with carcinoma of the breast. The pain may be at the site of the lesion, as occurs with rib tumors, or it may be referred to a distant area of the body, e.g., deep pain associated with metastatic hip disease. The pain, which is constant and usually progressive

in severity, is probably due to noxious stimulation of nociceptors in the perios-
teum and production of prostaglandin and lowering of nociceptors' threshold.

Compression or Infiltration of Nerve Roots, Nerve Trunks, and Plexuses

Sudden compression by metastatic fractures of bone adjacent to nerve roots
or nerves results in a radiculopathy or neuropathy accompanied by fairly sharp
neuralgic pain projected to the distribution of the nerve structure involved
(12,13). Progressive compression of nerve structures by an enlarging tumor,
enlarged lymph nodes, or both also produces neuralgic pain and sensory and
motor disturbances. Infiltration of peripheral nerves by tumor tissue causes
constant burning pain associated with hyperesthesia and dysesthesia in the area
of sensory loss. Tumor infiltration of the brachial plexus produces radicular
pain in the shoulder and arm often associated with paresthesia in the C8-T1
distribution (31). Eventually the paresthesia progresses to numbness and weakness. Tumor infiltration of the lumbar and sacral plexuses usually is seen in
patients with cancers of the genitourinary organs or the colon in which the
local tumor extends into adjacent lymph nodes and bones. The pain may be
felt initially in the low back and thigh and then progress to the calf and heel;
it is associated with paresthesia followed by numbness and dysesthesia as well
as progressive motor and sensory loss. Infiltration of the lower sacral plexus
produces dull, aching pain in the midline of the perineum associated with sensory
loss.

On the basis of current neurophysiological evidence (20,85), one may speculate
that these various etiologic factors may cause persistent mechanical noxious
stimulation of high threshold nociceptors and possibly partial damage of axons
and nerve membrane, which become extremely sensitive to norepinephrine and
pressure. Some of these patients develop causalgia-like pain and other symptomatology of reflex sympathetic dystrophy that can be dramatically relieved by
regional sympathetic block (12,44).

Infiltration of Blood Vessels

Infiltration of blood vessels and lymphatics by tumor cells results in vasospasm
and lymphangitis, with probable consequent irritation of nociceptors or nociceptive afferents in perivascular nerves (12). This process produces a diffuse burning
or aching pain that does not have a peripheral nerve distribution. Many of
these patients also develop causalgic pain and other signs of reflex sympathetic
dystrophy that can also be promptly eliminated by regional sympathetic block
(12,44).

Obstruction of a Hollow Viscus or the Ductal System in a Solid Viscus

It is well known that obstruction of the stomach, intestine, biliary tract, ureters,
uterus, or urinary bladder causes intense contraction of the smooth muscles

under isometric conditions (i.e., when the exit of the viscus is obstructed), with consequent increased tension and ischemia. These in turn produce visceral pain which is characteristically diffuse and poorly localized and referred to dermatomes supplied by the same spinal cord segments that supply the affected viscus (12). A similar mechanism is probably operative in oncologic processes which obstruct that outflow of ductal systems of the pancreas, liver, and other solid viscera. In all of these conditions, persistent obstruction produces greater contractions and finally intense distention with consequent progressively greater pain.

Occlusion of Blood Vessels

Occlusion of blood vessels, either partial or complete, by an adjacent tumor produces venous engorgement, arterial ischemia, or both (12,13). Venous engorgement results in edema of all the structures supplied by the obstructed vessels. The edema in turn causes distention of fascial compartments and other pain-sensitive structures, resulting in progressively more severe pain. Examples are the progressively more severe headache consequent to obstruction of the veins draining from the head, the pain and edema in upper limbs seen with cancer of the breast, or lower limb pain and edema caused by obstruction of the venous outflow by tumor and enlarged lymph glands in the pelvis. Ischemia produced by obstruction of a major artery may cause cellular breakdown with production of "pain-producing substances" which lower the threshold of nociceptors. The pain generated by these mechanisms is usually diffuse, does not follow any particular nerve distribution, and becomes progressively worse.

Tumefaction and Swelling in a Structure Invested Snugly by Fascia, Periosteum, or Other Pain-Sensitive Structures

The type of process wherein there is tumefaction and swelling in a tissue close to a pain-sensitive structure is probably responsible for the pain associated with growing tumors of liver, spleen, and certain types of kidney tumors or growing tumor of bone. Each of these processes produces distention of the investing pain-sensitive structure with consequent stimulation of mechanical nociceptors. If the pain-inducing tumor is in a superficial somatic structure, the pain is sharp and relatively well localized; whereas if the tumor is situated in deep somatic structures or the viscera, the pain is dull, poorly localized, and usually referred to dermatomes which receive the same nerve supply as the involved structure.

Necrosis, Infection, Inflammation, and Ulceration of Mucous Membranes and Other Pain-Sensitive Structures

Pathologic processes such as necrosis, infection, inflammation, and ulceration in pain-sensitive structures produce pain that is frequently excruciating. It is most likely to occur with cancer of the lips, mouth, oropharynx, and face, and tumors of the gastrointestinal and genitourinary tracts. It is likely that the inflammatory reaction lowers the threshold of nociceptors so that innocuous stimuli produce excruciating pain usually localized to the region.

Pain Syndromes Associated with Cancer Therapy

Pain that develops as a complication of cancer therapy can be further subdivided into three etiologic subgroups (31): (a) pain that develops after certain surgical operations; (b) pain that develops following chemotherapy; and (c) postradiation pain.

Postsurgical Pain

Pain following thoracotomy and mastectomy is usually due to damage of the nerves during the surgical operation. The nerves may be partially injured or completely severed. The pain becomes evident 1 to 2 months following the operation; it is characteristically constant in the area of sensory loss, with occasional intermittent shock-like pains. Dysesthesia in the scar area with hyperesthesia in the surrounding zone are often prominent symptoms. The proximal portions of severed nerves regenerate and produce small neuromas, and in partially damaged nerves there is damage to the nerve membrane (85). The neuroma and damaged membrane are hypersensitive to pressure and norepinephrine (85). Consequently, light touch and movement of the part or emotional stress, which usually increases catecholamine release, exacerbate the pain. As a result, some of these patients may develop a concomitant frozen shoulder and consequent limitation of motion, disuse atrophy of the arm, and occasionally a true reflex sympathetic dystrophy.

A number of patients who undergo radical neck dissection develop constant burning pain, dysesthesia, and lancinating pain in the region of the neck. The physiopathologic process is similar to that of other postsurgical neuropathies.

Postamputation pain in the severed limb may be of two types: pain in the stump and pain in the phantom limb (12). The stump pain is usually constant and burning in character, and the pain in the phantom limb may be either a burning pain or cramping "proprioceptive" pain characterized by abnormal position of the missing distal part of the limb.

In all of these postsurgical pain syndromes, peripheral–central mechanisms are probably operative. Initially, the peripheral nociceptive dysfunction predominates, but eventually the disturbance in the neuraxis plays the most important role. The clinical implication of this is that interruption of peripheral nociceptive pathways, sympathetic blocks, or both, done early, may relieve the pain, but when done late very likely will produce little or no relief.

Postchemotherapy Pain

Painful dysesthesia following treatment with the vinca alkaloid drugs such as vincristine and vinblastine occurs as part of a symmetrical polyneuropathy which usually develops with the doses of the drug required to achieve an antineoplastic effect (69). Dysesthesias are commonly localized to the hands and feet and are characterized by burning pain exacerbated by noxious stimuli. Children frequently develop more diffuse generalized myalgia and arthralgia, often beginning with jaw pain and progressing to a symmetrical polyneuropathy that includes cranial nerve dysfunction.

Steroid pseudorheumatism can follow withdrawal of steroid medications (71). Some patients develop diffuse myalgia and arthralgia with muscle and joint pain that is a dull aching with tenderness on palpitation but without objective inflammatory signs. These symptoms regress with reinstitution of steroid therapy.

Aseptic necrosis of the head of the femur or humerus, or both, with consequent pain in the hip and reference to the knee or shoulder joint, respectively, occurs as a complication of cancer therapy, specifically chronic steroid therapy (45). The pain is a deep dull aching that is constant and often severe.

Mucositis occurs after the administration of certain chemotherapeutic agents which apparently produce biochemical changes in mucous membranes and other pain-sensitive structures with consequent severe pain particularly in the lips, mouth, pharynx, and nasal passages.

Postradiation Therapy Pain

Following radiation therapy to the region of the brachial plexus or the lumbosacral plexus, fibrosis of the surrounding connective tissue occurs with secondary injury to the nerve structures (77). The condition is progressive with consequent increasing pain in part of the entire upper limb. The pain is often associated with numbness or paresthesia in the structures supplied by the affected nerves, lymphedema in the arm, and radiation skin changes and induration of the supraclavicular and axillary areas present with brachial plexus fibrosis. Similarly, fibrosis of the lumbosacral plexus produces pain associated with progressive motor and sensory changes and lymphedema in the lower limb. The fibrosis, which is a slow progressive process, produces injury to the nerves with consequent abnormal firing that eventually produces abnormal function in the somatosensory system in the neuraxis. Consequently, peripheral–central mechanisms produce the pain, which is not likely to respond to interruption of peripheral pathways.

Postherpetic neuralgia is a complication of radiation therapy or may occur following herpes zoster that develops in the area of tumor pathology (12). The patient usually experiences severe continuous burning pain in the area of sensory loss, painful dysesthesia, and intermittent lancinating pain. This condition involves peripheral–central mechanisms and is one of the most difficult pain syndromes to treat.

Radiation myelopathy produces pain localized to the area of the spinal cord involved, or it may be referred to peripheral somatic structures associated with dysesthesia below the level of injury (46). These patients usually develop neurologic symptomatology of the Brown-Séquard syndrome. Another complication of radiation therapy is the production of peripheral nerve tumors characterized by a painful enlarging mass in the area of previous irradiation (32).

THERAPEUTIC MODALITIES FOR CANCER PAIN

The management of intractable pain of malignant diseases revolves around three main methods of approach: (a) completely eliminating the tumor with anticancer modalities; (b) symptomatic relief of pain without affecting the neoplasm; and (c) a combination of a and b. Anticancer modalities include the use of: (a) chemotherapy; (b) endocrine therapy; (c) radiation therapy; (d) radioisotope therapy; and (e) palliative surgery, including excision of the tumor, bypass operation, and destruction or excision of endocrine organs such as hypophysectomy, adrenalectomy, and castration. In properly selected cases these are often effective in reducing the size or eliminating the tumor, or bypassing it and thus removing the cause of the pain (1,22,41,42,56,65). Discussion of anticancer modalities is beyond the scope of this presentation.

When the aforementioned measures prove totally or partially ineffective or not feasible, it is necessary to control pain symptomatically without affecting the neoplasm (12,18,22). The modalities in current use include: (a) systemic drugs consisting of nonnarcotic analgesics, sedatives, ataractics, psychotropic drugs, and narcotics; (b) therapeutic nerve blocks, which can be achieved either temporarily with a local anesthetic or for a prolonged period by injecting neurolytic agents; (c) neurosurgical operations, which may either be ablative (intended to interrupt pain pathways) or augmentative (which entail stimulation of pain-modulating mechanisms including transcutaneous stimulation, peripheral nerve stimulation, dorsal column stimulation, and stimulation of the brain); (d) psychologic methods, which include traditional psychotherapy, hypnosis, biofeedback, and operant conditioning. Many patients with cancer pain also need rehabilitation programs, which may include physical therapy, occupational therapy, exercise, and support by psychologists, nurses, theologians, etc.

As previously mentioned, when determining the best therapeutic modality or combination of therapies to effectively relieve the pain, it is essential to consider the etiology, intensity, and other characteristics of the pain, as well as the associated emotional reactions, physical condition of the patient, prognosis of the disease, possible extension and metastases of the tumor, and importantly the desires of the patient and his/her obligation to the family and the community. Obviously this requires a detailed history, comprehensive examination, and psychologic and psychosocial evaluation. Knowledge of various therapeutic modalities available and practical for the relief of cancer pain is crucial to the selection of the most effective therapy. The following brief discussion is intended to give a superficial overview of each major method of therapy. Only a few key references are given. A more detailed and comprehensive consideration of each of these methods is found in the monograph containing the proceedings of the International Symposium on Pain of Advanced Cancer (22).

Systemic Analgesics and Related Drugs

The administration of systemic analgesics, psychotropic drugs, anti-inflammatory agents, and hypnotics constitute the most practical and widely used methods of relieving cancer pain. These drugs are readily available, inexpensive, simple to administer, and if properly used, reasonably effective in relieving pain. As previously mentioned, in many instances they are unfortunately not administered in the most effective way, and consequently the patient does not derive optimal benefit and indeed may incur serious side effects.

Nonnarcotic Analgesics

In patients with mild to moderate cancer pain, nonnarcotic analgesics given in adequate doses are effective (35,43,81) and should be used before considering the administration of narcotic analgesics. These include aspirin, salicylamide and other derivatives of salicylic acid, paracetamol, metamizol, phenylbutazone, indomethacin, mefenamic acid, ibuprofen, and nefopam. Since many osseous metastases produce or induce the production of a prostaglandin which causes osteolysis and also lowers the "peripheral pain threshold" by sensitizing free nerve endings, aspirin and other nonsteroidal anti-inflammatory drugs are effective in relieving bone pain (29,81).

The generally prescribed doses and interval of administration of these drugs is totally inadequate for optimal cancer pain relief. Usually, two to three times the so-called optimal dose must be given at frequent intervals in order to obtain analgesic ceiling effect (35). For example, aspirin or salicylamide must be given in doses of 700 to 1,000 mg every 3 to 4 hr so that the total daily dose is 4 to 6 g. Moreover, the drug must be given continuously for a prolonged period of time to obtain optimal results.

Corticosteroids

Corticosteroids enhance or produce analgesia by preventing the release of prostaglandins and in other ways improve an inflammatory process and commonly stimulate appetite and elevate mood (80). Although these agents are not as effective as aspirin in relieving bone pain, they seem to be more effective in relieving pain associated with extensive soft tissue infiltration in relatively circumscribed areas such as head and neck cancers, pelvic malignancies, or massive hepatic metastases. Sometimes greater relief is obtained by using aspirin plus a corticosteroid. These drugs are also effective in partially or completely relieving pain caused by nerve compression and severe headache caused by increased intracranial pressure (31).

Psychotropic Drugs

Antidepressant tricyclic drugs have been used to elevate mood, increase sedation, and potentiate analgesia, and they may have an analgesic action of their own (36). Several selected phenothiazines, particularly hydroxyzine, have been used to increase sedation, decrease nausea and vomiting, and possibly potentiate the analgesic action of narcotics (36). Some phenothiazines can also be used for the treatment of confusion, delirium, or psychotic manifestations should these occur (80). Recently interest has centered on cannabis and several of its derivatives for use in the management of radiation/chemotherapy nausea and emesis and as antianxiety agents and to promote weight gain in cachectic patients (66).

Narcotic Analgesics

When pain becomes moderate to severe and persistent, and other more aggressive methods are not available or are contraindicated, the proper use of morphine or another potent long-acting narcotic is a great blessing to the patient and the family. Whatever the narcotic drug given and the route of administration, a cardinal rule is to give the patient sufficient amounts of narcotics to provide satisfactory pain relief with minimal side effects. This requires that an effective dose of the drug be given at fixed intervals to produce continuous pain relief. The dose required to achieve this may range from 5 to 100 mg morphine every 3 to 4 hr (80,82).

It is best to start potent narcotics by mouth (43,80,82). In this regard it is important to realize that oral equianalgesic doses of potent narcotics are two to five times the intramuscular doses. A baseline evaluation is carried out by noting the duration of effectiveness of each of the first two or three doses; the drug is then prescribed at regular intervals which are about one-half to three-quarters of an hour shorter than the average duration of analgesia. This provides even analgesia and avoids the peaks-and-valleys effect that causes the patient to have intervals of pain and discomfort.

To determine the optimal dose and frequency of administration, it is necessary to titrate the patient's pain with the drug over a period of days and carefully monitor and evaluate the analgesic action of each dose. This responsibility cannot be left to the nurse, but must be assumed by the physician or the pain therapy team. It deserves emphasis that "the optimal dose" of 10 mg morphine per 70 kg body weight, as determined years ago by Beecher and his associates (6) in patients with postoperative pain, may be totally ineffective in patients with cancer pain. In some patients the effective oral dose of morphine may be as much as 100 mg given every 3 to 4 hr. Since the pain counteracts the respiratory depressant effects of narcotics, there is minimal danger of respiratory depression even with such large doses, provided the patient is carefully titrated. Moreover, there is evidence that giving narcotics at regular intervals to provide sustained analgesia decreases the incidence of tolerance to the narcotic (80,82). It also deserves re-emphasis that addiction should not be considered a contraindication in patients with recurrent or metastatic cancer, especially during preterminal and terminal stages of the disease.

Analgesic (Nerve) Blocks

Nerve blocks, or analgesic blocks, achieved by injection of a local anesthetic or neurolytic agent near or into a nerve or nerve roots or into pain-sensitive structures, can be used as diagnostic or prognostic tools or for definitive therapy of cancer pain (12,13,21,74). Diagnostic blocks properly applied are very useful in: (a) helping to ascertain the specific nociceptive pathways; (b) helping to define the mechanisms of cancer pain; and (c) aiding the differential diagnosis of the site of nociceptive noxious stimuli.

Prognostic blocks are useful for predicting the analgesic efficacy and side effects of neurolytic blocks or neurosurgical section of peripheral nociceptive pathways for cancer pain. Moreover, prognostic blocks afford the patient an opportunity to experience the numbness and other side effects that follow the procedure and thus help him or her decide whether to have the operation.

Therapeutic Blocks

In a patient whose physical condition or prognosis contraindicates major neurosurgical operations and in whom narcotic therapy is ineffective, therapeutic nerve blocks should be used (12,13). Although there are certain limitations, properly applied nerve blocks can produce a greater degree of pain relief than narcotics and are associated with less stress and risk than most neurosurgical operations. A disadvantage of nerve blocks is that sometimes inadequate relief results, but since the block can be readily repeated this is not significant. A more important disadvantage is development of complications during or following nerve blocks, but, again, these can be minimized by skillful administration. Therapeutic blocks can be achieved with local anesthetics or with neurolytic agents such as alcohol or phenol.

Local anesthetic blocks

Local anesthetic blocks are used to provide patients with prompt relief of excruciating pain for hours or days and occasionally longer. For example, continuous segmental epidural block of the affected segments can be used for several weeks and thus relieve patients of cancer pain while they are receiving radiation or other anticancer modalities. In some instances it is desirable to combine a local anesthetic with a corticosteroid preparation injected into the extradural space where significant pain improvement can be achieved for weeks and at times months by decreasing the swelling of entrapped nerves.

Local anesthetic injection of trigger areas eliminates myofascial pain syndromes which sometimes develop in association with cancer pain (12). Local anesthetic blocks of sympathetic pathways may help relieve the burning pain which is present with certain types of cancer of the head, chest, and abdomen. Moreover, repeated sympathetic blocks are effective in eliminating the symptomatology of reflex sympathetic dystrophy which occasionally develops in cancer patients (44). In such instances the relief of pain and associated symptomatology usually outlasts pharmacologic effects of the block; moreover, if initiated early, a series of blocks produces prolonged and permanent relief. Finally, repeated blocks with local anesthetics initiated promptly after onset of postsurgical pain may prevent the development of peripheral–central mechanisms.

Neurolytic blocks

Neurolytic block, achieved by the injection of alcohol or phenol, involves intentional destruction of a nerve or nerves for a period of time to produce prolonged interruption (12,13,78). Subarachnoid neurolysis or chemical rhizotomy, achieved by injecting small amounts of alcohol or phenol into the subarachnoid space, is one of the most effective methods for relieving severe intractable cancer pain below the neck. The pain relief lasts for several days to several months and sometimes longer. Not infrequently it is necessary to do several blocks to effect prolonged relief. Numerous reports suggest that neurolytic subarachnoid block produces complete relief in about 50 to 60% of cancer patients, partial relief in about 20 to 25%, and no relief in the rest (12,13,48,61,77). These results compare favorably with those achieved with neurosurgical procedures, particularly as they are applied to patients with advanced or terminal cancer (12,13). This procedure is particularly useful and effective in relieving cancer pain of the trunk because involvement of somatic motor nerves is of no consequence and there is little or no risk of producing significant visceromotor dysfunction. In contrast, if the block involves nerves of the upper limb, there is risk of muscle weakness in about 15 to 20%, whereas if the block is done to relieve pain in the pelvis and lower limbs there is a 20 to 25% incidence of bladder and/or rectal dysfunction and lower limb muscle weakness (12,13, 48,61,77).

Neurolytic gasserian ganglion block is particularly useful if the lesion involves structures supplied by more than one of the major branches of the trigeminal nerve (12,13,21). In such cases it is preferable to carry out gasserian ganglion block at the onset to produce a widespread field of analgesia into which the cancer can spread without producing more pain subsequently. Because of the short life expectancy, the risk of corneal ulcer from block of the ophthalmic branches is not as significant as in patients with nonmalignant pain. Properly done, alcohol block of the gasserian ganglion produces pain relief in over 85% of patients with cancer pain in the anterior two-thirds of the head (12,13,21). In addition to the severe sharp somatic pain, some tumors of the face and head cause a burning discomfort which requires complementary neurolytic block of the cervical sympathetic chain (12,13,21).

Chemical Neuroadenolysis

Another related procedure is chemical neuroadenolysis achieved by injecting alcohol into the pituitary gland through needles placed transnasally and transsphenoidally. This procedure, first described by Moricca (55) in Rome, has been given trial by several other groups with encouraging results (52,54). Although originally used to reduce hormonal stimulation of specific hormone-dependent tumors in the body (e.g., carcinoma of the breast, carcinoma of the prostate, or endometrial carcinoma), a significant number of patients with non-hormone-dependent tumors derive prompt relief with neuroadenolysis. The procedure is especially useful when the pain is widespread and is not amenable to nerve block therapy or neurosurgical intervention.

Neurosurgical Procedures for Cancer Pain

For patients having severe intractable pain of inoperable or recurrent cancer, for whom palliative procedures cannot be done or have been ineffective, and who are still in fairly good health, prolonged relief can often be obtained by neurosurgical operations (12,58,88). Although this form of therapy is often considered a last resort because many of the procedures are major interventions, it should not be postponed unduly as this will result in unnecessary suffering. Moreover, once the decision to use this method has been made, a procedure to produce optimum and certain results should be carried out. The various neurosurgical operations for the management of cancer pain fall into two categories: ablative and augmentative (stimulating) techniques. Ablative techniques are intended to interrupt nociceptive (pain) pathways in peripheral nerves or at certain sites in the neuraxis. Stimulating techniques entail the application of electrical stimulation through the skin to a major peripheral nerve or via electrodes around the spinal cord or in certain sites in the brain.

Ablative Neurosurgical Procedures

Peripheral nerve sections

Resection of peripheral spinal or cranial nerves, although simple, is rarely indicated in cancer pain because the procedure produces only very limited analgesia for a short period followed by regeneration with possible consequent pain. Moreover, it can be done only in purely sensory nerves (e.g., the branches of the trigeminal nerve) or in mixed nerves in which interruption of motor pathways is insignificant (e.g., the intercostal nerves). In such circumstances, neurolytic block is preferable because it is simpler and produces less morbidity.

Splanchnicectomy

Section of afferent (pain) fibers supplying the upper abdominal viscera may be indicated in cancer of the pancreas and other visceral tumors which do not involve parietal peritoneum. In such instances, neurolytic block of the splanchnic nerves or the celiac plexus is equally effective; moreover, it is simpler and produces much less morbidity than the open operation.

Rhizotomy

Spinal dorsal rhizotomy entails section of the sensory roots of spinal nerves and might be considered in patients with cancer involving the thorax or abdomen; it should never be considered for extremity cancer pain because extensive deafferentation results in a virtually useless limb. The procedure has the disadvantage of requiring an extensive laminectomy in order to carry out section of multiple roots (because of the sensory overlapping) to produce a wide enough band of analgesia to assure persistent pain relief in the event tumor spreads beyond its original site. A recent modification, called "radiculotomy," which entails sections of the fine afferents in the lateral division of the dorsal root leaving the larger afferents in the medial division intact, produces loss of pain and temperature sensations without eliminating feelings of touch and pressure (74). This affords obvious advantages over standard rhizotomy and could prove useful in relieving pain limited to a discrete region. However, because only a limited number of cancer patients have undergone the procedure, it is difficult to evaluate its role.

Cranial sensory rhizotomy is a highly effective procedure to relieve pain in the face and the anterior two-thirds of the head (59,79,86). Depending on the site of the pain and the potential growth of the tumor, the roots of cranial nerves V, IX, and part of X, and the nervus intermedius portion of VII, can be sectioned; when indicated, these can be combined with section of the upper cervical sensory nerve roots. The disadvantage of the technique is that it requires a major intracranial operation, and so the patient must be in good physical condition. Patients with terminal cancer and those in poor physical condition are best managed with neurolytic blocks.

Tractotomy

Spinothalamic tractotomy, commonly known as anterolateral cordotomy, is probably the best and most widely used neurosurgical operation for cancer pain (86). Open cordotomy achieved through a laminectomy and section of the tract at the upper thoracic segments has been used for more than half a century, and in the hands of a skilled neurosurgeon it produces relief in 80 to 85% of patients for periods of 1.5 to 2 years and sometimes longer (86). It has the advantage of producing relief of pain with loss only of temperature sensation and without affecting other sensory modalities. In a varying percentage of patients, motor deficits occur as a complication of the operation owing to inadvertent interruption of motor tracts. Moreover, a small percent of patients develop sensory abnormalities, e.g., dysesthesia and paresthesia following the operation. During recent years the open operation has often been replaced by percutaneous cordotomy, achieved by introducing the needle with stereotactic control so that its tip is in the anterolateral quadrant of the upper cervical spinal cord and then applying radiofrequency current to destroy the tissue (49,70). This procedure has the distinct advantages of being a relatively minor operation with an extremely low mortality rate and a lower complication rate than open cordotomy. In skilled hands good pain relief is achieved in 80 to 95% of the cancer patients immediately after the operation; this persists for several months but then the percent drops with time (49,70,86).

Medullary tractotomy entails section of the descending trigeminal tract in the medulla to produce analgesia (and loss of temperature sensation) in the face and anterior two-thirds of the head. The operation—which interrupts the sensory fibers of the V and those of the VII, IX, and X, which are adjacent thereto—is analogous to section of the spinothalamic tract in the spinal cord. It has proved to be highly effective but requires a craniotomy (47,86). A percutaneous technique was described by Hitchcock, who reported pain relief in 75% of a small group of patients (40).

Mesencephalic tractotomy, done through a craniotomy, has been shown to have a high incidence of serious side effects and is not used.

Cranial stereotactic operations

In contrast, mesencephalic tractotomy or mesencephalotomy under stereotactic control carried out by a skilled and experienced surgeon produces long-term pain relief (37). Disadvantages of the technique are that only a few surgeons are sufficiently experienced to do the procedure effectively and safely, and the procedure is frequently followed by abnormalities in extraocular muscle movements. Hypothalamotomy, which entails a lesion of the posterior medial hypothalamus, was reported by Fairman (28) to provide long-term relief of cancer pain in a group of 125 patients and by Sano (72) in a smaller group of patients. Thalamolaminotomy, which entails a lesion in the internal medullary lamina of the thalamus, was reported by Sano (72) to be effective in relieving severe cancer pain in a majority of a small group of patients. However, pain relief usually lasts little more than 6 months to 1 year; therefore, the procedure should be limited to patients with short life expectancy.

Augmentative (Stimulating) Procedures

Peripheral stimulation

Transcutaneous nerve stimulation (TNS) has been tried in several relatively small groups of cancer pain patients with moderate success (84). The advantages of the technique, which include absence of side effects, low cost, and simplicity, suggest that it should be tried before more radical procedures are used. Direct application of the electrode on a peripheral nerve with the use of an implanted stimulator was used in approximately 300 pain patients, 60% of whom derived relief, although only a small number of these had pain caused by cancer (50). This procedure is limited to patients with very severe pain in a limb.

Spinal cord stimulation

Dorsal column stimulation (DCS) has been used for a decade in the treatment of chronic pain due to a variety of procedures, but very few of these patients had cancer pain (50,57). Because it requires a laminectomy and the long-term pain relief is less than 50%, it has no place in the management of the patient with cancer pain.

A percutaneously inserted spinal cord electrode system (PISCES) consists of implanted electrodes to stimulate the spinal cord. It can be instituted without performing a major operation and therefore has broadened the potential applicability of electrical stimulation of the spinal cord (81). Although its use in cancer pain has been very limited, its relative simplicity and theoretical advantages indicate that it may have a definite role.

Deep brain stimulation

Stereotactic placement of stimulating electrodes into the internal capsule, thalamus, and hypothalamus are procedures which appear to have promise in the management of pain due to cancer (28,72,86). Unfortunately only a small number of patients have been studied, and the data are very difficult to interpret. Electrical stimulation of the periaqueductal gray (PAG) region in the posterior hypothalamus or the mesencephalon produces complete abolition of pain by activating the descending supraspinal antinociception system, which involves increased liberation of endorphins. The procedure was used in a small group of patients and produced effective pain relief (67,68). At present this procedure must be considered experimental and restricted to those centers with personnel who have expertise in the technique.

Psychologic and Sociologic Methods

Many patients with unrelieved cancer pain and the associated anxiety, depression, and other complex psychologic, emotional, and behavioral problems also require aggressive psychologic therapy (7,8). Psychologic methods that can and should be used to relieve pain and emotional distress associated with cancer include: (a) psychologic support and psychotherapy; (b) biofeedback; and (c) hypnosis.

Psychotherapy

The health care team should provide ready, simple, and direct communication with all cancer patients and maintain compassion at all times regardless of what other pain-relieving procedure is being used (8,80). Many patients with severe cancer pain and the associated emotional distress, anxiety, and depression require more aggressive therapy with psychotropic drugs and traditional psychotherapeutic techniques (8). The main purpose of therapy is to help the patient accept the reality of the threats his or her illness poses in a positive way and to encourage the living of a full, emotional life with new and limited—but obtainable—goals during the remaining months (7). The use of anxiolytic drugs must be combined with counseling designed to remove as much anxiety as possible (8). These psychologic techniques and psychotropic drugs can be part of a comprehensive therapy program which includes nerve blocks or neurosurgical procedures.

Hypnosis

During the past two decades the successful use of hypnosis in managing cancer pain has been reported by a number of workers, but unfortunately the number of patients in each group has been relatively small. Hilgard and Hilgard (38,39) and others (23,24) found hypnosis quite effective in the treatment of severe chronic pain associated with terminal cancer. The clinical application of hypnosis in this area is directed toward two issues: controlling the pain and relieving the emotional distress the pain can cause. Its proponents consider that this modality has two principal advantages over other methods of managing cancer pain: (a) Hypnosis can control pain without unpleasant or destructive side effects—it does not affect body functions or mentally incapacitate the individual; and (b) hypnosis can create life-enhancing attitudes in the patient. Apparently, the degree of pain relief achieved varies from minimal to total relief.

Biofeedback

Biofeedback for the treatment of cancer pain is a new and untried procedure. In other conditions feedback for muscle tension has been widely and successfully applied to reduce stress, anxiety, and tension. Because cancer pain includes stress, tension, and anxiety, electroencephalographic (EEG) feedback should be a potentially useful technique for this management of cancer pain. Unfortunately there is only one report on this method: a series of 12 cancer patients who obtained significant benefit with muscle tension feedback combined with EEG feedback (34). Obviously, much more work needs to be done to evaluate the role of this technique in cancer pain.

REFERENCES

1. Ackerman, L. V., and Del Regato, J. A. W., editors (1970): *Cancer Diagnosis, Treatment and Prognosis,* 4th ed. Mosby, St. Louis.
2. Akil, H., Watson, S. J., Berger, B. A., and Barcha, J. D. (1978): Endorphins, β-LPH, and ACTH: Biochemical, pharmacological, and anatomical studies. In: *The Endorphins,* edited by E. Costa and M. Trabucchi, pp. 125–140. Raven Press, New York.
3. Almay, B. G. L., Johansson, F., von Knorring, L., Terenius, L., and Wahlstrom, L. A. (1978): Endorphins in chronic pain. 1. Differences in CSF endorphine levels between organic and psychogenic pain syndrome. *Pain,* 5:153–162.
4. American Cancer Society (1978): *Cancer Facts and Figures.* American Cancer Society, New York.
5. American Cancer Society—Massachusetts Division (1968): *Cancer: A Manual for Practitioners.* American Cancer Society, Boston.
6. Beecher, H. K. (1959): *Measurement of Subjective Responses,* p. 45. Oxford University Press, New York.
7. Bellak, L., and Small, L. (1965): *Emergency Psychotherapy and Brief Psychotherapy.* Grune & Stratton, New York.
8. Bond, M. R. (1979): Psychologic and psychiatric techniques for the relief of pain of advanced cancer. In: *Advances in Pain Research and Therapy, Vol. 2,* edited by J. J. Bonica and V. Ventafridda, pp. 215–222. Raven Press, New York.
9. Bond, M. R. (1979): Psychologic and emotional aspects of cancer pain. In: *Advances in Pain Research and Therapy, Vol. 2,* edited by J. J. Bonica and V. Ventafridda, pp. 81–88. Raven Press, New York.
10. Bond, M. R. (1971): The relation of pain to the Eysenck Personality Inventory, Cornell Medical Index and Whitely Index of Hypochondriasis. *Br. J. Psychiatry,* 119:671–678.
11. Bond, M. R., and Pearson, I. B. (1969): Psychologic aspects of pain in women with advanced cancer of the cervix. *J. Psychosom. Res.,* 13:13–19.
12. Bonica, J. J. (1953): *The Management of Pain.* Lea & Febiger, Philadelphia.
13. Bonica, J. J. (1954): The management of pain of malignant disease with nerve blocks. *Anesthesiology,* 15:134, 280–301.
14. Bonica, J. J. (1974): Organization and function of a pain clinic. In: *Advances in Neurology, Vol. 4,* edited by J. J. Bonica, pp. 433–443. Raven Press, New York.
15. Bonica, J. J. (1976): Introduction to First World Congress on Pain. In: *Recent Advances in Pain Research and Therapy, Vol. 1,* edited by J. J. Bonica and D. Albe-Fessard, pp. xxvii–xxxix. Raven Press, New York.
16. Bonica, J. J. (1978): Cancer pain: A major national health problem. *Cancer Nurs. J.,* 4:313–316.
17. Bonica, J. J. (1979): Cancer pain: importance of the problem. In: *Advances in Pain Research and Therapy, Vol. 2,* edited by J. J. Bonica and V. Ventafridda, pp. 1–12. Raven Press, New York.
18. Bonica, J. J. (1979): Introduction to the management of cancer pain. In: *Advances in Pain Research and Therapy, Vol. 2,* edited by J. J. Bonica and V. Ventafridda, pp. 115–130. Raven Press, New York.
19. Bonica, J. J. (1979): Important clinical aspects of acute and chronic pain. In: *Mechanisms of Pain and Analgesic Compounds,* edited by R. F. Beers, Jr., and E. G. Bassett, pp. 15–29. Raven Press, New York.
20. Bonica, J. J., and Albe-Fessard, D., editors (1976): *Recent Advances in Pain Research and Therapy, Vol. 1.* Raven Press, New York.
21. Bonica, J. J., and Madrid, J. L. (1979): Therapy of cancer pain in the head and neck: role of nerve blocks. In: *Advances in Pain Research and Therapy, Vol. 2,* edited by J. J. Bonica and V. Ventafridda, pp. 537–542. Raven Press, New York.

22. Bonica, J. J., and Ventafridda, V., editors (1979): *Advances in Pain Research and Therapy,* *Vol. 2.* Raven Press, New York.
23. Butler, B. (1954): The use of hypnosis in the care of the cancer patient. *Cancer,* 8:1–8.
24. Cangello, V. M. (1962): Hypnosis for the patient with cancer. *Am. J. Clin. Hypnosis,* 4:215–226.
25. Cartwright, A., Hockey, L., and Anderson, A. B. M. (1973): *Life Before Death.* Routledge & Kegan Paul, London.
26. Chapman, C. R. (1979): Psychologic and behavioral aspects of pain. In: *Advances in Pain Research and Therapy, Vol. 2,* edited by J. J. Bonica and V. Ventafridda, pp. 45–56. Raven Press, New York.
27. Committee on Professional Education of U.I.C.C. (1973): *Clinical Oncology (A Manual for Students and Doctors),* p. 322. International Union Against Cancer. Springer-Verlag, Berlin.
28. Fairman, D. (1976): Neurophysiological basis for the hypothalamic lesion and stimulation by chronic implanted electrodes for the relief of intractable pain in cancer. In: *Recent Advances in Pain Research and Therapy, Vol. 1,* edited by J. J. Bonica and D. Albe-Fessard, pp. 843–847. Raven Press, New York.
29. Ferreira, S. H., and Vane, J. R. (1974): New aspects of the mode of action of non-steroid anti-inflammatory drugs. *Annu. Rev. Pharmacol.,* 40:57–73.
30. Fink, D. (1978): Director of Division of Cancer Rehabilitation and Control, National Cancer Institute. *Personal communication.*
31. Foley, K. M. (1979): Pain syndromes in patients with cancer. In: *Advances In Pain Research and Therapy, Vol. 2,* edited by J. J. Bonica and V. Ventafridda, pp. 59–75. Raven Press, New York.
32. Foley, K. M., Woodruf, J. M., Ellis, F., and Posner, J. B. (1975): Radiation-induced malignant and atypical schwannomas. *Neurology (Minneap.),* 25:354.
33. Ford, G. (1979): Terminal care from the viewpoint of the National Health Service. In: *Advances in Pain Research and Therapy, Vol. 2,* edited by J. J. Bonica and V. Ventafridda, pp. 653–661. Raven Press, New York.
34. Fotopoulos, S. S., Graham, C., and Cook, M. R. (1979): Psychophysiological control of cancer pain. In: *Advances in Pain Research and Therapy, Vol. 2,* edited by J. J. Bonica and V. Ventafridda, pp. 231–243. Raven Press, New York.
35. Gerbershagen, H. U. (1979): Non-narcotic analgesics for cancer pain. In: *Advances in Pain Research and Therapy, Vol. 2,* edited by J. J. Bonica and V. Ventafridda, pp. 255–262. Raven Press, New York.
36. Halpern, L. M. (1979): Psychotropics, ataractics and related drugs. In: *Advances in Pain Research and Therapy, Vol. 2,* edited by J. J. Bonica and V. Ventafridda, pp. 275–283. Raven Press, New York.
37. Helfant, M. H., Leksell, L., and Stange, R. R. (1965): Experience with intractable pain treated by stereotaxic mesencephalotomy. *Acta Chir. Scand.,* 129:573–580.
38. Hilgard, E. R. (1975): The alleviation of pain by hypnosis. *Pain,* 1:213–231.
39. Hilgard, E. R., and Hilgard, J. R. (1975): *Hypnosis in the Relief of Pain.* Kaufmann, Los Altos, Calif.
40. Hitchcock, E. (1970): Stereotactic trigeminal tractotomy. *Ann. Clin. Res.,* 2:131–135.
41. Holland, J. F., and Frei, E., III, editors (1973): *Cancer Medicine,* p. 2018. Lea & Febiger, Philadelphia.
42. Horton, J., and Hill, G. J., editors (1977): *Clinical Oncology,* p. 819. Saunders, Philadelphia.
43. Houde, R. W. (1974): The use and misuse of narcotics in the treatment of chronic pain. In: *Advances in Neurology, Vol. 4,* edited by J. J. Bonica, p. 527. Raven Press, New York.
44. Hubert, C. (1978): Recognition and treatment of causalgic pain occurring in cancer patients. In: *Abstracts of the Second World Congress on Pain,* p. 47. International Association for the Study of Pain, Seattle.
45. Ihde, D. C., and DeVita, V. T. (1975): Osteonecrosis of the femoral head in patients with lymphoma treated with intermittent combination chemotherapy (including corticosteroids). *Cancer,* 36:1585–1588.
46. Jellinger, K., and Strum, K. W. (1971): Delayed radiation and myelopathy in man. *J. Neurol. Sci.,* 14:389–408.
47. Kunc, Z. (1964): *Tractus Spinalis Nervi Trigemini. Fresh Anatomic Data and Their Significance for Surgery.* Makladatelstvì Ceskoslovenské Akademie. Vêd, Prague.

48. Lifschitz, S., Debacker, L. J., and Buchsbaum, H. J. (1976): Subarachnoid phenol block for pain relief in gynecologic malignancy. *Obstet. Gynecol.,* 48:316–320.
49. Lipton, S., Dervin, E., and Heywood, O. B. (1974): A stereotactic approach to the anterior percutaneous electrical cordotomy. In: *Advances in Neurology, Vol. 4,* edited by J. J. Bonica, pp. 689–694. Raven Press, New York.
50. Loeser, J. D. (1979): Dorsal column and peripheral nerve stimulation for relief of cancer pain. In: *Advances in Pain Research and Therapy, Vol. 2,* edited by J. J. Bonica and V. Ventafridda, pp. 499–507. Raven Press, New York.
51. MacInnes, C. (1976): Cancer ward. *New Society,* April 29:232–234.
52. Madrid, J. (1979): Chemical hypophysectomy. In: *Advances in Pain Research and Therapy, Vol. 2,* edited by J. J. Bonica and V. Ventafridda, pp. 381–391. Raven Press, New York.
53. Marks, R. M., and Sochar, E. J. (1973): Undertreatment of medical inpatients with narcotic analgesics. *Ann. Intern. Med.,* 78:173–181.
54. Miles, J., and Lipton, S. (1976): Mode of action by which pituitary alcohol injection relieves pain. In: *Advances in Pain Research and Therapy, Vol. 1,* edited by J. J. Bonica and D. Albe-Fessard, pp. 867–969. Raven Press, New York.
55. Moricca, G. (1974): Chemical hypophysectomy for cancer pain. In: *Advances in Neurology, Vol. 4,* edited by J. J. Bonica. p. 707–714. Raven Press, New York.
56. Najerian, J. S., and Delaney, P., editors (1976): *Advances in Cancer Surgery,* p. 608. Stratton Intercontinental, New York.
57. Nielson, K. D., Adams, J. E., and Hosobuchi, Y. (1975): Experience with dorsal column stimulation for relief of chronic intractable pain. *Surg. Neurol.,* 4:148–152.
58. Pagni, C. A. (1979): General comments on ablative neurosurgical procedures. In: *Advances in Pain Research and Therapy, Vol. 2,* edited by J. J. Bonica and V. Ventafridda, pp. 405–423. Raven Press, New York.
59. Pagni, C. A., and Maspes, P. E. (1970): Problems in the surgical treatment of pain in malignancies of the head and neck. In: *Current Problems in Neurosciences,* edited by H. T. Wycis, pp. 138–153. Karger, Basel.
60. Pannuti, E., Martoni, A., Rossi, A. P., and Piana, E. (1979): The role of endocrine therapy for relief of pain due to advanced cancer. In: *Advances in Pain Research and Therapy, Vol. 2,* edited by J. J. Bonica and V. Ventafridda, pp. 145–165. Raven Press, New York.
61. Papo, I., and Visca, A. (1976): Intrathecal phenol in the treatment of pain and spasticity. *Prog. Neurol. Surg.,* 7:56–130.
62. Parkes, C. M. (1978): Home or hospital? Terminal care as seen by surviving spouse. *J. R. Coll. Gen. Pract.,* 28:19–30.
63. Pilowsky, I., Chapman, C. R., and Bonica, J. J. (1977): Pain, depression and illness behavior in a pain clinic population. *Pain,* 4:183–192.
64. Quattlebaum, J. (1978): President of the National Committee for the Treatment of Intractable Pain. *Personal communication.*
65. Raven, R. W., editor (1977): *Principles of Surgical Oncology,* p. 510. Plenum, New York.
66. Regelson, W., Butler, J. R., Schulz, J., Kirk, J., Peek, L., Green, M. L., and Zalis, M. O. (1976): Δ9-Tetrahydrocannabinol as an effective antidepressant and appetite stimulating agent in advanced cancer patients. In: *Pharmacology of Marihuana, Vol. 2,* edited by M. C. Braude and S. Szara, pp. 763–776. Raven Press, New York.
67. Richardson, D. E., and Akil, H. (1977): Pain reduction by electrical brain stimulation in man. I. Acute administration in periaqueductal and periventricular sites. *J. Neurosurg.,* 47:178–183.
68. Richardson, D. E., and Akil, H. (1977): Pain reduction by electrical brain stimulation in man. II. Chronic self-administration in periventricular gray matter. *J. Neurosurg.,* 47:184–194.
69. Rosenthal, S., and Kaufman, S. (1974): Vincristine neurotoxicity. *Ann. Intern. Med.,* 80:733–737.
70. Rosomoff, H. L. (1974): Percutaneous radiofrequency cervical cordotomy for intractable pain. In: *Advances in Neurology, Vol. 4,* edited by J. J. Bonica, pp. 683–688. Raven Press, New York.
71. Rotstein, J., and Good, R. A. (1957): Steroid pseudorheumatism. *Arch. Intern. Med.,* 99:545–555.
72. Sano, K. (1977): Intralaminar thalamotomy (thalamolaminotomy) and posterior medial hypo-thalamotomy in the treatment of intractable pain. In: *Pain—Its Neurosurgical Management.*

Part II. *Central Procedures,* edited by H. Krayenbuhl, P. E. Maspes, and W. H. Sweet, pp. 50–103. Karger, Basel.

73. Saunders, C. (1979): The nature and management of terminal pain and the hospice concept. In: *Advances in Pain Research and Therapy, Vol. 2,* edited by J. J. Bonica and V. Ventafridda, pp. 635–651. Raven Press, New York.
74. Sindow, M., Fischer, G., Goutelle, A., and Mansuy, L. (1974): La radicellotomie postérieure sélective. Premiers résultats dans la chirurgie de la douleur. *Neurochirurgie,* 20:391–408.
75. Sternbach, R. H. (1974): *Pain Patients, Traits and Treatments,* p. 17. Academic Press, New York.
76. Stoll, B. A., and Andrews, J. T. (1966): Radiation-induced peripheral neuropathy. *Br. Med. J.,* 1:834–837.
77. Stovner, J., and Endresen, R. (1972): Intrathecal phenol for cancer pain. *Acta Anaesthesiol. Scand.,* 16:17–21.
78. Swerdlow, M. (1978): *Relief of Intractable Pain,* 2nd ed. Elsevier/North-Holland, Amsterdam.
79. Tasker, R. R. (1975): Neurological concepts of pain management in head and neck cancer. *Can. J. Otolaryngol.,* 4:480–484.
80. Twycross, R. G. (1979): Continuing in terminal care: an overview. In: *Advances in Pain Research and Therapy, Vol. 2,* edited by J. J. Bonica and V. Ventafridda, pp. 617–633. Raven Press, New York.
81. Twycross, R. G. (1978): Bone pain in advanced cancer. In: *Topics in Therapeutics, Vol. 4,* edited by D. W. Vere, pp. 94–110. Pitman Medical, London.
82. Twycross, R. G. (1977): Choice of strong analgesic in terminal cancer: Diamorphine or morphine? *Pain,* 3:94–104.
83. Twycross, R. G. (1974): Clinical management with diamorphine in advanced malignant disease. *Int. J. Clin. Pharmacol.,* 93:184–198.
84. Ventafridda, V., Sganzerla, E. P., Fochi, C., Pozzi, G., and Cordini, G. (1979): Transcutaneous nerve stimulation in cancer pain. In: *Advances in Pain Research and Therapy, Vol. 2,* edited by J. J. Bonica and V. Ventafridda, pp. 509–515. Raven Press, New York.
85. Wall, P. D., and Gutnick, M. (1974): Ongoing activity in peripheral nerves: the physiology and pharmacology of impulses originating from a neuroma. *Exp. Neurol.,* 43:580–593.
86. White, J. C., and Sweet, W. H. (1969): *Pain and the Neurosurgeon.* Charles C Thomas, Springfield, Ill.
87. Wilkes, F. (1974): Some problems in cancer management. *Proc. R. Soc. Med.,* 67:23–27.
88. Wood, K. M. (1978): The use of phenol as a neurolytic agent: A review. *Pain,* 5:205–229.
89. Woodforde, J. M., and Fielding, J. R. (1975): Pain and cancer. In: *Pain, Clinical and Experimental Perspectives,* edited by M. Weisenburg, pp. 332–336. Mosby, St. Louis.

Medical Complications in Cancer Patients,
edited by J. Klastersky and M. J. Staquet.
Raven Press, New York © 1981.

The Responsibilities of Physicians Toward Dying Patients

Harold Y. Vanderpool

Institute for the Medical Humanities, University of Texas Medical Branch, Galveston, Texas 77550

Physicians have not always been responsible for the care of chronically ill and slowly dying persons. Indeed, throughout much of human history the roles of physicians with regard to those suffering prolonged death were highly restricted. With the rise of modern medicine during the nineteenth century, however, physicians became more and more responsible for the circumstances surrounding the deaths of a growing number of their fellow human beings. This trend has increased dramatically during the twentieth century (from approximately 8% in 1910 to 62% in 1975) (11,25) and inevitably raises a host of questions regarding the duties of physicians toward the patients who entrust themselves to their care. What are the responsibilities required of the physician with respect to slowly dying patients?

We can seek to determine what a physician's responsibilities ought to be in a variety of ways. For example, we can assume that these responsibilities consist of all the things physicians need to do in order to satisfy patient desires. The assumption that the physician's responsibilities to dying persons consist of positive responses to their needs and longings may be very well intentioned, but in my opinion leads to an unfair placing of yet another set of external requirements or burdensome obligations on physicians.

We could also assume that a doctor's responsibilities consist of various obligations rooted in social, legal, and medical precedent. Precedents and pragmatic realities require that someone be "in charge" of basic operational procedures and decisions, and since so many of the responsibilities in the hospital belong to the physician, we could try to give a logical and complete listing of these.

Although I take into consideration patient desires and social precedent, I work here with another fundamental understanding of responsibility. Here the term is understood in a moral sense: it refers to the actions and decisions inherent to the occupational roles assumed by physicians and accepted or expected by patients and their families. Moral responsibilities are meaningless or nonexistent if they are not inextricably linked to roles chosen by physicians and approved of by patients and families. They arise out of the implicit and explicit contracts between physician and patient.

In order to speak meaningfully about what physicians ought to do for terminally ill patients, I employ the disciplines of history and ethics. History enables us to define the nature of the contracts between physicians and patients. It permits us to identify the implicit and explicit roles undertaken by physicians and accepted by patients. Did these roles arise by accident? Did physicians reluctantly acquiesce to the pleas for aid and comfort by patients? Or did doctors attempt purposefully to expand their control by seeking to supervise how persons die? What degrees of control or influence were accepted or seized by physicians—social and psychological as well as medical? Did they undertake the supervision of families as well as patients? How has the ferment over the nature of terminal care during the last 15 years reshaped past roles and responsibilities?

Once we obtain these data, we draw on the discipline of ethics in order to identify responsibilities required of physicians with respect to terminally ill patients. This historical and ethical inquiry should in turn raise a number of provocative questions about new forms of medical training or new types of policy guidelines which may be called for.

THE DRAMA OF HUMAN DYING

Unless we use a concept such as "drama" to describe the feelings and actions surrounding death, we fail to capture the degree to which the prolonged deaths of humans throughout history are surrounded with the strongest of human emotions and give rise to intense social and psychological conflict. Human dying is a drama not because it always represents the enactment of a stylized tragedy in the Greek sense, or because it overly dramatizes human loves and losses as in soap operas, but because it grips us with its ultimate seriousness. Grief, hope, fear, courage, and innumerable other emotions accompany human dying; and each human society seeks to control and channel the force of these emotions by developing distinctive, patterned social rituals which surround this inescapable human experience. In addition, death as a fact of human biological existence profoundly shapes human thought and culture, including systems of religious belief, the ways humans are taught to behave and think from childhood to old age, and even why fortunes are made and why university chairs are endowed in the names of those desiring to be remembered (5).

To speak of gradual human dying as a drama is not to say that all deaths are dramatic, for this is surely not the case. Osler (30) rightly observed 75 years ago that most persons fade calmly and quietly from the scene of human existence. That the moment of death for the great majority of humans is not dramatic, however, should not diminish our awareness of its immense social and emotional significance. One of the questions before us is the degree to which the drama of human dying continued to be manifest in the hospital, for the responsibilities of physicians are very different depending on whether it continued or largely ceased once humans were hospitalized during the last months, weeks, or days of their lives.

DYING PERSONS BECOME PATIENTS

Except for bringing drugs that relieved pain—drugs which could be administered by the family (6)—most physicians in the West before the nineteenth century could do little for the care of the dying. It was widely assumed in early and Revolutionary America, for example, that any sensible person (the others being "damn fools") would know when he or she would die, making a physician's diagnosis superfluous in most cases (36). Furthermore, because of the stigma attached to too close an association between death and the questionably effective medicine in those days, most physicians, before the advent of the modern hospital, were counseled to avoid scenes of death and dying whenever possible, and especially to shun the funerals of former patients (10). So when did physicians begin to believe that, owing to unique professional expertise, they should preside over humans who were suffering prolonged death? When did they and the public become convinced that essential medical functions could positively contribute to the care of the terminally ill?

Not until the middle of the nineteenth century did educated physicians in America agree that they "ought not to abandon a patient because the case is deemed incurable." Specific moral duties of physicians toward terminally ill patients and their families were outlined as part of the rules unanimously accepted by the American Medical Association (AMA) in 1847 (35). The dying were referred to as "patients," and the AMA Code of 1847 stipulated that if at all possible the physician should "revive expiring life" and should in any case maintain life as long as possible. If life could not be revived, the physician should "soothe the bed of death" by relieving "mental anguish" and "comforting the relatives." The soothing and comforting offered by the physician must be circumscribed by his primary role as a "minister of hope" in regard to the reviving and extending of life. The physician was therefore admonished to avoid telling the patient about the severity of his condition. He was never to make statements that could "discourage the patient" or "depress his spirits," for such statements might so alarm the patient as to cut his life short. Indeed, not only the words but also the actions and manner of the physician must be controlled lest the patient's life be shortened.

Most of the responsibilities regarding the care of the incurably ill in the 1847 AMA Code were taken verbatim from a treatise on medical ethics by the famous English physician Thomas Percival (31). Through this treatise and the Code—which was regarded virtually as scripture by American physicians for the next 60 years and was used and adopted in several other nations—these duties were widely disseminated and accepted among physicians in England, Canada, and the United States.

The writings of other midnineteenth century physicians (e.g., the highly respected, widely read American, Worthington Hooker) give us a more precise definition of the new roles being assumed by physicians. Hooker and other physicians were opposed to the previous and apparently dominant style of noble dying in America. This style or ideal included several elements. First, sensible persons were expected to know when they were dying—surely due in part to their many experiences with dying adults and children. Second, terminally ill persons should accept or resign themselves to death, for this was a sure sign of faith that God would give them eternal life. Third, dying persons, families, and friends should pray and sing together, testify regarding their faith in God, and read from the Bible and devotional books (6). These settings clearly gave physicians roles secondary to the predominant roles assumed by ministers, relatives, and dying persons themselves.

Hooker could not have disagreed more with this style of dying. Aware of the most recent studies of human physiology, Hooker and his colleagues believed that predictions of death by laymen were often inaccurate and could result in early, untimely death (18). Hooker also espoused a form of "psychosomatic medicine" and believed that depressing and discomforting thoughts would shorten human existence. He furthermore believed that fervent prayers and worship services could strain and exhaust weak patients who otherwise might live, and considered such ceremonies as largely ineffective anyway. He claimed that most dying patients were so weak that they hardly knew what was being said by others or, for that matter, even what they themselves were saying (19).

Hooker and other American and Continental physicians believed they had a mandate to set forth and supervise a new style of terminal care in America, a style characterized by new social and psychological dynamics, and supervised by physicians. Their greater knowledge of human physiology led them to believe that they could predict whether and when death would ensue far more accurately than physicians or lay persons could do previously. Their convictions about the influence of mental states on the body led them to disagree strongly with previous family and religious styles of dying, which they viewed as either harmful or misdirected. Imbued with the moral mandate of reviving and prolonging life, they believed that the ethos of human dying should be characterized by quietude, sweet pleasantries, and hopefulness. Physiological knowledge, psychosomatic theory, and a sense of moral virtue were just grounds, they believed, for influencing, even dictating, how humans should die. Dying persons were to become patients.

HOSPITALIZED PATIENTS

Although many physicians presumed that they were responsible for the medical and emotional well-being of terminally ill patients by the middle of the nineteenth century, several developments after 1850 further increased the physician's power over terminally ill persons and the number of persons dying under direct medical supervision. Within medicine these developments included great advances in the physician's scientific knowledge and skill, as well as the evolution of the most characteristic of medical institutions, the modern hospital. Outside of medicine, major social, intellectual, and institutional shifts brought on by urbanization, secularization, and, perhaps surprisingly, the development of funeral directing greatly strengthened these internal changes.

The germ theory of disease and the accompanying new developments in pathology, antisepsis, and surgery enabled physicians to treat numerous diseases and injuries which before had been regarded as terminal. Instead of resignation in the face of death, patients by the hundreds of thousands were rushed to hospitals where physicians often were able to revive them or extend their lives. Advances in the diagnosis and control of infectious diseases after 1890 had dramatic and far-reaching effects on the capacity of medicine to rescue the sick and dying.

The development of new medical specialities also brought new populations of patients into the hospital either to be cured or to die. Obstetrics/gynecology, pediatrics, and geriatrics (after 1919) were notable examples of this trend. By the 1930s, due partly to changing patterns of disease and partly to the development of new medical techniques, campaigns to cure chronic illnesses were begun (7). The number of hospitals and the types of service they offered increased dramatically, and of course they changed accordingly.

These developments within modern medicine were intricately related to major social and intellectual changes occurring at the same time. With a greater percentage of the population moving into often overcrowded and unsanitary urban areas, and with more and more husbands and wives working away from their homes, hospitals became the natural place in which the sick, injured, and terminally ill were cared for. Greater skepticism toward literal religious beliefs in eternal life after death accompanied by the increased comforts and pleasures of urban and suburban living surely supplemented earlier tendencies to regard medical science as a means of secular salvation (34). Furthermore, even as the modern hospital kept fewer and fewer humans from dying in their homes, so also the funeral industry made it far less likely that family members would care for the bodies of the dead. Nonprofessionals were becoming less and less familiar with dying and the dead, which in turn gave all the more credence to professional opinion and probably made dying all the more awesome and mystifying (17). Terminal care under the supervision of physicians thus came into being because of the explicit efforts of physicians as well as broader changes and needs of society.

Although the trek from home to the hospital at or near the end of human life represents a major change in Western history, this change occurred gradually, and until about a decade ago it was not seriously challenged or questioned. Physicians, patients, and families alike regarded the hospital in very positive terms. Here life might be extended, health possibly recovered; and death—should it occur—was at least familiar.

PHYSICIANS' DUTIES, 1890 TO 1960: FOUR PRIORITIES

Physicians consciously sought to supervise the medical, social, and psychological milieu of dying patients in the hospital by developing a list of responsibilities with the following priorities: First, if at all possible, physicians were to employ their knowledge and utmost skill to cure the critically ill. Second, as devotees of medical science, they were to use their experiences to develop better methods of diagnosis and therapy. Third, they were to comfort the dying. Fourth, they were to counsel and comfort family and friends.

The first of these priorities needs little elaboration. American hospital physicians between 1880 and 1960 assumed that the reason for the hospital's existence lay in the ability of its physicians to diagnose and cure. Soothing and comforting were not to be avoided or forgotten but clearly were considered secondary to healing and curing.

Speaking in 1900, Baldwin (3) recounted a conversation between a physician and the relative of a patient. The patient told the relative that she wanted to die. The relative asked if the case was hopeless. "Yes," said the physician. Was the patient suffering? "Yes." Then why was it necessary to try so hard to keep her alive? "It is my duty to keep her living as long as possible." Baldwin then indicated that various heroic measures were used on wealthy patients to keep them alive. These included the forced drinking of special nutrients, hypodermic injections of various types of fluid, and even injecting strychnine in order to shake the body into activity for yet a few more hours (3). Writing in 1938, 3 years after the beginning of the campaign to cure chronic illness, Bluestone (7) said that one of the problems with the chronically ill was that some of them were resigned to dying. Resignation toward death had been regarded as the ultimate achievement of good dying during the nineteenth century, but was regarded as a negative sign by numerous hospital physicians. Resisting the tide of normal hospital procedures, the physician Worcester (44) wrote in 1935 that "all of these modern methods of resuscitation" were often "most decidedly out of place. . . . Too many of our profession seem to believe themselves duty bound to do their utmost" to revive the dying, he added.

The second duty, contributing to progress in medical science, was carried out in a variety of ways. Believing that sophisticated medicine required scientific pathology, most physicians believed that securing the permission for an autopsy was crucially significant even if the "feelings of bereaved relatives" were sometimes interfered with (12). Occasionally physicians also became interested in the phenomenon of human dying and sought to correct popular misunderstandings. For example, several writers said that popular beliefs about the pain of death as evidenced in "death throes" were inaccurate and argued that what appears to be a death struggle is far more painful to the witnesses than to the dying person. Osler had reported that the majority of humans die "unconscious and unconcerned"; but other well-known physicians including Worcester and Cabot disagreed with Osler, claiming that near the end of life their patients only appeared to be "unconscious." In fact, they were still aware of what was being said and done around them (8,44).

A key set of presuppositions which linked twentieth century hospital physicians to their nineteenth century forebears was held with respect to the third duty of physicians, the comforting of the dying. Physicians generally agreed that their responsibilities did not end when curing and healing were no longer possible. What then was the character of the care they felt bound to give?

Between 1890 and 1960, those who wrote about the care for the dying assumed two values as primary: (a) extending pain-free life as long as possible and (b) enabling patients to die in peace (26,44). These values gave rise to two standardized policies regarding ideal care: Hope must be maintained, and patients must not be disturbed. In moral terms, maintaining hope was viewed as a display of benevolence or kindness; and not disturbing was understood as an expression of the longstanding medical mandate of not harming. In turn, these policies call into play a third policy which was to be honored whenever possible: Physicians and other hospital personnel should conceal the severity of the patient's medical condition. Blatant lying to patients (but not always to family members) was to be avoided, but "white lying" and pretending were so thoroughly accepted that elaborate social games designed to conceal the diagnostic truth from patients were developed (16,29).

The duties of maintaining hope (29) and of concealing and optimistically embellishing the diagnosis were viewed as complementary policies designed to comfort and shield patients from the singular, overwhelming harm—knowledge of death. Physicians agreed almost unanimously that knowledge of death leads to deep despair, to alarming terror, to dark and distorted thoughts, very possibly even to psychopathology and suicide (2,8,10,29). Since ideal care consisted of enabling patients to live as peacefully as possible to the very end, it became imperative that they be shielded from knowledge about the eminence of death which might lead directly to despair and early death. Two physicians wrote that "in almost every case" a diagnosis of cancer carries with it the "real possibility" of suicide. Severe cases of "cancerphobia" may require multiple electric shock treatments; and if these do not work, a prefrontal lobotomy will relieve intractable pain and result in "the loss of this preoccupation with self and future" (21).

These beliefs and values apparently became almost universally honored in American hospitals from 1890 through 1960. Regarded as "medical judgments," they were transcribed into explicit social policies, leading physicians and nurses to "manage" or supervise patients according to these norms. As institutions molded by and reflecting predominant medical values, hospitals became an ideal setting in which such control could be maintained. "There is a hardened convention, a conspiracy of silence," reported one hospital chaplain in 1955, "that makes it difficult if not impossible for the critically ill person to talk about his impending death" (4). When the sociologists Glaser and Strauss conducted their famous study concerning the social exchanges between dying patients, health care professionals, and relatives, they discovered that only in a Veterans Administration (VA) hospital was it a normal procedure to tell patients about the nature of their illnesses. Moreover, this policy appeared to have been instituted because of the low social status and destitute circumstances of VA patients, not because it was regarded as innovative or virtuous (16). Very few physicians recommended exceptions to these policies (1).

Fourth and finally, physicians between 1880 and 1960 regarded the counseling and comforting of the relatives of dying patients as one of their responsibilities. The stipulations set forth in the AMA Code of 1847 became normative as a course of action for the next 120 years. Physicians were to give family and friends of the patient a "timely notice of danger," although this information should be kept from patients if at all possible. Like the duties designed to comfort patients, the responsibility "to steady and comfort the stricken family" led to explicit types of social control in the hospital (16,44). Physicians were responsible for seeing that family members control their emotions, muffle their grief, and maintain "cheerful" countenances (8,10,26,44). Displays of emotion disrupt hospital routines, and hospitals can hardly tolerate grieving relatives "dashing through the corridors" (26).

To summarize, our sources reveal that between 1890 and 1960 an elaborate and normative set of interrelationships between physicians, patients, relatives, and other hospital personnel were consciously developed within the hospital in order to manage dying patients and their families in accordance with physician's theories and values. As "medical opinion" these viewpoints were institutionalized in hospitals as explicit guidelines for the supervision of patients. They resulted in the development of an elaborate social ritual, a unique human drama designed to pacify patients, maintain peaceful hospital routines, and comfort relatives (16). The drama of human dying was never lost; it had been revised according to the medical values and judgments operative in the modern hospital. This new form of terminal care was not merely the product of medical professionals—it was compatible with broader social, ideological, and institutional changes within American and Western culture. Medical opinion molded and satisfied broader human needs.

A CRITIQUE OF THE PAST

Medicine's historical legacy, however, also includes the very recent period of great turmoil over the nature of appropriate terminal care. In fact, during the last approximately 15 years we have witnessed an extensive re-evaluation of the priorities and presuppositions that were assumed as valid between 1890 and 1960. It is imperative that we know something about the character and causes for this wholesale reassessment before we can set forth clearly and concisely the responsibilities of contemporary physicians. The four priorities of 1890 to 1960 are now reviewed in the light of these recent debates and revisions.

In the first place, the responsibility of reviving or prolonging life is no longer uncritically valued. Nor is it assumed that physicians alone can make all decisions about which lives should be prolonged and how long intensive care equipment should be used. Patients, families, the courts, and new state laws are insisting that other parties become involved in a number of decisions involving resuscitation and prolongation.

Surely numerous factors are responsible for the debates and dilemmas regarding the responsibility to prolong life and the assumption that such prolongation is a "medical" and, *ipso facto,* a physician's decision. It was only a matter of time before such a decision disagreed with the wishes of family members and exposed the dehumanizing, even ghastly effects of intensive care technology. The case of Karen Quinlin symbolizes these problems. In addition, other technological developments within medicine caused certain decisions involving the prolongation of life to become exceedingly complex. Procedures associated with the transplantation of human organs, for example, caused other interested parties—scientists, physicians, patients, and families—to become deeply concerned with when and why the bodies of patients should be kept alive and what definitions of death would be endorsed. Finally, a wholesale review of terminal care has been under way, a review surely influenced by the questioning of traditional forms of authority which characterized the 1960s, by a franker realism concerning the limits of science and the hopelessness of even extremely sophisticated medical technology, and surely also by the great expenses involved in a world increasingly aware of its limited resources.

Fewer questions have been raised about the second traditional medical priority, advancing medical knowledge. In fact, the great resurgence of interest in death and dying has led to an increased concern about physical aspects of death, the development of better pain therapy, and probably a greater desire on behalf of many relatives to know the medical causes of death. Nevertheless, the widespread movement to monitor and regulate human experimentation has set limits on the way scientific data can be collected.

A storm of controversy, however, has arisen over the third and fourth sets of responsibilities assumed previously by physicians, i.e., the care and comfort of dying patients and their relatives. First, given the dilemmas associated with prolonging life, there is great concern about making appropriate decisions as to when to stop trying to cure and when to begin giving only personalized care and pain relief. One of the first of the new wave of books on medical ethics highlighted this as a crucially significant issue in the care of the dying (33), and subsequent studies investigated in great detail the issues associated with this criticial decision. These issues include the need to determine reasonable and unreasonable treatments, to understand the rights of patients (e.g., their right to refuse treatment), to distinguish between competent and incompetent adults as well as between adults and children, and to set forth the characteristics of moral and workable public policies (42,43).

Second, numerous questions have been raised regarding the traditional pattern of comfort and control which had become institutionalized in the modern hospital. Although many patients, families, physicians, and nurses still regard the traditional pattern of patient care (characterized by peacefulness, hope, and concealment) as meaningful and useful (whether it is moral is quite another matter), numerous health care professionals and others have begun to question thoroughly the major presuppositions of this care. These criticisms and questions can be grouped under three headings: images of death, truthtelling, and conformity.

Meaningful questions and debates over images of death must include an understanding of death and human psychology. The social rituals developed within the modern hospital between 1890 and 1960 were constructed on the presupposition that news of impending death was so psychologically catastrophic that in the great majority of cases it must be concealed from the patient. An uncritical acceptance of this presupposition is no longer possible. Major studies and even intellectual movements within philosophy and religion, history and anthropology, and psychology show that death need not be viewed as an "unrelieved calamity" (4). News about impending death can be known, talked about, and endured. The issues here involve fundamental questions, only the bare outlines of which can be suggested.

The writings of philosophers and theologians indicate the degree to which Judaism and Christianity value life and regard death as a great and evil enemy— even if these traditions also affirm that it can be overcome (32). Perhaps, then, the horror of death became particularly acute after the rise of post-Darwinian secularism when negative images of death were retained while the solace of resurrection and eternal life was significantly lost, and when the majority of the dying and dead were removed from homes into hospitals and funeral parlors. At any rate, during the last decade, numerous philosophers and theologians attempted either to recover less alarming images of death from Greek philosophy (14,28) or to view a forthright struggle with death as the ultimate sign of courage and humanism (27).

History and anthropology also undermine the notion of death as an unrelieved calamity, the news of which always causes terror and cuts life short. In other eras of Western history and in non-Western cultures, humans have adjusted to death in numerous ways other than by fear or terror or by pretending that medical science can somehow offer miraculous hope (15,22).

A vast amount of writing and research has been done on the psychological dimensions of death, dying, and grieving. Much of this thinking disagrees with past perspectives. The philosopher–psychologist Ernst Becker, for example, calls into question certain fundamental presuppositions of Sigmund Freud. Indicating that Freud was seeking to secure his own form of immortality by vindicating the centrality of his theories of sexuality in the face of backsliding peers and students, Becker underlines the degree to which death more than sex shapes the human psyche, molds human culture, and serves as the ultimate test for human greatness and creativity (5). On a more practical level, the famous studies of Elisabeth Kübler-Ross indicate how hospitalized patients can consciously cope with death, and she proposes that their coping occurs according to patterned psychological reactions—by the five stages of denial, anger, bargaining, depression, and acceptance (23). Her work presupposes a now widely accepted understanding of adult psychology, i.e., that instead of reaching a uniform psychological plateau after adolescence, adults go through numerous psychological stages throughout their lives (37).

Truth-telling has been no less thoroughly reviewed. To be sure, on numerous hospital wards, some family members still maintain that their dying relatives do not want to hear about and cannot cope with the truth about their condition. Yet the great majority of persons expect and request franker, more explicit information (9,29,42), and in some studies indicate that the families of patients who are told the truth cope far better than those who are "shielded" from it (9).

Why many patients and family members desire more explicit truth-telling is a complicated and intriguing question. Surely this change is connected in part to the emergence of numerous human rights movements between the mid-1950s and the present, and these movements have sponsored an increased public scrutiny of every major social institution, be it governmental, legal, economic, or medical. Medicine is not the sole subject of such intense scrutiny.

Dying quietly and in conformity with traditional hospital routines is also being reassessed. Quoting the poet R. M. Rilke, Aronson, as late as 1959, observed that in hospitals it was rare indeed for anyone to desire "to have a death of one's own" (2). The emergence and growth of the hospice and home-care movements indicate how and why many persons now disagree with this once orthodox perspective. Countless individuals now wish to spend the last weeks and months of their lives according to their own style of living—on their own social turf, among family and friends, in the midst of their possessions, and with the celebrations of their own choosing.

CONTEMPORARY RESPONSIBILITIES

Given the penetrating critique of traditional medical responsibilities and practices, we might well be tempted to despair from searching for clear answers. Why not conclude that we are in a period of drift, a period when it may be best vaguely to counsel individuals and groups to be "as thoughtful and responsible as possible" in the midst of difficult and uncertain times? Neither history nor ethics supports this reaction.

The historical sketches above and the very recent writings of a number of physicians indicates that a majority of patients and families want and need comprehensive care (pain relief, psychological counseling, social support, and even curative therapy if it stands a chance to work), but they increasingly do not want this care according to the traditional model which predominated within hospitals between 1890 and 1960. This is precisely in keeping with one of the central themes of this essay, i.e., that human dying *includes* physiological processes and calls for uniquely "medical" expertise and decision-making, but that it has not and cannot be reduced to these. Slow, prolonged dying is a physiological and a deeply emotional process. It is also an individual and communal process, the community in the hospital consisting of patient, family, friends, and a variety of health professionals. Dying is a drama fraught with profound emotional and social significance. It was a drama before dying patients were ushered into the hospital; it became an elaborate drama when they were brought there; and it remains one today. The great popularity of innumerable personal accounts of grappling with fatal illness underlines this fundamental perspective (20).

In the light of the human needs associated with prolonged dying and the implicit and explicit beliefs, expectations, and roles of patients, families, and physicians, what morally required actions should be observed by physicians? The very fact that patients and families turn to physicians when death threatens or approaches pinpoints the crucial significance of medical expertise. Yet patients seek this expertise as a means of realizing fundamental values or ends, ends such as an extension of conscious life, freedom from pain, and a continued recognition of their significance as persons. What ethical principles will suffice for displaying the physician's responsibilities?

I propose the following: First, there are responsibilities regarding medical means, i.e., regarding medical expertise and judgments. Second, there are responsibilities associated with the preservation of certain fundamental human values. These values are best summarized by the concept of the worth of persons, a concept which captures the comprehensive dynamics of human dying far more adequately than the ideal of "death with dignity" (39). Humans are endowed or credited with worth if their rights are respected, if they are sustained by a caring community, and if their bodily needs are cared for (39).

An upholding of these essential elements of human worth by health professionals helps to compensate for the low priority and lack of worth so easily attributed to dying patients in hospitals, particularly teaching hospitals where attention focuses on saving lives and learning from interesting, treatable cases (22). A respecting of these values also counterbalances the lack of worth attributed to inactive, nonproductive persons in an industrial society. If these principles are upheld, some of the deepest fears associated with dying will be defused, i.e., the fears of being a burden rather than autonomous, being abandoned rather than being cared for and communicated with, and becoming disfigured and suffering from pain rather than being groomed and set free from pain (9,22).

We thus arrive at four sets of responsibilities: those pertaining to (1) medical expertise and judgment, (b) patient rights, (c) the patient's community or milieu, and (d) bodily care. Attention is given here only to the broadest, most basic of these morally required actions.

Medical Expertise and Judgment

Physicians hardly need reminding that there is no substitute for first-rate medical competence, including drug therapy, knowledge about the growing body of literature dealing with the psychological dimensions of patient care, and the development of counseling and communicating skills.

The famous work by Kübler-Ross can serve as a beginning point for understanding the psychological processes of terminally ill persons, but only as a beginning point. Her outline of the stages of shock and denial, anger, bargaining, depression, and acceptance is extremely useful in working with terminally ill patients or with other persons enduring major physical or emotional losses. Nevertheless, as Kübler-Ross herself later notes, it is questionable whether these are five stages or step-like processes proceeding one after another. These are best understood not as stages but as types of normal reactions which "may be present simultaneously, disappear and reappear, or occur in any order" (9,24). How or whether patients manifest these reactions depends on a variety of factors, including age, social circumstance, and past experiences with separations (40). Furthermore, fixing on five "stages," ignores such reactions as confusion, fear, guilt, envy, grief, anxiety, courage, and trust (20). Finally, there is a need not to confuse "is" with "ought," i.e., not to confuse a description of staged psychological phenomena with the therapeutic necessity of needing to usher patients through the first four "stages" to the last.

The ability to communicate effectively is another ingredient in responsible care for dying patients. The development of skill in communication does not require that physicians become articulate speakers, but rather that they develop effective listening skills, learn to "read" what patients are saying, know how to ask questions which encourage patients to speak of their primary concerns, and remember to communicate through touch.

Patient Rights

One of the beginning points for ethical behavior is the regarding of other persons as means in themselves, as persons who define their own ends, rather than as individuals who can be used as a means for another's ends. Patients must therefore be regarded as autonomous individuals rather than passive creatures who are managed by others. This requires the defining of an ethically responsible physician–patient relationship in which the physician is neither parent nor priest (unless perhaps the patient specifically and strongly requests it) but is a concerned fellow human who informs the patient and receives his or her consent for every major clinical decision (13). These decisions include the following: telling the truth about diagnosis and prognosis, beginning and ending of therapeutic regimens, initiating any form of biomedical experimentation, determining where the patient should be cared for, and terminating life support procedures. Forms of coercion should be avoided. These include policies which presume that all patients must be told the truth or that all should not be told the truth, that patients should be ushered through "earlier" psychological "stages" to an acceptance of death, or that patients should be required to live with life-prolonging technology or to die without it.

The accent here is on valuing patients to the extent that they are given appropriate medical information and are endowed with the right to make decisions concerning what they wish to know about their medical condition; whether they would rather spend their final days or weeks at home, in the hospital, or in a hospice; or if they wish life-prolonging procedures to be used when they lose consciousness. Without question, the institution of this approach to patient care is one of the most challenging of moral and professional responsibilities. Does this call for a major revision of medical practice? Yes, if these decisions are being made unilaterally by physicians who are relying on habits and hunches to determine "what the patient wants." No, if it is assumed that this approach calls for an idealistic obliviousness to the ever-present time constraints of medical practice, or that this approach necessarily entails a lengthy conference with patient and family at every juncture in the patient's care. What is called for is special attention to and training in this aspect of care so that the physician can determine what the patient wants skillfully and briefly—even if what is determined is that the patient and family want the physician to make the decision.

A conscientious honoring of the right to decide is what counts, although this becomes especially complex and sensitive for children or "incompetent" patients (42). On the practical level, health professionals should think of ways to enhance the choices, self-control, and even minor contributions which can be made by terminally ill patients (39).

The Patient's Milieu

With respect to sustaining the worth of persons, responsibilities associated with the patient's social and psychological milieu are of equal or greater importance to those dealing with the patient's rights. Empirically, human worth is not so much achieved as received. We are valued and view ourselves as valued because others have shown affection for us, cared for us, and communicated with us—not merely because we are autonomous individuals who have the ability to think and act on our own. We are denigrated or devalued if we are dealt with thoughtlessly, foolishly, or outrageously. Human worth, therefore, is grounded in communal and relational experiences. It is also rooted in religious and philosophical views of human nature, including the beliefs that we are created, loved, and redeemed by God, or that we are endowed with reason and a moral sense.

Because of these dimensions of human worth, physicians should give great attention to the social, psychological, and "spiritual" milieu of the hospital, for the hospital environment can either augment or undermine a sense of human worth. The community consists of physicians, patients, families, other members of the health care team, and chaplains. The traditional and legal authority of physicians means that they are ultimately responsible for much of the purpose and *esprit de corps* of the health care team; the emotional, and sometimes the physical, needs of family members; the presence or absence of chaplains (22); and the degree of empathy and regular communication afforded to patient and family.

Bodily Care

As I observed elsewhere, "a person's sense of worth or well-being is reflected by his bodily carriage and is affected by personal grooming, by the presence or absence of pain, and by disfigurement or mutilation" (39). Self-worth, therefore, has extremely important physiological and aesthetic dimensions. It is by no means painless for patients to decide to undergo a chemotherapeutic regimen knowing that their hair will fall out (41). Disfigurement and a loss of personal attractiveness easily lead to a sense of shame and denigration. Odor, excretion, incontinence, drooling, and hemorrhaging are often accompanied by a loss of self-esteem. Attending to these problems enables patients to retain a sense of pride and well-being. These forms of bodily care can make life still pleasurable and meaningful (9). It is easily and falsely assumed that tastes, smells, sights, and sounds are not at times exquisitely moving to persons who are terminally ill. One terminal patient confided recently, "I don't take nothin' for granted anymore; I never realized how much I could enjoy just the common things." Pain relief, of course, is of central importance in the care of body and psyche.

TRAINING AND POLICY FORMATION

For almost a century, comprehensive care of dying persons under the direction of medical professionals has steadily increased. Whether this trend is continuing at the present time, however, is very much in question. The rapid growth of hospice and home care movements—growth which has occurred simultaneously with the thoroughgoing critique of traditional medical care—suggests that we are in a time of transition when medical supervision is being revised and alternative forms of care which view medical expertise as essential but auxiliary are developing and expanding. Factors such as shifting cultural and personal values, economic circumstances, the power of professional organizations, the willingness of medical professionals to review and revise their care, and the way medical professionals place limits on their roles will ultimately determine the shape of the future. I offer here some final observations on the last two of these factors.

In the first place, it is clear that numerous physicians and several innovative hospital programs are presupposing that medical supervision of dying persons is desired, meaningful, and effective. The responsibilities outlined above indicate how this type of care can be meaningful, effective, and moral.

The responsibilities displayed here, however, are best understood as a point of departure for medical professionals and planners. As I indicated elsewhere, explicit public and institutional policies are always founded on moral and philosophical perspectives, whether those forming such policies realize it or not (38). Physicians and health care planners are charged with the responsibility of establishing specific criteria and policies for the care of terminally ill adults and children in the light of the beliefs, values, and norms identified above. Certain precedents for such policy formation already exist (13).

The deficits of the past cannot be remedied easily. Conscientious care of terminally ill persons calls for new levels of knowledge, expertise, and training in such areas as psychological knowledge, counseling and communicating skills, and new therapeutic procedures. Answers to the fundamental question are called for: What does "medical competence" consist of with respect to expert and humane medical care for fatally ill and slowly dying patients? Policy and training must be built on the answers to this question.

Although in my opinion unlikely, it is still conceivable that physicians will wish to delimit their roles by divesting themselves of many of the personal, psychological, and social responsibilities surrounding human death. One physician remarked recently that he wants to limit his decisions and attention to cost-effective biomedical procedures. Another, predicting that greater specialization is inevitable, said that physicians will and should excuse themselves "from those in slow death." Only time will tell whether doctors will seek to limit their interactions to curative procedures and pain medication. If they do place these limits on their practice, their interventions must be supplemented by the care of other professionals who are trained to attend to the other essential needs of dying persons. The drama of death will not go away. The worth of persons is at stake.

REFERENCES

1. Alvarez, W. C. (1952): The care of the dying. *JAMA,* 150:86–91.
2. Aronson, G. J. (1959): Treatment of the dying person. In: *The Meaning of Death,* edited by H. F. Feifel, pp. 251–258. McGraw-Hill, New York.
3. Baldwin, S. E. (1904): *The Natural Right to a Natural Death,* pp. 3–6. Frank H. Vehr, Cincinnati.
4. Beatty, D. C. (1955): Shall we talk about death? *Pastoral Psychol.,* 6:11–14.
5. Becker, E. (1973): *The Denial of Death.* Free Press, New York.
6. Beecher, L. (1961): *The Autobiography of Lyman Beecher,* edited by B. M. Cross, pp. 215–221. Harvard University Press, Cambridge, Mass.
7. Bluestone, E. M. (1938): Unfinished business—Chronic patients. *Mod. Hosp.,* 55:82–84.
8. Cabot, R. C., and Dicks, R. L. (1936): *The Art of Ministering to the Sick,* pp. 298–314. Macmillan, New York.
9. Cassem, N. H., and Stewart, R. (1975): Management and care of the dying patient. *Int. J. Psychiatr. Med.,* 6:293–304.
10. Cathell, D. W. (1890): *Book on the Physician Himself,* pp. 113–121. F. A. Davis, Philadelphia.
11. DePorte, J. V. (1929): Where do people die—at home or in hospitals? *Mod. Hosp.,* 34:68–73.
12. Development in autopsies in the hospital field: a report by the American Hospital Association Committee on Post-Mortem Examinations. *Mod. Hosp.,* 36:61–70 (1931).
13. Duff, R. S. (1979): Guidelines for deciding care of critically ill or dying patient. *Pediatrics,* 64:17–23.
14. Engelhardt, T., Jr. (1975): The counsels of finitude. In: *Death Inside Out,* edited by P. Steinfels et al., pp. 115–128. Harper & Row, New York.
15. Fabian, J. (1973): How others die—Reflections on the anthropology of death. In: *Death in American Experience,* edited by A. Mack, pp. 177–201. Schocken Books, New York.
16. Glaser, B. G., and Strauss, A. L. (1965): *Awareness of Dying.* Adline, Chicago.
17. Gorer, G. (1976): The pornography of death. In: *Death: Current Perspectives,* edited by E. S. Shneidman, pp. 71–75. Mayfield, Palo Alto, Calif.
18. Hooker, W. (1872): *Human Physiology.* Sheldon, New York.
19. Hooker, W. (1849): *Physician and Patient,* pp. 352–401. Baker & Scribner, New York.

20. Jaffe, L., and Jaffe, A. (1975): Terminal candor and the coda syndrome. In: *New Meanings of Death*, edited by H. Fiefel, pp. 196–211. McGraw-Hill, New York.
21. Kline, N. S., and Sobin, J. (1951): The psychological management of cancer cases. *JAMA*, 146:1547–1551.
22. Krant, M. J., and Sheldon, A. (1971): The dying patient—Medicine's responsibility. *J. Thanatol.*, 1:1–24.
23. Kübler-Ross, E. (1969): *On Death and Dying*. Macmillan, New York.
24. Kübler-Ross, E. (1974): *Questions and Answers on Death and Dying*. Collier, New York.
25. Lerner, M. (1975): When, why, and where people die? In: *The Dying Patient*, edited by O. G. Brim, Jr., et al., pp. 22–23. Russell Sage Foundation, New York.
26. Love, E. (1944): Do all hands help ease the sting of death by tact and kindliness? *Hospitals*, 18:47–48.
27. May, W. (1975): The metaphysical plight of the family. In: *Death Inside Out*, edited by P. Steinfels et al., pp. 49–60. Harper & Row, New York.
28. Morison, R. S. (1975): The dignity of the inevitable and necessary. In: *Death Inside Out*, edited by P. Steinfels et al., pp. 97–100. Harper & Row, New York.
29. Oken, D. (1961): What to tell cancer patients: A study of medical attitudes. *JAMA*, 175:1120–1128.
30. Osler, W. (1906): *Science and Immortality*, pp. 18–20. Archibald Constable, London.
31. Percival, T. (1979): *Percival's Medical Ethics*, edited by C. D. Leake, pp. 90–93. Robert E. Krieger, New York.
32. Ramsey, P. (1974): The indignity of "death with dignity." In: *Death Inside Out*, edited by P. Steinfels et al., pp. 81–96. Harper & Row, New York.
33. Ramsey, P. (1970): *The Patient as Person*. Yale University Press, New Haven, Conn.
34. Ranney, G. E. (1892): Death a universal law. *Transact. Mich. State Med. Soc.*, 16:9–29.
35. Reiser, S. J., et al. (1977): *Ethics in Medicine: Historical Perspectives in Contemporary Concerns*, pp. 26–34. MIT Press, Cambridge, Mass.
36. Saum, L. O. (1974): Death in the popular mind of pre-civil war America. *Am. Q.*, 24:477–495.
37. Sheehy, G. (1974): *Passages*. Dutton, New York.
38. Vanderpool, H. Y. (1978): B. F. Skinner on ethics and the control of retarded persons. *Linacre Q.*, 45:135–151.
39. Vanderpool, H. Y. (1978): The ethics of terminal care. *JAMA*, 239:850–852.
40. Vanderpool, J. P. (1976): Understanding death and the dying patient. *Cont. Educ. Family Physician*, 5:77–85.
41. Vaughn, E. G. (1979): My mother breathing light. *New Yorker*, Sept. 10:48–53.
42. Veatch, R. M. (1976): *Death, Dying, and the Biological Revolution*, Chap. 3–5. Yale University Press, New Haven, Conn.
43. Veatch, R. M. (1977): Death and dying: The legislative options. *Med. Commun.*, 6:23–29.
44. Worcester, A. (1935): *The Care of the Aged, the Dying, and the Dead*, pp. 33–71. Charles C Thomas, Springfield, Ill.

Medical Complications in Cancer Patients,
edited by J. Klastersky and M. J. Staquet.
Raven Press, New York © 1981.

Nephropathy as a Consequence of Neoplasms or Their Treatment

*Bernard S. Kaplan, **Mathew H. Gault, and †Juergen Knaack

*Nephrology Service, The Montreal Children's Hospital, and Department of Pediatrics, McGill University, Montreal, Quebec H3H 1P3, Canada; **Department of Medicine (Nephrology), Memorial University of Newfoundland, St. Johns, Newfoundland A1B 3V6, Canada; and †Department of Pathology, Institute of Pathology and McGill University, Montreal, Quebec H3H 1P3, Canada

Extrarenal neoplasms can inflict renal injury through a variety of mechanisms (46,47,57,84,87,92,107,118,119), including thrombosis or compression of the inferior vena cava or renal vein, amyloidosis, glomerular injury, direct invasion of the parenchyma, obstruction of urine flow, and damage by calcium, uric acid, or phosphate. Practically every kind of neoplasm, whether solid or leukemic, malignant or benign, has the potential to damage the kidneys through any or all of these mechanisms and give rise to clinical syndromes of renal disease such as acute renal failure, chronic renal failure, nephrotic syndrome, glomerulonephritis, or obstructive uropathy.

The association of neoplasia–nephropathy has important implications for optimal patient care and provides an experiment of nature that allows insights into the pathogenesis of aspects of each condition. Furthermore, the treatment of neoplasia is fraught with potential danger to the patient's kidneys because of the nephrotoxic effects of antibiotics, chemotherapeutic agents, and irradiation (4,13,29,103,168).

ACUTE RENAL FAILURE IN PATIENTS WITH CANCER

Acute renal failure frequently occurs in patients with cancer (47,57,107). Once such prerenal factors as dehydration, shock, or congestive heart failure have been excluded, obstructive and intrinsic renal causes should be considered. Obstruction to urine output (87) can be caused by tumors of the prostate, bladder, pelvis, or abdomen and by retroperitoneal fibrosis. Renovascular compression, or obstruction, by thrombus or tumor occasionally causes renal failure (45,140).

Radiotherapy (103), chemotherapy (13,29,168), and many antibiotics (4) are potentially nephrotoxic. Acute tubular necrosis can occur as a result of shock secondary to sepsis, blood loss, or disseminated intravascular coagulation. Pyelonephritis is an important cause of acute renal failure in immunocompromised individuals (127).

Hyperuricemia, a frequent cause of acute renal failure in patients with lymphoproliferative disorders (75,89,127), also occurs with other neoplasms (34,171). Hyperuricemia can damage the kidney before and after chemotherapy. Treatment with allopurinol has reduced the prevalence of this complication; uric acid precursors, however, can also cause renal injury (8). Hyperphosphatemia secondary to rapid cell lysis was recently recognized as a cause of acute renal failure (8,12,23,49,83).

Bence-Jones proteins in patients with myeloma (36) and mucoproteins derived from pancreatic carcinoma (74) have induced acute renal failure by obstructing renal tubules.

Patients with non-Hodgkin's lymphoma, especially those with American Burkitt's lymphoma, have been identified as being at greater risk for the occurrence of acute renal failure (107). These large, rapidly growing tumors sensitive to cytolytic agents have the potential of producing loads of uric acid and phosphate, which can cause renal failure, and potassium, which can cause death. In addition, patients with some degree of renal failure at presentation have a greater potential for further deterioration, and mechanical urinary tract obstruction is more likely in patients with abdominal tumors (107).

CHRONIC RENAL FAILURE IN CANCER PATIENTS

Progression to chronic renal failure has occurred in some patients with neoplasia and glomerular injury (153) and in others after irradiation, chemotherapy, or subtotal nephrectomy. Gradual ureteral obstruction by tumor lymph nodes or retroperitoneal fibrosis has reduced renal function, and uremia has occurred as a result of massive (114,149,159) or selective (161) infiltration of the kidneys by solid tumor (114,149,159), leukemia (102), or malignant histiocytosis (161). Amyloid deposits have resulted in chronic renal failure with and without nephrotic syndrome (7,87).

GLOMERULAR INJURY AND NEOPLASIA

Estimates of the prevalence of the nephrotic syndrome in patients with neoplasia range from 6% (76) to 11.0% (92,153). A chance association is often difficult to exclude except perhaps in cases in which glomerular deposits of tumor-derived antigen are demonstrated (31,33,95,133,147,177). Circumstantial evidence favoring malignancy as a cause of the nephrotic syndrome includes the relatively large numbers of patients who have had Hodgkin's disease and a minimal-change form of the nephrotic syndrome (lipoid nephrosis), remission of the nephrotic syndrome with treatment of the neoplasm, relapse of nephrotic syndrome with recurrence of the tumor, and the synchronous occurrence of the two conditions (84).

PERSONAL CASES

We have studied six men and one woman aged 47 to 74 years in whom glomerular injury appeared to have been associated with a neoplastic disease (58) (Table 1). The duration of symptoms ranged from 1 to 36 months. In six patients the presenting symptoms were those of the glomerular injury: six had microscopic and/or macroscopic hematuria, six had edema, and four had mildly elevated blood pressure. The primary carcinoma involved the lung in two, the adrenal in two, and the colon and kidney in one patient each. One man had a lymphosarcoma. None had systemic lupus, diabetes mellitus, cryoglobulinemia, antecedent streptococcal infection, amyloidosis, or main renal vein thrombosis.

All had BUN levels greater than 39 mg/dl, serum creatinine concentrations over 2.2 mg/dl, and urine protein excretion in excess of 3.5 g/24 hr.

The VDRL was negative in each case, and the antinuclear factor or lupus erythematosus (LE) cell phenomenon was negative in six patients. Cryoglobulins were not detectable, and ASO titers were normal in four patients tested. All had low serum albumin levels, but only three had elevated cholesterol values (128). One of six tested had a persistently reduced B_{1C} globulin concentration.

The time interval between the diagnosis of the glomerulopathy and the malignancy was brief, averaging 8 months. Renal disease was diagnosed before the malignancy was found in five patients. Urinalysis and renal function were documented as normal in two patients 2 years before diagnosis of renal disease. The tumor was first found at autopsy in two cases and was the cause of death in two; three died from renal failure and one of cardiac failure. Renal failure progressed rapidly in three patients (cases 3, 6, 7), and the intervals from the diagnosis of renal disease until the institution of dialysis were 1, 2, and 4 months, respectively.

A renal biopsy was performed on six patients and an autopsy on five. The major feature of the glomerular injury in six cases was an increase in mesangial cells and matrix, especially the latter. One patient had an epimembranous glomerulonephritis. The characteristic findings of membranoproliferative glomerulonephritis were demonstrated by light, immunofluorescence, and ultrastructural studies of glomeruli from the patient with lymphosarcoma and nephrotic syndrome.

Patient 1 was treated with prednisone and cyclophosphamide for 2 months without apparent improvement in proteinuria or renal function. The lymphosarcoma of case 7 was treated with vincristine, prednisone, and cyclophosphamide before the onset of renal disease and again with cyclophosphamide and prednisone for the renal disease for 2 months, without improvement in proteinuria or renal function.

CARCINOMA AND GLOMERULOPATHY

The following sequence has been proposed to account for the pathogenesis of glomerular lesions in patients with carcinoma and glomerulopathy (76): Tumor

TABLE 1. *Features of seven patients with neoplasms and glomerular injury*

Case	Sex	Age (years)	Presentation	Duration of symptoms (months)	Time from diagnosis of renal disease to death (months)	Site of malignancy	Renal histology
1	F	66	Edema	4	4	Colon	Membranoproliferative glomerulonephritis
2	M	68	Edema	1	1	Kidney	Mesangial cell proliferation
3	M	61	Hematuria	3	2	Lung	Proliferation of mesangial cells and matrix
4	M	47	Edema	6	6	Adrenal	Epimembranous glomerulopathy
5	M	72	Edema	3	3	Lung	Proliferation of mesangial cells and matrix
6	M	64	Flank pain, edema	2	1	Adrenal	Proliferation of mesangial cells and matrix
7	M	74	Lymphadenopathy	36	4	Lymphosarcoma	Membranoproliferative glomerulonephritis

products, perhaps viruses acting as antigens, possibly induce antibody responses which activate the complement system and create immune complexes capable of causing glomerular injury. Many kinds of neoplastic disease can cause glomerular injury, but most of the observations which have verified the association have been derived from patients with carcinomas.

The most frequent sites of origin of the carcinomas are the lung, colon/rectum, and stomach, although tumors are also reported from skin, head, neck, breast, gallbladder, kidney, adrenal, cervix uteri, vulva, and ovary (20,22,30, 31,33,40,43,46,58,61,72,73,77,84,85,92,95,99,126,133,145–147,153,173,174, 177,178). Few cases have occurred in patients with breast or uterine cancers (59).

Histologic types of carcinoma (46) include adenocarcinoma, squamous cell carcinoma, unclassified carcinoma of the lung, and less frequently, basal cell carcinoma, melanoma, and hypernephroma. More males are affected than females, but this could be a reflection of the higher incidence of lung cancer in the former. The prevalence of carcinoma in patients with epimembranous glomerulopathy, 11% (153), is similar to that found with all forms of cancer and glomerular injury (76,92).

The nephrotic syndrome may manifest clinically before the carcinoma is diagnosed (176); the two conditions may present at the same time; or in some cases, the tumor is recognized before the onset of the nephrotic syndrome. The prognosis for both conditions is dismal, with most patients dying soon after diagnosis of the carcinoma. In relatively few cases does the renal disease respond to therapy, although a few patients have been reported in whom removal of the tumor resulted in remission of the nephrotic syndrome (20,145).

Three-fourths of the reported patients with carcinoma and glomerular injury had renal histologic findings of membranous (epimembranous) glomerulonephritis; the remainder had either membranoproliferative glomerulonephritis (58) or crescentic glomerulonephritis (77,179). Circulating immune complexes are rarely detected, and serum C3 concentrations are usually normal (58).

The establishment of a link between carcinoma and glomerular injury depends mainly on the demonstration of tumor-derived antigen and specific antitumor antibody in the glomerular immune deposits (46). This evidence has accrued from a few careful studies. Eluates of immunoglobulins from glomeruli of patients with nephrotic syndrome and bronchogenic carcinoma were found to react specifically with tumor cell membrane antigens (95) and nonspecifically with normal lung and lung tumor tissue (147). Carcinoembryonic antigen (CEA), immunoglobulins, and complement were found in a granular distribution along the glomerular capillary walls of a patient with nephrotic syndrome and adenocarcinoma of the colon (31). Although this important observation has not been reproduced (33,78), an antigen with similar biological, but different immunological, properties than those of CEA was identified in the glomeruli of a patient with colon carcinoma, nephrotic syndrome, and a high serum CEA concentration (33). Granular deposits of melanoma antigen, IgG, B_1C-globulin, properdin, and C_3PA were detected on the glomerular capillary walls of a patient with malignant melanoma, nephrotic syndrome, and a low serum C3 concentration (177).

A different mechanism invoking antibody production against normal DNA with resultant DNA/anti-DNA complex deposition in the glomeruli has been invoked to explain the finding of antinuclear activity in the eluate of kidney from a patient with oat cell carcinoma of the lung and nephrotic syndrome (53). This patient also had elevated titers of antinuclear antibodies and glomerular deposits of C3 and IgG. It was not clear whether the DNA originated from tumor cells or normal tissue (53).

Renal cell carcinoma has induced glomerular injury presumably in a manner akin to that of extrarenal neoplasia (37,58,60,92,133,170,179). Ozawa et al. (133) found renal tubular epithelial antigen and antibody to normal proximal tubular brush borders, the glomeruli, and proximal tubules of their patient, and cross reactivity among patients with similar tumors. The significance of these findings is difficult to evaluate as the cases had the minimal-change form of nephrotic syndrome in which glomerular immune-complex deposits could not be demonstrated. These findings have not been confirmed, however (85).

We are aware of only one animal model of carcinoma-induced epimembranous glomerulonephritis (42). Normal rats, transplanted with the Walker 256 adenocarcinoma, developed circulating antitumor antibodies, proteinuria, and membranous glomerulopathy (42). The glomerular lesion was not well defined, as neither immunofluorescence nor ultrastructural studies were done. Glomerular injury has also been produced in mice with virus-induced mammary tumors (136) and in hamsters transplanted with tumors from human benign prostatic adenoma (148), and proliferative forms of glomerulonephritis have occurred in mice with spontaneous liver cancer (125). In two of these models tumor-specific antibody (136,148) or viral antigen (136) have been eluted from the glomerular immune complex deposits.

HODGKIN'S DISEASE AND THE NEPHROTIC SYNDROME

The nephrotic syndrome has occurred in patients with Hodgkin's disease in association with three broad categories of glomerular injury: amyloidosis, minimal-change nephrotic syndrome (lipoid nephrosis), and immune complex glomerulonephritis. Some 50 cases of Hodgkin's disease, renal amyloidosis, and nephrotic syndrome have been reported (50,62,93,157,175,180), but this complication appears to have become exceedingly uncommon in recent years (50).

Although there are many reports of nephrotic syndrome and Hodgkin's disease (1,10,14,21,52,55,60,68,69,80,81,88,91,98,100,115,134,137,142,151,152,158,167, 169,181) (aside from amyloidosis), this association is based largely on circumstantial evidence and speculative musings (156). In contrast to some patients with carcinoma in whom immunological studies have revealed a relationship, similar findings have not been forthcoming in Hodgkin's disease–nephrotic syndrome.

Nor has it been possible to demonstrate a role for factors released by circulating T-cells in mediating the nephrotic syndrome associated with Hodgkin's disease (32). In several animal models viruses seem to cause lymphoproliferative disease and glomerular injury (3,63,123,129,130,135), and this may yet prove to be true for Hodgkin's disease and nephrotic syndrome (172).

The nephrotic syndrome has occurred as a prodrome to the clinical manifestation of Hodgkin's disease (60) and has also signaled a recurrence of the malignancy. Resection of the tumor has been followed by rapid remission of the nephropathy (68,169), and relapse of the Hodgkin's disease has been accompanied by relapse of the renal disease (142).

Patients with this association ranged in age from 2 to 62 years, and males predominated in a ratio of 2:1. Most of the patients had proteinuria, hypoalbuminemia, and hypercholesterolemia; hematuria, hypertension, and azotemia were uncommon findings.

Many regimens induce remission of the nephrotic syndrome: radiotherapy, radiotherapy and prednisone, radiotherapy and chemotherapy, prednisone, chemotherapy, surgical excision. One case, resistant to prednisone, responded to radiotherapy (158). Spontaneous remission of the nephrotic syndrome has also been documented (25).

The most common histologic type of Hodgkin's disease is the mixed cellular type, but nodular sclerosis, lymphocyte depletion, and granulomatous thymoma have also been encountered (101).

Most of the patients with Hodgkin's disease–nephrotic syndrome have had the minimal-change type of nephrotic syndrome with no immunological or ultrastructural evidence of immune-complex injury (119). There have also been reports, however, of cases with glomerular immune deposits and proliferative, membranous, or membranoproliferative glomerulonephritis (55,69,80,98, 100,167).

Additional evidence favoring an immune-complex pathogenesis of the glomerular lesion was provided by the finding of gamma globulin and complement in the glomeruli of 13% of patients with Hodgkin's disease; none had clinical or laboratory evidence of renal disease (166). Antiglomerular basement membrane antibody glomerulonephritis was also reported in a patient with Hodgkin's disease and herpes zoster infection, but the significance of these findings in the context of Hodgkin's disease–nephrotic syndrome is unclear (108).

GLOMERULAR INJURY IN PATIENTS WITH LEUKEMIA AND NON-HODGKIN'S LYMPHOMA

There have been no reports of glomerular injury associated with acute leukemia. However, subclinical glomerular immune complex disease (6 of 37 patients) with an antigen related to the interspecies (gs-3) antigen of mammalian oncornovirus was detected in the kidneys of two patients with acute myelocytic leukemia (165).

Chronic lymphocytic leukemia, however, has been reported in association with the nephrotic syndrome in six patients aged 49 to 64 years, again with a marked predominance of men to women (5:1) (19,35,94,112,155). In four cases the nephrotic syndrome and leukemia were diagnosed at approximately the same time, and in the remainder the leukemia occurred years before the onset of the renal disease. The nephrotic syndrome improved with treatment in only two cases. Various types of glomerular injury were found with histologic studies, with no one type predominating.

The nephrotic syndrome has also occurred in association with lymphosarcoma (58,64,143), lymphocytic lymphoma (56,154), reticulum cell sarcoma (122), and Burkitt's lymphoma (80). The renal histopathology encountered in these cases was most often that of the membranoproliferative types (58) as exemplified by case 7 in our series. Strong evidence has been adduced from studies of renal glomeruli in patients with Burkitt's lymphoma in favor of an immune-complex pathogenesis in which Epstein-Barr virus has an antigenic role (131). Immunological evidence of glomerular disease was found in 60% of patients with retroperitoneal lymphoma (lymphosarcoma, seven cases; reticulum cell type, two; Hodgkin's disease, one) (66); each patient had clinical or laboratory features of renal disease.

The association of crescentic glomerulonephritis with renal failure and lymphocytic lymphoma has also been reported (138).

MULTIPLE MYELOMA

Clinical manifestations of kidney disease in patients with multiple myeloma include proteinuria (132), acute renal failure (36,117), chronic renal failure (36), the Fanconi syndrome (111), and, rarely, crescentic glomerulonephritis (41). Insidious, progressive renal failure is a common complication in multiple myeloma and may be the single most important factor in its prognosis (27). Many causes have been defined to account for the renal failure: hyperuricemia, hypercalcemia, plasma hyperviscosity, severe dehydration, intravenous urography, amyloid, plasma cell infiltration, urinary tract obstruction, and pyelonephritis (36). Tubulointerstitial changes consist of dilated distal tubules containing casts of whole immunoglobulins, light chains, or amyloid. Crystals have been demonstrated in lumens and epithelial cells (182). The prognosis, with rare exceptions, is ominous (15), although complete recovery from acute renal failure has been reported. In addition to prednisolone and cyclophosphamide (117), plasmapheresis (51) and renal transplantation (79) have been used successfully in a few cases.

The occurrence of the Fanconi syndrome in patients with Bence-Jones proteinuria is of interest because the features of renal tubular dysfunction can antedate the diagnosis of multiple myeloma (111).

Renal failure and myeloma-like kidney lesions were also reported in a patient with malignant lymphoma (16) and in one with acinic cell adenocarcinoma of the pancreas (116).

WALDENSTROM'S MACROGLOBULINEMIA

Despite the frequency with which pathological changes are seen in the kidneys of patients with Waldenstrom's macroglobulinemia, clinical manifestations of renal disease are uncommon (120). Glomerular injury occurs either as a result of massive deposition of IgM within glomerular capillaries (120) or as a consequence of immunologically mediated mechanisms (96,113). Severe dehydration may result in the accumulation of proteinaceous material in the renal tubules and the production of acute renal failure (5). Improvement of the nephrotic syndrome with a combination of corticosteroid and chlorambucil has been reported (113).

WILMS' TUMOR, GENITAL ANOMALIES, AND GLOMERULAR INJURY

Various combinations of genital abnormalities, Wilms' tumor, and glomerular injury have been reported (9,30,39,44,54,67,97,153,160,162,183). The concurrence of these disorders implies that they originate during embryogenesis at the same time as pseudohermaphroditism. The glomerular injury and tumor may become clinically obvious only months or years after birth (9). Many of these infants had sclerotic glomeruli or the renal histologic features of congenital nephrotic syndrome (Finnish type) with dilated proximal renal tubules (9).

Benign Tumors and Glomerular Injury

There is an exciting possibility that benign tumors may be associated with the nephrotic syndrome (30,101)—exciting from a nephrologist's viewpoint because of the potential of reversal of the renal disease with removal of the tumor (30,101). Remission of the nephrotic syndrome has occurred following excision of a carotid body tumor (101), removal of a benign mesenteric lymphoid tumor (78), evacuation of a hydatidiform mole and coexistent fetus (26), and excision of a pheochromocytoma (150).

RADIATION THERAPY AND RENAL INJURY

Radiation nephritis is usually the result of irradiation of the abdominal cavity, particularly for testicular and ovarian neoplasms, Wilms' tumor, neuroblastoma, and lymphoma of the gastrointestinal tract (110). Large series of cases in man may have been reported (105,106,121). In 1975 it was suggested (11) that the syndrome of radiation-induced nephritis had all but disappeared because of limitation of the total radiation dose delivered to the kidneys. However, this form of nephritis continues to be reported (6,24,25,86,163), which may be due in part to the more recently used combination of radiation and chemotherapy (6,24,25,163).

In a follow-up report of 58 cases, Luxton (106) classified the lesions into five types: (a) acute radiation nephritis; (b) chronic radiation nephritis; (c) asymptomatic proteinuria; (d) benign hypertension; and (e) late malignant hypertension.

Acute radiation nephritis may be caused by a homogeneous dose of as little as 2,300 rads delivered to the whole of both kidneys over 5 weeks. However, the risk of renal failure can be decreased by ensuring that one-third of the volume of the kidneys is outside the treatment portals (90).

Acute radiation nephritis usually develops after a latent period of 6 to 13 months in adults and sometimes after shorter periods in children. Clinically there is frequently proteinuria, microscopic hematuria, moderate to severe hypertension, varying degrees of renal insufficiency, and anemia. Perhaps one-third of the patients develop seriously impaired renal function. The prognosis is dependent to a large degree on the severity of the hypertension in terms of renal function and other complications. Intravascular coagulation may be another complication (25,164). Of 20 patients who suffered from acute nephritis (104), 6 died within 12 months of the onset from malignant hypertension and 3 died of chronic uremia 7 to 21 years after radiotherapy; 9 were alive after an average of 10 years, but all had mild chronic renal failure, hypertension, or proteinuria.

The use of chemotherapy during or after radiation may predispose to the development of radiation nephritis (6,24,25,164) and may lead to earlier presentation which in various studies occurred 5 weeks (24), 3.5 months (164), and 3.25 and 4 months (6) after commencement of irradiation. Bleomycin and vinblastine were used in two patients (24,25); actinomycin and vincristine in two (6); and vincristine, cyclophosphamide, and dacarbazine in one (164). Whether one or more of these drugs act in an additive or synergistic manner with renal irradiation in man remains to be clearly established. However, both bleomycin and vinblastine have increased radiation-induced tissue damage in the mouse (139), and bleomycin was found to enhance pulmonary injury when given with pulmonary radiotherapy (48).

Chronic radiation nephritis may develop with or without a previous acute episode. The prognosis is better in those without a history of acute nephritis. The disorder is characterized by one or more of the following: proteinuria, hypertension, anemia, hyposthenuria, and impaired renal excretory function which is rarely progressive. Benign and occasionally malignant hypertension are believed to have developed 2 to 11 years after irradiation. Occasionally it results from injury to one kidney, with potential cure by nephrectomy (110).

With regard to the pathology and pathogenesis, the critical target tissue is most often stated to be endothelium and perhaps also connective tissue. Damage to the endothelium of glomerular capillaries has been found on light and electron microscopy in man (25,86) with subendothelial deposition of electron-lucent material along with splitting of basement membranes and increased basement membrane-like material. Somewhat similar changes have been reported in cases with the hemolytic uremic syndrome and in renal allograft rejection. There could also be damage to the endothelium of larger vessels. It has been postulated (86) that endothelial cell damage or death could lead to local activation of the coagulation system with consequent thrombosis of small renal vessels. Two patients with acute radiation nephritis and evidence of disseminated intravascular coagulation were recently reported (25,164), supporting this hypothesis.

NEPHROTOXICITY WITH CHEMOTHERAPEUTIC AGENTS

Chemotherapeutic agents reported to cause impairment of renal function include cisplatin, methyl CCNU (1,2-chlorethyl-3,4-methylcyclohexyl-1-nitrosourea), methotrexate, dacarbazine, doxorubicin, bleomycin, mitomycin, and streptozocin (2). Renal damage due to cisplatin may occur after a single dose, is dose related, and can be severe (109). Autopsy and animal experimental data suggest that nephrotoxicity is analogous to the acute tubular necrosis caused by heavy metal poisoning (163). Aminoglycosides may aggravate nephrotoxicity (38); and treatment associated with gentamicin and cephalothin, beginning as long as 13 days after cisplatin therapy, was associated with acute progressive renal failure that persisted until death in four patients (65). Nevertheless, in a prospective study of renal function in 19 patients who received a divided dose schedule and moderate hydration, the only renal abnormality was a small decrease in glomerular filtration rate (163). Another report (71) indicates that nephrotoxicity can be ameliorated by concomitant use of mannitol and furosemide, along with large infusions of fluid.

Methyl CCNU has been used for more than 6 years to treat a variety of solid tumors, but its potential for serious nephrotoxicity was only recently appreciated (70). Although the administration of the drug as an adjuvant makes the response difficult to assess, all six children who received more than 1,500 mg/m² over 17 months had a decrease in kidney mass and severe renal damage. Renal biopsies showed marked interstitial fibrosis, moderate lymphocytic infiltration, focal tubular atrophy and tubular loss, and sclerotic and partly sclerotic glomeruli. There was no hypertension, and urinalysis was normal during and after treatment. The authors recommended that use of the drug should be limited to lower doses for shorter periods until its potential for toxicity has been clarified.

Methotrexate is completely filtered and also actively secreted by the tubules (53). There is a pH-dependent solubility with formation of a precipitate as the pH falls to 5.7, and it is believed that precipitation in the renal tubules is a major cause of nephrotoxicity with high-dose methotrexate therapy (53). Jaffe and Traggis (82) reported that 6 of 41 patients who received 542 high-dose treatment courses developed nephrotoxicity, enhanced by dehydration related to nausea and vomiting, infection, and retention of methotrexate in effusions.

However, it was also reported that nephrotoxicity could be prevented by maintaining hydration, alkalinization with sodium bicarbonate to maintain the urine pH above 7, draining effusions before therapy, and adjusting dosage if renal function is impaired (141). Hemodialysis is potentially of value in the management of acute renal failure as toxic blood levels of methotrexate can be reduced (28).

Streptozotocin has been reported to cause tubulointerstitial nephritis and renal spindle cell "tumors" in man (124) and renal adenocarcinoma with metastases in rats (144).

Daunorubicin was shown to be nephrotoxic in rats (18); and doxorubicin (adriamycin), a structural analog, was reported to cause acute interstitial nephritis with crescentic glomerulonephritis and renal failure in man (17).

CONCLUSION

A neoplasm should be looked for in all older patients with apparent idiopathic glomerular injury. Recurrence of nephrotic syndrome may indicate recurrence of the tumor. Hyperuricemia and hyperphosphatemia are important causes of acute renal failure in patients with leukemia or solid tumors, especially after rapid induction of therapy. Dehydration and/or intravenous urography can precipitate renal failure in patients with myeloma. Radiation, drug doses, and their combinations must be carefully monitored in patients with malignancies.

REFERENCES

1. Aach, R., and Kissane, J. (1971): Clinicopathologic conference: Hodgkin's disease complicated by thrombocytopenia and nephrotic syndrome. *Am. J. Med.,* 51:109–120.
2. Abramowicz, M., editor (1978): The medical letter on drugs and therapeutics. *Cancer Chemother.,* 20:81–88.
3. Anderson, L. J., and Jarret, W. F. (1971): Membranous glomerulonephritis associated with leukemia in cats. *Res. Vet. Sci.,* 12:179–180.
4. Appel, G. B., and Neu, H. C. (1977): The nephrotoxicity of antimicrobial agents. *N. Engl. J. Med.,* 296:663–670, 722–728, 784–787.
5. Argani, I., and Kipkie, G. F. (1964): Macroglobulinemic nephropathy. Acute renal failure in macroglobulinemia of Waldenström. *Am. J. Med.,* 36:151–157.
6. Arneil, G. C., Emmanuel, I. G., Flatman, G. E., Harris, F., Young, D. G., and Zachery, R. B. (1974): Nephritis in two children after irradiation and chemotherapy for nephroblastoma. *Lancet,* 1:960–963.
7. Azzopardi, J. G., and Lehner, T. (1966): Systemic amyloidosis and malignant disease. *J. Clin. Pathol.,* 19:539–548.
8. Band, P. R., Silverberg, D. S., Henderson, J. F., Ulan, R. A., Wensel, R. H., Banerjee, T. K., and Little, A. S. (1970): Xanthine nephropathy in a patient with lymphosarcoma treated with allopurinol. *N. Engl. J. Med.,* 283:354–357.
9. Barakat, A. Y., Papadopoulou, Z. L., Chandra, R. S., and Hollerman, C. E. (1974): Pseudohermaphroditism, nephron disorder and Wilm's tumor: A unifying concept. *Pediatrics,* 54:366–369.
10. Bichel, J., and Bjørn Jensen, K. (1971): Nephrotic syndrome and Hodgkin's disease. *Lancet,* 2:1425–1426.
11. Bloomer, W. D., and Hellman, S. (1975): Normal tissue responses to radiation therapy. *N. Engl. J. Med.,* 293:80–83.

12. Breneton, H. D., Anderson, T., Johnson, R. E., and Schein, P. S. (1975): Hyperphosphatemia and hypocalcemia in Burkitts' lymphoma. *Arch. Intern. Med.,* 135:307–309.
13. Broder, L. E., and Carter, S. K. (1973): Pancreatic islet cell cancer. II. Results of therapy in 52 patients. *Ann. Intern. Med.,* 79:108–118.
14. Brodovsky, H. S., Samuels, M. L., Migliore, P. J., and Howe, C. D. (1968): Chronic lymphocytic leukemia, Hodgkin's disease, and the nephrotic syndrome. *Arch. Intern. Med.,* 121:71–75.
15. Brown, W. W., Herbert, L. A., Piering, W. G., Pisciotta, A. V., Lemann, J., and Garancis, J. C. (1979): Reversal of chronic end-stage renal failure due to myeloma kidney. *Ann. Intern. Med.,* 90:793–794.
16. Burke, J. F., Flis, R., Lasker, N., and Simenhoff, M. (1976): Malignant lymphoma with "myeloma kidney" acute renal failure. *Am. J. Med.,* 60:1055–1060.
17. Burke, J. F., Laucius, J. F., Brodovsky, H. S., and Soriano, R. Z. (1977): Doxorubicin hydrochloride-associated renal failure. *Arch. Intern. Med.,* 137:385–388.
18. Buss, H., and Lamberts, B. (1973): The kidney glomerulus of the rat during experimental daunomycin nephrosis: a comparative transmission and electron microscopic study. *Beitr. Pathol.,* 148:360–387.
19. Cameron, S., and Ogg, C. S. (1974): Nephrotic syndrome in chronic lymphatic leukemia. *Br. Med. J.,* 4:164.
20. Cantrell, E. G. (1969): Nephrotic syndrome cured by removal of gastric carcinoma. *Br. Med. J.,* 2:739–740.
21. Carpenter, C. B., Castleman, B., Scully, R. E., and McNeely, B. U. (1973): Case records of the Massachusetts General Hospital. Weekly clinicopathological exercises: Case 49–1973. *N. Engl. J. Med.,* 289:1241–1247.
22. Catane, R., Kaufmann, J. H., Douglass, H. D., Jr., Kim, U., and Mittelman, A. (1977): Nephrotic syndrome associated with gastric cancer. *J. Surg. Oncol.,* 9(2):207–211.
23. Chu, J., O'Connor, D. M., Roodman, S. T., and Ahrens, R. C. (1977): Tetany and renal failure prior to chemotherapy in acute lymphocytic leukemia. *Am. J. Dis. Child.,* 131(8):925.
24. Churchill, D. N., Hong, K., and Gault, M. H. (1978): Radiation nephritis following combined radiation and chemotherapy (bleomycin–vinblastine). *Cancer,* 41:2162–2164.
25. Cogan, M. G., and Arieff, A. L. (1978): Radiation nephritis and intravascular coagulation. *Clin. Nephrol.,* 10:74–78.
26. Cohen, A. W., and Burton, H. G. (1979): Nephrotic syndrome due to preeclamptic nephropathy in a hydatidiform mole and coexistent fetus. *Obstet. Gynecol.,* 53(1):130–4.
27. Cohen, H. J., and Rundles, R. W. (1975): Managing the complications of plasma cell myeloma. *Arch. Intern. Med.,* 135:177–184.
28. Collett, P., Raghavan, D., Salasoo, S., Tattersall, M., and Tiller, D. (1977): Successful treatment of methotrexate-induced renal failure by hemodialysis. *Aust. NZ J. Med.,* 7:441.
29. Condit, P. T., Changes, R. E., and Joel, W. (1969): Renal toxicity of methotrexate. *Cancer,* 23:126–131.
30. Cosby, R., Yamauchi, H., Lee, J. C., and Hopper, J., Jr. (1974): Tumor related renal lesions— Reversal following tumor excision. *Clin. Res.,* 22:136A.
31. Costanza, M. E., Pinn, V., Schwartz, R. S., and Nathanson, L. (1973): Carcinoembryonic antigen–antibody complexes in a patient with colonic carcinoma and nephrotic syndrome. *N. Engl. J. Med.,* 289:520–522.
32. Couser, W., Badger, A., Cooperband, S., Stilmand, M., Jermanovich, N., Aurora, S., Doner, D., and Schmitt, G. (1977): Hodgkin's disease and lipoid nephrosis. (Letter). *Lancet,* 1:912–913.
33. Couser, W. G., Wagonfeld, J. B., Spargo, B. H., and Lewis, E. J. (1974): Glomerular deposition of tumor antigen in membranous nephropathy associated with colonic carcinoma. *Am. J. Med.,* 57:962–970.
34. Crittenden, D. R., and Ackerman, G. L. (1977): Hyperuricemic acute renal failure in disseminated carcinoma. *Arch. Intern. Med.,* 137(1):97–99.
35. Dathan, J. R. E., Heyworth, M. F., and MacIver, A. G. (1974): Nephrotic syndrome in chronic lymphatic leukemia. *Br. Med. J.,* 4:655–658.
36. DeFronzo, R. A., Humphrey, R. L., Wright, J. R., and Cooke, C. R. (1975): Acute renal failure in multiple myeloma. *Medicine,* 54:209–223.
37. Denis, J., Mignon, F., Ramee, M.-P., Morel-Maroger, L., and Richet, G. (1978): Glomérulites extra-membraneuses associées aux tumeurs viscérales. *Nouv. Press. Med.,* 7:991–996.
38. Dentino, M., Luft, F. C., Yum, M. N., Williams, S. D., and Einhorn, L. H. (1978): Long-

term effect of *cis*-diamminedichloride platinum (CDDP) on renal function and structure in man. *Cancer,* 41:1274–1281.

39. Denys, P., Malraux, P., Van Der Berghe, H., Tanghe, W., and Proesmans, W. (1967): Association d'un syndrome anatomo-pathologique: De pseudohermaphrodisme masculin, d'une tumeur de Wilms, d'une nephropathie parenchymateuse et d'un mosaicisme XX/XY. *Arch. Fr. Pediatr.,* 24:729–739.

40. De Swiet, J., and Wells, A. L. (1975): Nephrotic syndrome associated with renal venous thrombosis and bronchial carcinoma. *Br. Med. J.,* 1:1341–1343.

41. Dhar, S. K., Smith, E. C., and Fresco, R. (1977): Proliferative glomerulonephritis in monoclonal gammopathy. *Nephron,* 19:288–294.

42. Dinh, B.-L., and Brassard, A. (1968): Renal lesions associated with the Walker 256 adenocarcinoma in the rat. *Br. J. Exp. Pathol.,* 49:145–151.

43. Domant, A., Hazard, J., Modaï, J., Gubler, J., and Kleinknecht, D. (1965): Syndrome néphrotique apparement primitif associé à un cortico surrénalone malin. *Bull. Soc. Med. Hop. (Paris),* 116:1161–1173.

44. Drash, A., Sherman, F., Hartmann, W. H., and Blizzard, R. M. (1970): A syndrome of pseudohermaphroditism, Wilm's tumor, hypertension, and degenerative renal disease. *J. Pediatr.,* 76:585–593.

45. Dumbadze, I., Crawford, E. D., and Mulvaney, W. P. (1979): Lymphomatoid tumor infiltration of renal veins. *J. Urol.,* 121:88–89.

46. Eagen, J. W., and Lewis, E. J. (1977): Glomerulopathies of neoplasia. *Kidney Int.,* 11:297–306.

47. Eckman, L. N., and Lynch, E. C. (1978): Acute renal failure in patients with acute leukemia. *South. Med. J.,* 71:382–385.

48. Einhorn, L., Krause, M., Hornback, N., and Furnas, B. (1976): Enhanced pulmonary toxicity with bleomycin and radiotherapy in oat-cell cancer. *Cancer,* 37:2414–2416.

49. Ettinger, D. S., Harker, W. G., Gerry, H. W., Sanders, R. C., and Saral, R. (1978): Hyperphosphatemia, hypocalcemia, and transient renal failure. Results of cytotoxic treatment of acute lymphoblastic leukemia. *JAMA,* 23:2472–2474.

50. Falkson, G., and Falkson, H. C. (1973): Amyloidosis in Hodgkin's disease. *S. Afr. Med. J.,* 47:62–64.

51. Feest, T. G., Burge, P. S., and Cohen, S. L. (1976): Successful treatment of myeloma kidney by diuresis and plasmaphoresis. *Br. Med. J.,* 1:503–504.

52. Foth, R., Bader, K., and Kark, R. (1964): Development of nephrotic syndrome secondary to renal vein thrombosis with bronchogenic carcinoma and Hodgkin's disease. *Ill. Med. J.,* 125:505–509.

53. Fox, R. M. (1979): Methotextrate nephrotoxicity. *Clin. Exp. Pharmacol. Physiol.,* [*Suppl.*], 5:43–45.

54. Frasier, S. D., Bashore, R. A., and Mosier, H. D. (1964): Gonadoblastoma associated with pure gonadal dysgenesis in monozygous twins. *J. Pediatr.,* 64:740–745.

55. Froom, D. W., Franklin, W. A., Hano, J. E., and Potter, E. U. (1972): Immune deposits in Hodgkin's disease with nephrotic syndrome. *Arch. Pathol.,* 94:547–553.

56. Gagliano, R. G., Costanzi, J. J., Beathard, G. A., Sarles, H. E., and Bell, J. D. (1976): The nephrotic syndrome associated with neoplasia: an unusual paraneoplastic syndrome. Report of a case and review of the literature. *Am. J. Med.,* 60:1026–1031.

57. Garnick, M. B., and Mayer, R. J. (1978): Acute renal failure associated with neoplastic disease and its treatment. *Semin. Oncol.,* 5(2):155–165.

58. Gault, M. H., Kaplan, B. S., Chirito, E., Klassen, J., and Knaack, J. (1973): Glomerulopathy associated with neoplasia. *Am. Soc. Nephrol.,* p. 39 (abstract).

59. Germuth, F. H., Jr., and Rodriguez, E. (1973): *Immunopathology of the Renal Glomerulus,* p. 90. Little, Brown, Boston.

60. Ghosh, L., and Muehrcke, R. C. (1970): The nephrotic syndrome: A prodrome to lymphoma. *Ann. Intern. Med.,* 72:379–382.

61. Glassock, R. J., and Bennett, C. M. (1976): The glomerulopathies. In: *The Kidney, Vol. 2,* edited by B. M. Brenner and F. Rector, pp. 1013–1014. Saunders, Philadelphia.

62. Gledhill, R. C., and Shillitoe, A. J. (1952): Purpura and amyloidosis in Hodgkin's disease. *Br. Med. J.,* 1:1336–1337.

63. Glick, A. D., Horn, R. G., and Holscher, M. (1978): Characterization of feline

glomerulonephritis associated with viral-induced hematopoietic neoplasms. *Am. J. Pathol.,* 92(2):321–332.

64. Gluck, M. C., Gallo, G., Lowenstein, J., and Baldwin, D. S. (1973): Membranous glomerulonephritis. Evolution of clinical and pathological features. *Ann. Intern. Med.,* 78:1–12.
65. Gonzalez-Vitale, J. C., Hayes, D. M., Cvitkovic, E., and Sternberg, S. S. (1978): Acute renal failure after *cis*-dichlorodiammineplatinum (II) and gentamicin–cephalothin therapies. *Cancer Treat. Rep.,* 62:693–698.
66. Gupta, R. K. (1973): Immunohistochemical study of glomerular lesions in retroperitoneal lymphomas. *Am. J. Pathol.,* 71:427–433.
67. Habib, R., and Kleinknecht, C. (1971): The primary nephrotic syndrome of childhood. In: *Pathology Annual,* edited by S. C. Sommers, p. 417. Appelton-Century-Crofts, New York.
68. Hansen, E. H., Skov, P. E., Askjaer, S. A., and Albertsen, K. (1972): Hodgkin's disease associated with the nephrotic syndrome without kidney lesion. *Acta Med. Scand.,* 191:307–313.
69. Hardin, J. G., Jr., Coker, A. S., and Blanton, J. H. (1969): Medicine grand rounds from the University of Alabama Medical Center. *South. Med. J.,* 62:1111–1118.
70. Harmon, W. E., Cohen, H. J., Schneeberger, E. E., and Grupe, W. E. (1979): Chronic renal failure in children treated with methyl CCNU. *N. Engl. J. Med.,* 300:1200–1203.
71. Hayes, D. M., Cvitkovic, E., Golbey, R. B., Scheiner, E., Helson, L., and Krakoff, I. H. (1977): High dose *cis*-platinum diamminedichloride amelioration of renal toxicity of mannitol diuresis. *Cancer,* 39:1372–1381.
72. Heaton, J. M., Menzin, M. A., and Carney, D. N. (1975): Extrarenal malignancy and the nephrotic syndrome. *J. Clin. Pathol.,* 28:944–946.
73. Higgins, M. R., Randall, R. E., and Still, W. J. S. (1974): Nephrotic syndrome with oat-cell carcinoma. *Br. Med. J.,* 3:450–451.
74. Hobbs, J. R., Evans, D. J., and Wrong, O. M. (1974): Renal tubular obstruction by mucoproteins from adenocarcinoma of pancreas. *Br. Med. J.,* 2:87–89.
75. Holland, J. F., Sharpe, W., Mamrod, L. M., David, E., and Hartstock, M. (1959): Urate excretion in patients with acute leukemia. *J. Natl. Cancer Inst.,* 23:1097–1105.
76. Hopper, J., Jr. (1974): Tumor related renal lesions. *Ann. Intern. Med.,* 81:550–551.
77. Hopper, J., Jr., Biava, C. B., and Naughton, J. L. (1976): Glomerular extracapillary proliferation (crescentic glomerulonephritis) associated with non-renal malignancies. *Kidney Int.,* 10:544, (abstract).
78. Humpherys, S. R., Holley, K. E., Smith, L. H., and McIlrath, D. C. (1975): Mesenteric angiofollicular lymph node hyperplasia (lymphoid hamartoma) with nephrotic syndrome. *Mayo Clin. Proc.,* 50:317–321.
79. Humphrey, R. L., Wright, J. R., Zachary, J. B., Sterioff, S., and De Fronzo, R. A. (1975): Renal transplantation in multiple myeloma. A case report. *Ann. Intern. Med.,* 83:651–653.
80. Hyman, L. R., Burkholder, P. M., Joo, P. A., and Segar, W. E. (1973): Malignant lymphoma and nephrotic syndrome: a clinicopathologic analysis with light, immunofluroescence, and electron microscopy of the renal lesions. *J. Pediatr.,* 82:207–217.
81. Jackson, R. H., and Oo, M. (1971): Nephrotic syndrome with Hodgkin's disease. *Lancet,* 2:821–822.
82. Jaffe, N., and Traggis, D. (1975): Toxicity of high dose methotrexate (NSC-740) and citrovorum factor (NSC-3590) in osteogenic carcinoma. *Cancer Chemother. Rep.,* 6:31–36.
83. Kanfer, A., Roland, J., Chatelet, F., and Richet, G. (1979): Hyperphosphatemic acute renal failure (ARF) following therapy of lymphosarcoma. *Kidney Int.,* 15:450 (abstract).
84. Kaplan, B. S., Klassen, J., and Gault, M. H. (1976): Glomerular injury in patients with neoplasia. *Annu. Rev. Med.,* 27:117–125.
85. Kerpen, H. O., Bhat, J. G., Feiner, H. D., and Baldwin, D. S. (1978): Membranous nephropathy associated with renal cell carcinoma. Evidence against a role of renal tubular or tumor antibodies in pathogenesis. *Am. J. Med.,* 64:863–867.
86. Keane, W. F., Crosson, J. T., Staley, N. A., Anderson, W. R., and Shapiro, F. L. (1976): Radiation-induced renal disease. A clinicopathologic study. *Am. J. Med.,* 60:127–137.
87. Kiely, J. M., Wagoner, R. D., and Holley, K. E. (1969): Renal complications of lymphoma. *Ann. Intern. Med.,* 71:1159–1175.

88. Kiy, Y. (1967): Sindrome nefrótica associade à doença de Hodgkin. *Rev. Hosp. Clin. Fac. Med. Sao Paulo*, 22:186–191.
89. Kritzler, R. A. (1958): Anuria complicating treatment of leukemia. *Am. J. Med.*, 25:532–538.
90. Kunkler, P. B., Farr, R. F., and Luxton, R. W. (1972): The limit of renal tolerance to X-rays. *Br. J. Radiol.*, 25:190–201.
91. Larson, L. S., and Fritz, R. D. (1976): Nephrotic syndrome in association with Hodgkin's disease. *Wis. Med. J.*, 75:14–17.
92. Lee, J. C., Yamauchi, H., and Hopper, J., Jr. (1966): The association of cancer and the nephrotic syndrome. *Ann. Intern. Med.*, 64:41–51.
93. Lehman, R. G. (1943): Hodgkin's disease complicated by amyloidosis and a nephrotic syndrome: Case report. *Ohio State Med. J.*, 39:232–233.
94. Leonard, B. J. (1957): Chronic lymphatic leukemia and the nephrotic syndrome. *Lancet*, 1:1356–1357.
95. Lewis, M. G., Loughridge, L. W., and Phillips, T. M. (1971): Immunological studies in nephrotic syndrome associated with extrarenal malignant disease. *Lancet*, 2:134–135.
96. Lin, J. H., Orofino, D., Sherlock, J., Letteri, J., and Duffy, J. L. (1973): Waldenstrom's macroglobulinemia, mesangiocapillary glomerulonephritis, angiitis and myositis. *Nephron*, 10:262–270.
97. Lines, D. R. (1968): Nephrotic syndrome and nephroblastoma. *J. Pediatr.*, 72:264–265.
98. Lokich, J. J., Galvanek, E. G., and Moloney, W. C. (1973): Nephrosis of Hodgkin's disease. *Arch. Intern. Med.*, 132:597–600.
99. Loughridge, L. W., and Lewis, M. G. (1971): Nephrotic syndrome in malignant disease of non-renal origin. *Lancet*, 1:256–258.
100. Lowry, W. S., Munzenrider, J. E., and Lynch, G. A. (1971): Nephrotic syndrome in Hodgkin's disease. *Lancet*, 1:1127.
101. Lumeng, J., and Moran, J. F. (1966): Carotid body tumor associated with mild membranous glomerulopathy. *Ann. Intern. Med.*, 65:1266–1270.
102. Lundberg, W. B., Cadman, E. D., Finch, S. C., and Capizzi, R. L. (1977): Renal failure secondary to leukemic infiltration of the kidneys. *Am. J. Med.*, 62:636–642.
103. Luxton, R. W. (1953): Radiation nephritis. *Q. J. Med.*, 22:215–242.
104. Luxton, R. W. (1962): The clinical and pathological effects of renal irradiation. In: *Progress in Radiation Therapy, Vol. 2*, pp. 15–34. Grune & Stratton, New York.
105. Luxton, R. W., and Baker, S. B. de C. (1969): Radiation nephritis. In: *Structural Basis of Renal Disease*, edited by E. L. Becker, pp. 620–656. Harper & Row, New York.
106. Luxton, R. W. (1971): Effects of irradiation on the kidney. In: *Diseases of the Kidney, Vol. 2*, 2nd ed., edited by M. B. Strauss and L. G. Welt, pp. 1040–1070. Little, Brown, Boston.
107. Lynch, R. E., Kjellstrand, C. M., and Coccia, P. F. (1977): Renal and metabolic complications of childhood non-Hodgkin's lymphoma. *Semin. Oncol.*, 4:325–334.
108. Ma, K. W., Golbus, S. M., Kaufman, R., Staley, N., Londer, H., and Brown, D. C. (1978): Glomerulonephritis with Hodgkin's disease and herpes zoster. *Arch. Pathol. Lab. Med.*, 102(10):527–529.
109. Madias, N. E., and Harrington, J. T. (1978): Platinum nephrotoxicity. *Am. J. Med.*, 65:307–314.
110. Madrazo, A., Schwarz, G., and Churg, J. (1975): Radiation nephritis: A review. *J. Urol.*, 114:822–827.
111. Maldonado, J. E., Velosa, J. A., Kyle, R. A., Wagoner, R. D., Holley, K. E., and Salassa, R. M. (1975): Fanconi syndrome in adults. A manifestation of a latent form of myeloma. *Am. J. Med.*, 58:354–364.
112. Mandalenakis, N., Mendoza, N., Pirani, C. L., and Pollack, V. E. (1971): Lobular glomerulonephritis and membranoproliferative glomerulonephritis: A clinical and pathologic study based on renal biopsies. *Medicine*, 50:319–355.
113. Martello, O. J., Schultz, D. R., Pardo, V., and Perez-Stable, E. (1975): Immunologically mediated renal disease in multiple myeloma. *Am. J. Med.*, 58:567–575.
114. Martinez-Maldonado, M., and Ramirez De Arellano, G. A. (1966): Renal involvement in malignant lymphomas: A survey of 49 cases. *J. Urol.*, 95:485–488.
115. Miller, D. G. (1967): The association of immune disease and malignant lymphoma. *Ann. Intern. Med.*, 66:507–521.
116. Min, K.-W., Cain, D., Györkey, P., and Györky, F. (1976): Myeloma-like lesions of the

kidney. Occurrence in a case of acinic cell adenocarcinoma of the pancreas. *Arch. Intern. Med.,* 136:1299–1302.

117. Misiani, R., Remuzzi, G., Bertani, T., Licini, R., Levoni, P., Crippa, A., and Mecca, G. (1979): Plasmapheresis in the treatment of acute renal failure in multiple myeloma. *Am. J. Med.,* 66:684–688.

118. Moorthy, A. V., Zimmerman, S. W., and Burkholder, P. M. (1978): Effects of extrarenal neoplasms on the kidney. In: *Pediatric Kidney Disease,* edited by C. M. Edelmann, pp. 811–828. Little, Brown, Boston.

119. Moorthy, A. V., Zimmerman, S. W., and Burkholder, P. M. (1976): Nephrotic syndrome in Hodgkin's disease. Evidence for pathogenesis alternative to immune complex disease. *Am. J. Med.,* 61:471–477.

120. Morel-Maroger, L., Basch, A., Danon, F., Verroust, P., and Richet, G. (1970): Pathology of the kidney in Waldenstrom's macroglobulinemia. *N. Engl. J. Med.,* 283:123–129.

121. Mostofi, F. K. (1966): Radiation effects on the kidney. In: *The Kidney—International Academy of Pathology,* Monograph 6, edited by F. K. Mostofi and D. E. Smith, p. 338. Williams & Wilkins, Baltimore.

122. Muggia, F. M., and Ultmann, J. E. (1971): Glomerulonephritis or nephrotic syndrome in malignant lymphoma, reticulum cell type. *Lancet,* 1:805.

123. Murray, M., and Wright, N. G. (1974): Morphologic study of canine glomerulonephritis. *Lab. Invest.,* 30:213–221.

124. Myerowitz, R. L., Sartiano, G. P., and Cavallo, T. (1976): Nephrotoxic and cytoproliferative effects of streptozotocin. *Cancer,* 38:1550–1555.

125. Nakopoulou, L., and Papacharalampous, N. (1978): Glomerulonephritis in malignant extrarenal neoplasms. Experimental study on mice using the method of immunofluorescence. *Res. Exp. Med.,* 172(1):1–6.

126. Nichols, G., Roth, S. I., Castleman, B., and Kibbee, B. U. (1963): Case records of the Massachusetts General Hospital. weekly clinicopathological exercises: Case 29. *N. Engl. J. Med.,* 268:943–953.

127. Norris, H. J., and Wiener, J. (1961): The renal lesions in leukemia. *Am. J. Med. Sci.,* 241:512–518.

128. Nydegger, U. E., and Butler, R. E. (1972): Serum lipoprotein levels in patients with cancer. *Cancer Res.,* 32:1756–1760.

129. Oldstone, M. B. A., Aoki, T., and Dixon, F. J. (1972): The antibody response of mice to murine leukemia virus in spontaneous infection: Absence of classical immunologic tolerance. *Proc. Natl. Acad. Sci. USA,* 69:134–138.

130. Oldstone, M. B. A., Tishon, A., Tonietti, G., and Dixon, F. J. (1972): Immune complex disease associated with spontaneous murine leukemia: Incidence and pathogenesis of glomerulonephritis. *Clin. Immunol. Immunopathol.,* 1:6–14.

131. Oldstone, M. B. A., Theofilopoulos, A. N., Gunven, P., and Klein, G. (1974): Immune complexes associated with neoplasia: Presence of Epstein-Barr virus antigen-antibody complexes in Burkitt's lymphoma. *Intervirology,* 4:292–302.

132. Ooi, B. S., Pesce, A. J., Pollak, V. E., and Mandalenakis, N. (1972): Multiple myeloma with massive proteinuria and terminal renal failure. *Am. J. Med.,* 52:538–546.

133. Ozawa, T., Pluss, R., Lacher, J., Boedecker, E., Guggenheim, S., Hammon, D. W., and McIntosh, R. (1975): Endogenous immune complex nephropathy associated with malignancy. I. Studies on the nature and immunopathogenic significance of glomerular bound antigen and antibody, isolation and characterization of tumor specific antigen and antibody and circulating immune complexes. *Q. J. Med.,* 44:523–541.

134. Papillon, J., Pinet, F., Bouvet, R., Pinet, A., and Chasshard, J. L. (1957): A propos de deux cas de manifestations urinaires de la maladie de Hodgkin (syndrome néphrotique, localization unétérale). *J. Radiol. Electrol. Med. Nucl.,* 38:974–976.

135. Pascal, R. R., Koss, M. N., and Kassal, R. L. (1973): Glomerulonephritis associated with immune complex deposits and viral particles in spontaneous murine leukemia. An electron microscopic study with immunofluorescence. *Lab. Invest.,* 29:159–165.

136. Pascal, R. R., Rollwagen, F. M., Harding, T. A., and Sciavine, W. A. (1975): Glomerular immune complex deposits associated with mouse mammary tumor. *Cancer Res.,* 35:302–304.

137. Perlin, E., Powers, J. M., Dickson, L. G., and Moquin, R. B. (1972): The nephrotic syndrome in Hodgkin's disease. *Med. Ann. DC,* 41:354–356.

138. Petzel, R. A., Brown, D. C., Staley, N. A., McMillen, J. J., Sibley, R. K., and Kjellstrand,

C. M. (1979): Crescentic glomerulonephritis and renal failure associated with malignant lymphoma. *Am. J. Clin. Pathol.,* 71:728–732.

139. Phillips, T. L., and Fu, K. K. (1976): Quantification of combined radiation therapy and chemotherapy effects on critical normal tissues. *Cancer,* 37:1186–1300.

140. Piessens, W. F., and Zeicher, M. (1970): Hodgkin's disease causing a reversible nephrotic syndrome by compression of the inferior vena cava. *Cancer,* 25:880–884.

141. Pitman, S. W., Parker, L. M., Tattersall, M. H. N., Jaffe, N., and Frei, E. (1975): Clinical trial of high dose methotrexate (NSC-740) with citrovorum factor (NSC-3590)—Toxicologic and therapeutic observations. *Cancer Chemother. Rep.,* 6:43–49.

142. Plager, J., and Stutzman, L. (1971): Acute nephrotic syndrome as a manifestation of active Hodgkin's disease: Report of four cases and review of the literature. *Am. J. Med.,* 50:56–66.

143. Rabkin, R., Thatcher, B. N., Diamond, L. H., and Eales, L. (1973): The nephrotic syndrome, malignancy and immunosuppression. *S. Afr. Med. J.,* 47:605–606.

144. Rakieten, N., and Gordon, B. S. (1975): Metastatic renal adenocarcinoma produced by streptozotocin (NSC-85998). *Cancer Chemother. Rep.,* 59:891–892.

145. Revol, L., Viala, J.-J., Revillard, J. P., and Manuel, Y. (1964): Protéinurie associée à des manifestations paranéoplastiques au cours d'un cancer bronchogenic. *Lyon Med.,* 212:907–916.

146. Richard, C., Dupont, E., Dupuis, F., Potvliege, P., and Toussaint, C. (1973): Syndrome néphrotique associé au cancer bronchique. *J. Urol. Nephrol.,* 79:745–748.

147. Richard-Mendes Da Costa, C., Dupont, E., Hamers, H., Hooghe, R., Dupuis, E., and Potvliege, R. (1974): Nephrotic syndrome in bronchogenic carcinoma: Report of two cases with immunochemical studies. *Clin. Nephrol.,* 2:245–251.

148. Richman, A. V., and Alexander, R. W. (1979): Immunity to cell surface antigens and immune complex glomerulonephritis in hamsters bearing human epithelial tumors. *Cancer Res.,* 29:459–464.

149. Richmond, J., Sherman, R. S., Diamond, H. D., and Craver, L. F. (1962): Renal lesions associated with malignant lymphomas. *Am. J. Med.,* 32:184–207.

150. Rizzuto, V. J., Mazzara, J. T., and Grace, W. J. (1965): Pheochromocytoma with nephrotic syndrome. *Am. J. Cardiol.,* 16:432–437.

151. Rohmer, P., and Sacrez, R. (1948): Un cas de nephrose lipoidique au cours d'une maladie de Hodgkin. *Strasbourg Med.,* 108:45–55.

152. Routledge, R. C., Hann, I. M., and Morris Jones, P. H. (1976): Hodgkin's disease complicated by the nephrotic syndrome. *Cancer,* 38:1735–1740.

153. Row, P. G., Cameron, J. S., Turner, D. R., Evans, D. G., White, R. H. R., Ogg, C. S., Chantler, C., and Brown, C. B. (1975): Membranous nephropathy: Long-term follow-up and association with neoplasia. *Q. J. Med.,* 44:207–239.

154. Sagel, J., Muller, H., and Logan, E. (1971): Lymphoma and the nephrotic syndrome. *S. Afr. Med. J.,* 45:79–80.

155. Scott, R. B. (1957): Chronic lymphatic leukemia. *Lancet,* 1:1162–1167.

156. Shalhoub, R. J. (1974): Pathogenesis of lipoid nephrosis; a disorder of T-cell function. *Lancet,* 2:556–559.

157. Sherman, M. J., Morales, J. B., Bayrd, E. D., and Schierman, W. D. (1955): Amyloid nephrosis secondary to Hodgkin's disease. *Arch. Intern. Med.,* 95:618–621.

158. Sherman, R. L., Susin, M., Weksler, M. E., and Becker, E. L. (1972): Lipoid nephrosis in Hodgkin's disease. *Am. J. Med.,* 52:699–706.

159. Siegel, M. B., Alexander, E. A., Weintraub, L., and Idelson, B. A. (1977): Renal failure in Burkitt's lymphoma. *Clin. Nephrol.,* 7:279–283.

160. Smith, N. J. (1946): Glomerulonephritis, Wilms' tumor, and horseshoe kidney in an infant. *Arch. Pathol.,* 42:549–554.

161. Sparling, T. G., Rosen, D. A., Corbett, W. E., and Galbraith, P. R. (1979): Microvascular closure in malignant histiocytosis. *Can. Med. Assoc. J.,* 120:47–48, 53–54.

162. Spear, G. S., Hyde, T. P., Gruppo, R. A., and Slusser, R. (1971): Pseudohermaphroditism, glomerulonephritis with the nephrotic syndrome, and Wilms' tumor in infancy. *J. Pediatr.,* 79:677–681.

163. Stark, J. J., and Howell, S. B. (1978): Nephrotoxicity of cisplatinum (II) dichlorodiammine. *Clin. Pharmacol. Ther.,* 23:461–466.

164. Steele, B. T., and Lirenman, D. S. (1979): Acute radiation nephritis and the hemolytic uremic syndrome. *Clin. Nephrol.,* 11:272–274.

165. Sutherland, J. C., and Mardinay, M. R. (1973): Immune complex disease in the kidneys of lymphoma-leukemia patients: The presence of an oncornovirus-related antigen. *J. Natl. Cancer Inst.,* 50:633–644.

166. Sutherland, J. C., Markham, R. V., Jr., Ramsey, H. E., and Mardiney, M. R., Jr. (1974): Subclinical immune complex nephritis in patients with Hodgkin's disease. *Cancer Res.,* 34:1179–1181.

167. Szabo, J., Lustyik, G. Y., Szabo, T., Erdei, I., and Szegedi, G. Y. (1974): Glomerulonephritis of immunocomplex origin associated with Hodgkin's disease. *Acta Med. Acad. Sci. Hung.,* 31:187–193.

168. Talley, R. W., O'Bryan, R. M., Gutterman, J. U., et al. (1973): Clinical evaluation of toxic effects of cis-diammine-dichloroplatinum (NSC-119875)—Phase I clinical study. *Cancer Chemother. Rep.,* 57:465–471.

169. Tapie, J., La Porte, J., and Ricalens, S. (1957): Syndrome néphrotique au cours de la maladie de Hodgkin-Sternberg. *Presse Med.,* 65:287–293.

170. Tydings, A., Weiss, R. R., Lin, J. H., Bennett, J., and Tejani, N. (1978): Renal-cell carcinoma. *NY State J. Med.,* 78:1950–1954.

171. Ultmann, J. E. (1962): Hyperuricemia in disseminated neoplastic disease other than lymphomas and leukemias. *Cancer,* 15:122–129.

172. Vianna, N. J., Greenwald, P., and Davies, J. N. (1971): Nature of Hodgkin's disease agent. *Lancet,* 1:733–736.

173. Vincent, F. M. (1978): Paraneoplastic CNS and renal syndromes. Simultaneous occurrence in a patient with bronchogenic carcinoma. *JAMA,* 240(9):862–863.

174. Volhard, F., cited by Revol, L., Viala, J.-J., Revillard, J. P., and Manuel, Y. (1964): Protéinurie associée à des manifestations paranéoplastiques au cours d'un cancer bronchogénique. *Lyon Med.,* 212:907–916.

175. Wallace, S. L., Feldman, D. J., Berlin, I., Harris, C., and Glass, I. A. (1950): Amyloidosis in Hodgkin's disease. *Am. J. Med.,* 8:552–557.

176. Weintraub, S., Stavorovsky, M., and Griffel, B. (1975): Membranous glomerulonephritis. An initial symptom of gastric carcinoma? *Arch. Surg.,* 110:833–838.

177. Weksler, M. E., Carey, T., Day, N., Susin, M., Sherman, R., and Becker, C. (1974): Nephrotic syndrome in malignant melanoma: Demonstration of melanoma antigen–antibody in kidney. *Kidney Int.,* 6:112A.

178. Whitworth, J. A., Unger, A., and Cameron, J. S. (1975): Carcinoembryonic antigen in tumour-associated membranous nephropathy. (Letter). *Lancet,* 2:611.

179. Whitworth, J. A., Morel-Maroger, L., Mignon, F., and Richet, G. (1976): The significance of extracapillary glomerulonephritis. *Nephron,* 16:1–19.

180. Winawer, S. J., and Feldman, S. M. (1959): Amyloid nephrosis in Hodgkin's disease. *Arch. Intern. Med.,* 104:793–796.

181. Yum, M. N., Edwards, J. L., and Kleit, S. (1975): Glomerular lesions in Hodgkin's disease. *Arch. Pathol.,* 99:645–649.

182. Zlotnik, A., and Rosenmann, E. (1975): Renal pathologic findings associated with monoclonal gammopathies. *Arch. Intern. Med.,* 135:40–45.

183. Zunin, C., and Soave, F. (1964): Association of nephrotic syndrome and nephroblastoma in siblings. *Ann. Pediatr.,* 203:29–38.

Medical Complications in Cancer Patients,
edited by J. Klastersky and M. J. Staquet.
Raven Press, New York © 1981.

Hypercalcemia of Malignancy

Brian P. First and Leonard J. Deftos

*Endocrine Section, University of California and San Diego Veterans Administration
Medical Center, La Jolla, California 92161*

Malignancy is the most common cause of hypercalcemia encountered in hospital practice (1,2). In the majority of cases (80 to 85%) the hypercalcemia is
caused by malignant invasion of the skeleton. In the remainder (15 to 20%)
no evidence of bone metastases is demonstrable, and in these patients one or
more humoral factors are thought to be responsible for the development of
hypercalcemia. Many of the symptoms of hypercalcemia (anorexia, nausea, vomiting, weight loss, and altered mental status) may be attributable to the underlying
malignancy. Unless the correct diagnosis is established, inappropriate therapy
may be administered with detrimental effects to the patient, whereas specific
treatment of the hypercalcemia may allow the patient many more months of
near-normal existence. It is therefore important to be familiar with the mechanisms of hypercalcemia in malignancy and with the regimens available for treating this life-threatening condition.

MECHANISMS OF THE HYPERCALCEMIA OF MALIGNANCY

Skeletal Metastases

Direct invasion of bone by tumor with subsequent destruction of bone mass
is the most common cause of hypercalcemia. Hypercalcemia can therefore be
encountered with almost any malignancy but is most frequently associated with
those tumors which have a high incidence of bone metastases (breast, lung,
kidney). The involvement of bone by malignancy may be demonstrable by appropriate X-ray studies. However, in many instances this is not the case, and invasion
of bone by the cancer may be demonstrated only after special procedures such
as bone scanning, bone biopsy, or both (3,4). The mere presence of bone metastases, however, does not ensure the development of hypercalcemia, and in fact
many patients with bone metastases remain normocalcemic. The extent of skeletal involvement necessary for the development of hypercalcemia is unknown;
some recent studies indicate that the manner by, and rate with which, bone is
destroyed may be more important than the apparent degree of bone involvement

by tumor (5). Available evidence indicates that enhanced bone resorption is the fundamental event in the production of cancer hypercalcemia (6), and recent investigations have begun to clarify the mechanism involved. It is the osteoclasts and not the metastatic cells which are active at the margin of the lesion resorbing the bone (7). Faccini (8) and Galasko (9) found that transplanted tumors in rabbits appear to induce osteoclastic bone resorption in the adjacent bone at an early stage of tumor growth. In multiple myeloma the increased bone resorption appears to be related primarily to the induction of osteoclasts adjacent to plasma cells (10). The appearance of increased numbers of osteoclasts adjacent to malignant lesions of the skeleton is probably mediated by at least two chemical factors, prostaglandin E_2 and osteoclast activating factor.

Increased Production of Parathyroid Hormone or Parathyroid Hormone-Like Factors

One proposed mechanism by which malignancy can cause hypercalcemia is through tumor production of parathyroid hormone (PTH) or a PTH-like substance, an idea first proposed by Albright in 1941 (11). The term pseudohyperparathyroidism was first used by Fry (12) in his description of a patient with bronchogenic carcinoma who had the chemical characteristics of hyperparathyroidism but no evidence of parathyroid disease or bone metastases at autopsy. Tashjian et al. (13) in 1964 were the first to demonstrate that extracts of nonparathyroid tumors from patients with hypercalcemia of malignancy may contain a PTH-like substance. During recent years immunoreactive PTH has been identified in malignant tumors and in the serum of patients who are hypercalcemic, hypophosphatemic, and without skeletal metastases (14). Many tumors, including epidermoid tumors of the head, neck, and esophagus (15); lymphomas (16); leukemias (17); hepatomas (18); and gastrointestinal or genitourinary (14) neoplasms may produce PTH or a PTH-like substance. The syndrome (termed ectopic or pseudohyperparathyroidism) is most common in patients with squamous cell carcinomas, particularly of the lung, or with hypernephroma (14,19). Breast carcinoma rarely produces the syndrome, although cases have been reported (20), and in one series of 14 patients with breast cancer and hypercalcemia, all had elevated serum levels of immunoreactive PTH (14). Benson and associates (14) demonstrated ectopic PTH in 95% of their patients with hypercalcemia of malignancy, indicating that most patients have parathormone-producing tumors. Powell and associates (21), on the other hand, in a study of 11 patients with tumor-associated hypercalcemia, were unable to demonstrate the presence of PTH by multiple immunoassay techniques designated to measure intact hormone as well as precursors and fragments in plasma samples and tumor tissues; they concluded that humoral factors other than PTH may be responsible for the development of hypercalcemia. There is some debate about the exact frequency of the syndrome which, in fact, stems from immunologic differences between native PTH and tumor PTH and differences in the radioimmunoassay methodology used to identify this peptide (22). It must be stressed that the mere finding of elevated values of plasma PTH in patients with hypercalcemia of malignancy is not sufficient evidence for the diagnosis of ectopic hyperparathyroidism, since cancer patients with coexistent primary hyperparathyroidism may also have elevated values. This is not an uncommon association, 118 cases having been noted by Heath in a recent review (23).

Differentiation between the two conditions can be extremely difficult, although the presence of at least one (and preferably more) of the following favors a diagnosis of ectopic hyperparathyroidism: demonstration of an arteriovenous difference in plasma PTH across the tumor bed; temporal correlation of plasma PTH and serum calcium concentrations with tumor growth or tumor therapy; extraction of large amounts of immunoreactive PTH from the tumor; absence of a plasma PTH gradient in parathyroid venous effluent; and observation of normal or atrophic parathyroid glands at surgery or autopsy (2). Many of these procedures are difficult to perform and are not readily available, and therefore more simple methods have been advocated to differentiate the two conditions. Patients with ectopic PTH syndrome rarely have osteitis fibrosa or kidney stones (24), usually have a normal chloride/phosphate ratio (25), and ordinarily have weight loss and anemia (19) to help distinguish them from patients with primary hyperparathyroidism.

Some investigators examined the use of nephrogenous cyclic AMP to differentiate the two conditions. Cyclic AMP is elevated in 95% of patients with primary hyperparathyroidism (26,27), whereas in a recent study of 15 patients with hypercalcemia and a malignancy, 6 with elevated nephrogenous cyclic AMP determinations were found to have primary hyperparathyroidism at surgery (10). The authors concluded that an elevated nephrogenous cyclic AMP in a patient with a malignancy strongly suggests the presence of primary hyperparathyroidism. However, this has not been confirmed in other studies.

Another indirect test of PTH activity is the acid–base status. Lafferty (19) stressed the surprising finding of hypochloremic alkalosis in patients with pseudohyperparathyroidism as compared to hyperchloremic acidosis in primary hyperparathyroidism. Finally, the radioimmunoassay for PTH may help in the differentiation of the two conditions. A study performed at the Mayo Clinic (28) demonstrated that, in general, for any given serum calcium concentration the level of PTH was higher when the patient had primary hyperparathyroidism. Also the patients with malignancy generally have a higher serum calcium level. When approaching this problem it must also be remembered that Berson and Yalow (29) found a significant percentage of patients with carcinoma of the lung who had elevated PTH levels in the absence of hypercalcemia. The problem of correct interpretation of PTH results in this condition were recently reviewed (29a).

Nonparathormone Hypercalcemic Factors

Prostaglandins

The finding of Klein and Raisz (30) in 1970 that prostaglandin E_2 (PGE_2) is a potent stimulator of bone resorption *in vitro* led to the consideration of prostaglandins as a humoral mediator of hypercalcemia. Tashjian et al (31) demonstrated in 1972 that the hypercalcemia caused by fibrosarcomas in mice could be reversed by administration of indomethacin, providing further evidence that prostaglandins might mediate tumor-associated hypercalcemia in man. Powell et al. (21) noted that many of their cancer patients with hypercalcemia and no bone metastases had no detectable PTH in peripheral blood or tumor tissue. Observing that tumor extracts from these patients had osteolytic activity in a bone culture system *in vitro,* they concluded that some humoral substance other than PTH was mediating the hypercalcemia in this group of patients.

Prostaglandins are extremely potent biogenic compounds and as such are formed in quite small amounts *in vivo*. The total body production of PGE_2 is less than 1 μmole/day (32). The prostaglandins are quite rapidly metabolized, making measurement of their metabolites a valuable approach for investigating clinical disorders of prostaglandin biosynthesis. The major initial step in the metabolism is 15-dehydrogenation followed by 13,14-reduction, yielding 15-keto-13,14-dihydro-PGE_2, the principal metabolite in the circulation (33). This compound is further metabolized, yielding the major urinary metabolite 7α-hydroxy-5,11-diketotetranorprostanedioic acid (PGE-M) (34). Measurement of this urinary metabolite may be employed as an indicator of total body PGE synthesis (35). During recent years there have been numerous animal and clinical studies that provided further evidence for the role played by prostaglandins in the pathogenesis of hypercalcemia of malignancy. In mice, transplantation of the fibrosarcoma $HSDM_1$ produces hypercalcemia within about 2 weeks of tumor implantation (31). The tumor neither metastasizes to bone nor appears to invade bone locally, and the hypercalcemia remits when the tumor is excised (36). In addition to hypercalcemia, mice bearing the $HSDM_1$ tumor have elevated plasma concentrations of PGE_2 and markedly raised concentrations of the longer-lived metabolite of PGE_2, 13,14-dihydro-15-keto-PGE_2 (31,37). Administration of indomethacin to these animals lowered the plasma concentration of calcium, PGE_2, and 15-keto-13,14-dihydro-PGE_2. Similar results were obtained in rabbits bearing the transplantable VX2 carcinoma.

In patients with hypercalcemia associated with solid tumors, the excretion of the major urinary metabolite of the E prostaglandins has been considerably increased in some studies (38). Of 14 patients with tumor-associated hypercalcemia, the excretion of PGE-M was normal in only 2. In patients with solid tumors and normocalcemia only slightly elevated levels for PGE-M are found, and in patients with primary hyperparathyroidism the levels are normal. In view of these findings, the therapeutic effects of indomethacin and aspirin on serum calcium were evaluated in relation to the PGE-M levels. In patients whose hypercalcemia was associated with elevated PGE-M, either indomethacin or aspirin reduced levels of serum calcium to the normal range when there were no clinically detectable bony metastases; they reduced calcium only slightly and not into the normal range when bony metastases were evident. When the hypercalcemia is not associated with an elevation of PGE-M, no reduction in serum calcium results from the inhibition of prostaglandin synthesis.

Prostanglandins appear to act by significantly increasing osteoclastic bone resorption. Santoro et al. (39) demonstrated an increase in osteoclast population after daily injections of a long-acting analog to PGE_2 to mice. They observed a maximum loss of 33% of trabecular bone volume, a 15% loss of bone calcium, and a 140% increase in osteoclast numbers. PGE infusion causes an increase in the number and extent of invaginations and evaginations of the ruffled border and the presence of large vacuoles. This is suggestive of a metabolically more active osteoclast engaged in resorbing bone (40).

Osteoclast Activating Factor

The presence of an osteoclast activating factor (OAF) was initially demonstrated in 1972 by Horton et al. (41). They found a soluble mediator of bone resorption in the culture media of normal human leukocytes stimulated by phytohemagglutinin or an antigen. The possibility that OAF is parathyroid hormone, a vitamin D metabolite, or a prostaglandin has been excluded by immunochemical studies, differential extraction procedures, and by comparing the dose-response curves of these substances in a bioassay utilizing fetal bone in organ culture (10). Results of subsequent experiments suggested that supernatant from a variety of cultured lymphoid cell lines from patients with multiple myeloma, Burkett's lymphoma, or malignant lymphoma spontaneously produced a similar factor that caused bone resorption *in vitro* (42). The unstimulated cultures of peripheral blood mononuclear cells from a hypercalcemic patient with lymphosarcoma cell leukemia produced a powerful bone resorbing factor (43) with activity that was either the same as or similar to the OAF produced by normal human peripheral blood leukocytes after mitogen activation. Dose-response curves for both were found to be identical, and, as with normal OAF, its effects were inhibited by the administration of corticosteroids in low concentrations. Thus it appears that a factor, presumably OAF, is elaborated that can induce osteoclastic resorption *in vitro*. This was demonstrated also in lymphocytes from women with operable breast cancer (6).

OAF is thought to be a lymphokine similar to macrophage inhibition factor. It is a peptide and may exist in two interconvertible forms with molecular weights of approximately 14,000 and 2,000 daltons (big and little OAF) (44). In some recent work by Luben et al. (45), highly sensitive and specific antibodies against OAF were produced in useful titers by means of somatic cell hybridization followed by selection of hybridoma clones with the desired characterics. These antibodies will be screened for their suitability for use in immunoassay and immunocytochemical tests for OAF in clinical samples. This is extremely important because even though OAF is strongly implicated as a mediator of hypercalcemia in some types of malignant disease, the extent of its importance cannot be assumed until the development of more satisfactory techniques for its measurement, e.g., a radioimmunoassay.

Osteolytic Phytosterols

Gordon and associates (46) demonstrated in 1966 that extracts of breast tumors can have an osteolytic effect on rat calvaria *in vitro;* they also presented evidence for the production of vitamin D-like sterols by breast tumors. Certain osteolytic phytosterols have been identified in carcinomatous breast tissue (46) in patients who presented with biochemical features of vitamin D intoxication (47). However, these phytosterols, stigmesterol acetate and 7-dihydrositosterol, may be found in plasma from healthy lactating and nonlactating women as well as in cancers of other tissues unassociated with hypercalcemia (48). In view of these findings, the significance of these substances in tumor-induced hypercalcemia has been questioned.

Vasoactive Intestinal Peptide

Verner and Morrison (49) were the first to describe the syndrome of copious watery diarrhea, hypokalemia, and non-β islet cell tumor of the pancreas. Hypercalcemia has been reported in a number of these cases (50,51), and although the exact relationship between vasoactive intestinal peptide (VIP) and hypercalcemia remains circumstantial, there is preliminary evidence suggesting a direct action of VIP on bone resorption with induction of hyeprcalcemia (51).

Associated Factors Aggravating the Hypercalcemia

Dehydration

Due to the anorexia, vomiting, and polyuria frequently present in patients with hypercalcemia, dehydration is usually present. Contraction of the intravascular compartment together with decreased glomerular filtration produces a further elevation in total plasma calcium.

Immobilization

Many patients with malignant disease are confined to bed, and the immobilization may worsen the hypercalcemia. The mechanism of this effect is not firmly established, and usually the hypercalcemia is only slightly aggravated.

Therapeutic Agents

There are a number of therapeutic agents used in breast carcinoma with bone metastases which have led to rapid progression of hypercalcemia. These agents—estrogens, androgens, progestins, and tamoxifen—apparently stimulate the growth of these tumors, resulting in greater destruction of bone (3). Other agents that can aggravate hypercalcemia include thiazide diuretics, vitamins A and D, and lithium.

Adrenal Insufficiency

Adrenal insufficiency due to adrenal gland metastases is an unusual mechanism for hypercalcemia of malignancy. It probably does not represent a true increase in ionized calcium but results from increased binding of calcium by serum proteins (3).

Hypergammaglobulinemia

High levels of gamma globulin as seen in multiple myeloma is another mechanism by which there may be an increase in the total calcium without increasing the ionized calcium.

TREATMENT OF THE HYPERCALCEMIA OF MALIGNANCY

A fairly large number of drugs are now available for the treatment of the hypercalcemia associated with malignancy. Not all of these are needed in every patient, therefore, before starting treatment the severity of the hypercalcemia should be determined. Mild hypercalcemia in an asymptomatic patient may be treated simply by increasing the amount of oral fluids, whereas severe hypercalcemia in a comatosed patient is a medical emergency requiring one or more of the therapeutic agents outlined below.

Hydration

As previously mentioned, dehydration due to anorexia, vomiting, and polyuria is an almost invariable accompaniment of moderate or severe hypercalcemia. Rehydration therefore represents the first step in the treatment of hypercalcemia. There is general agreement that isotonic saline is the agent of choice (3,4,6), although some authors have advocated the use of isotonic sodium sulfate (52). Replacement with saline not only restores the intravascular volume but promotes renal excretion of calcium. In many instances large amounts of saline (3 to 6 liters or more within 24 hr) are required for effective therapy, and so renal and cardiac status must be monitored closely particularly when these organs are known to be impaired. Rehydration with saline alone may control mild hypercalcemia, but in most cases of significant hypercalcemia additional therapy is necessary.

Calciuresis

A dramatic increase in urinary excretion of calcium may result from sodium diuresis induced by the simultaneous infusion of saline and administration of furosemide or ethacrynic acid (1,3,4). These drugs act by decreasing renal tubular reabsorption of sodium and calcium. Thiazides cannot be used as they may aggravate hypercalcemia (53) by depressing the urinary excretion of calcium. These diuretic agents are given intravenously: ethacrynic acid in doses of 20 to 40 mg/1 to 2 hr, and furosemide in doses of 80 to 100 mg/1 to 2 hr (3,4). Forced diuresis can be used effectively even in the presence of mild renal failure. However, patients must be monitored very closely and preferably in an intensive care unit. Urinary losses of large amounts of potassium and magnesium can be expected during the course of such therapy, so that frequent measurements of urine and serum electrolytes are necessary to guide further management; 20 to 40 mEq potassium chloride and 10 to 20 mg magnesium ion per liter of infusate should be adequate for replenishing electrolyte losses (54). Because of the degree of patient monitoring required during forced diuresis, such therapy should be used for the initial treatment of significant hypercalcemia, but should be followed by a more feasible and practical subsequent treatment plan (3).

As mentioned, sodium sulfate has been the preferred agent by some for initial treatment of hypercalcemia (52). Sodium sulfate is reported to be more effective than comparable amounts of saline in promoting calciuresis, presumably because sulfate complexes are formed with calcium in the urine (55). One liter of an isotonic solution of sodium sulfate can lower blood calcium by approximately 1 mg%, but nausea can occur with rapid infusion (3). Sodium sulfate administration is attended by the same complications as isotonic saline, including serious hypernatremia, volume overexpansion, and fluid overload. In addition, hypocalcemia can occur during the course of therapy (4). EDTA increases urinary calcium excretion by forming soluble, filtrable, and largely nonreabsorbable complexes with calcium. By chelating the calcium in blood, EDTA also directly reduces the ionized calcium concentration (1). Serious side effects include hypotension and renal failure (56), and in view of the many alternate regimens available this form of therapy is used only infrequently. Hemodialysis and peritoneal dialysis may be effective for rapid removal of calcium from extracellular fluid. Such extreme measures are seldom needed but may be considered in patients with oliguric renal failure and congestive heart failure.

Inorganic Phosphate

The calcium-lowering effects of inorganic phosphate have been known for many years; it is one of the most effective and reliable means of decreasing the serum calcium level (57). Inorganic phosphate may be administered orally, intravenously, and on occasion rectally as a retention enema (1). The administration of inorganic phosphate is associated with a fall in serum calcium levels, a reduction in urinary calcium levels, and a positive calcium balance. The effects of inorganic phosphate are probably due to a net movement of calcium and phosphate into the skeleton. Rasmussen and Bordier (58) suggested that phosphate acts *in vivo* by stimulating osteoblastic activity; Raisz and Niemann (59) found that an increasing phosphate concentration in the medium of bone cell cultures not only increases the rate of bone formation but also decreases the rate of resorption.

Orally administered phosphate is most useful for the chronic treatment of hypercalcemia. A dose of 2 g daily can lower serum calcium by several milligrams. However, several days are necessary for maximum effect; therefore, this form of treatment is not suitable for the acute management of hypercalcemic crisis. This form of therapy is usually well tolerated, although gastrointestinal intolerance with diarrhea may occur but can be minimized by gradually increasing the dose. Intravenous phosphate can be used for the acute control of hypercalcemia. The recommended dose is 1.5 g over 6 to 8 hr. The serum calcium level may fall within minutes after initiation of the infusion, and the maximum decline may be delayed for as long as 5 days (59).

Complications of phosphate therapy are fairly common, and this has led to their decreased use in many centers. These complications are far more likely with intravenous phosphate administration, but chronic oral use has also been associated with extraskeletal calcifications in the heart, kidneys, lens, and other soft tissues (60). Intravenous phosphate can cause a precipitous fall in serum calcium, hypotension, acute renal failure, and even death (61). In patients with impaired renal function, no more than 0.5 to 1 g of phosphate should be administered intravenously over 24 hr (62), and therapy should be discontinued or the dose greatly reduced if serum phosphate levels rise above 6.0 mg/dl (54). Phosphate therapy should be restricted in those patients who are already hyperphosphatemic.

Calcitonin

Calcitonin—the hypocalcemic, hypophosphatemic polypeptide hormone—has been used in various forms of hypercalcemia (63). Its action is attributed mainly to an inhibition of bone resorption, but it also increases the renal clearance of calcium (64). Of the three species of calcitonin (porcine, human, and salmon), the one derived from salmon is the most potent and has the longest duration of action (3). Calcitonin is effective only when given parenterally, and the hypocalcemic response is usually only moderate and unsustained. The usual dose is 3 to 6 MRC units/kg body weight/day given as a 24-hr infusion (64). The calcium decreases within a few hours, but after several days escape from the hypocalcemic effects of calcitonin can occur (3). Phosphate loading enhances, and phosphate depletion inhibits, the hypocalcemic effect of calcitonin in experimental animals, and there are isolated reports suggesting that the escape phenomenon may be averted by the concomitant use of phosphate (65) or steroids (66). Calcitonin, unlike the other drugs available, is not associated with any serious toxic reactions. This, together with its rapid onset of action, make it a useful adjunct to the therapy of hypercalcemia.

Mithramycin

Mithramycin, a cytotoxic antibiotic produced by the microorganism *Streptomyces plicatus,* has been used successfully in the treatment of certain testicular tumors. Its hypocalcemic effect was first observed in normocalcemic patients treated for such tumors and subsequently in hypercalcemic patients with neoplasia (67). Mithramycin exerts its effect by directly inhibiting bone resorption. It probably acts by forming a complex with DNA, thereby inhibiting DNA-directed RNA synthesis (68). Mithramycin must be given intravenously either as a rapid infusion or over 4 to 24 hr. The usual dose is 25 μg/kg body weight, and its hypocalcemic effect is manifest within 24 to 48 hr (69). Thereafter, serum calcium concentration may remain under adequate control for as long as 10 to 14 days before repeated administration becomes necessary. Repeated doses can be given when the serum calcium level begins to rise, although the serious side effects of mithramycin are more likely with repeated doses. The major side effects—thrombocytopenia (with normal megakaryocytes on bone marrow examination), hepatocellular necrosis, and hemorrhage—are more likely in patients with renal insufficiency (69). Nausea and vomiting are frequent but can be controlled by slowing down the infusion and by appropriate use of prochloroperazine (Compazine®) (70). Rare complications are sudden arterial occlusion (71) and toxic epidermal necrolysis (72). Symptomatic hypocalcemia may occur with mithramycin, particularly when it is used in combination with calcitonin (73). These toxic effects are rare if only one or two doses are used, and, with the exception of hemorrhage, can usually be reversed by stopping the drug (69). When used cautiously and conservatively, therefore, mithramycin can be a relatively safe and effective calcium-lowering agent.

Corticosteroids

The calcium-lowering action of glucocorticoids in the treatment of hypercalcemia is still incompletely defined in terms of their efficacy and mechanism of action. Although they do have a mild calciuretic effect, their primary mechanism of action appears to be an antitumor effect. Accordingly, steroids were thought to be effective only in those neoplasms whose growth is inhibited by their administration. These most commonly include myeloma, lymphoma, and carcinoma of the breast (3). However, there is now suggestive evidence (74) that glucocorticoids administered to rats in high doses can cause sufficient inhibition of osteoprogenitor cell proliferation to result in a reduction in the pool size of osteoblasts and osteoclasts. Therefore a direct action of glucocorticoids on bone cannot be clearly excluded. Recent studies also indicate that glucocorticoids may inhibit either prostaglandin synthesis (75) or prostaglandin release (76). For acute management of hypercalcemia very large doses of steroids—up to several hundred milligrams of cortisone or its equivalent (40 to 60 mg prednisone) daily—are required. The response is relatively slow, occurring usually over 3 to 4 days. The complications of chronic steroid therapy are well known and preclude prolonged treatment with these drugs.

Prostaglandin Synthesis inhibitors

Aspirin and indomethacin, both inhibitors of prostaglandin synthesis, have been shown to cause a variable and inconsistent decrease in serum calcium concentrations in hypercalcemic patients with malignancy (77). The recommended dosages for indomethacin and acetylsalicylic acid are 75 to 150 mg/day and 1.8 to 4.8 g/day, respectively, in divided doses for 5 to 7 days. Their hypocalcemic effect is somewhat slow to develop and becomes evident over a period of 1 to 2 days. Treatment with these drugs should still be considered experimental and perhaps should be reserved for use in patients with cancer hypercalcemia without bone metastases who have undetectable levels of serum immunoreactive PTH.

Ultimately those measures that are best suited to control the neoplasm are the best measures to treat the attending hypercalcemic patient, particularly those without bone metastases. This may mean surgical removal of the tumor or treatment with chemotherapy or radiation therapy, alone or in combination. All the treatment modalities discussed above are only supportive, pending successful treatment of the tumor.

SUMMARY

Hypercalcemia is a common complication of malignant disease, occurring in 10 to 20% of patients with this condition. It occurs most frequently when there are overt metastatic deposits of tumor in bone. Under these circumstances there is localized bone resorption, resulting in the excessive liberation of osseous calcium into the extracellular fluid and hence hypercalcemia. In a significant fraction of patients with cancer and hypercalcemia, no bone metastases can be demonstrated and the cause of the hypercalcemia appears to the humoral. In these cases removal of the bulk of the tumor leads to remission of the hypercalcemia. Parathyroid hormone, prostaglandin E, and osteoclast activating factor are the three important humoral factors thought to be involved in the pathogenesis of the hypercalcemia in these situations.

Hypercalcemic crisis is a medical emergency requiring prompt and effective therapy. The first line of treatment usually consists of rehydration with isotonic saline together with calciuretic dieuretics (furosemide or ethacrynic acid). This form of treatment requires careful monitoring, and its use is restricted in patients with renal or cardiac disease. Intravenous mithramycin effectively lowers the calcium level and is considered a very effective agent after rehydration and calciuresis. However, mithramycin is associated with severe side effects, particularly with repeated use. Intravenous phosphate can be used as an alternative to mithramycin. It, too, is associated with severe side effects, particularly in patients with impairment of renal function and pre-existing hyperphosphatemia. Calcitonin, on the other hand, is a relatively safe drug. However, it has only a moderate calcium-lowering effect, and "resistance" appears to develop after repeated use. Corticosteroids are especially effective with those tumors for which they are cytotoxic. Oral phosphate can be effective for chronic treatment of hypercalcemia, and indomethacin and aspirin may play a useful role in those cases of hypercalcemia thought to be mediated by increased levels of prostaglandin.

ACKNOWLEDGMENTS

CIBA-GEIGY provided generous support for these studies. Elaine Kimbler provided secretarial assistance. The studies were also supported by the American Cancer Society, the National Institutes of Health, and the Veterans Administration.

REFERENCES

1. Lee, D. B. N., Zawada, E. T., and Kleeman, C. R. (1978): The pathophysiology and clinical aspects of hypercalcemic disorders. *West. J. Med.,* 129:278–320.
2. Murray, T. M., Josse, R. G., and Heersche, J. N. M. (1978): Hypercalcemia and cancer: An update. *Can. Med. Assoc. J.,* 119:915–920.
3. Deftos, L. J., and Neer, R. (1974): Medical management of the hypercalcemia of malignancy. *Annu. Rev. Med.,* 25:323–331.
4. Mazzaferri, E. L., O'Dorisio, T. M., and LoBuglio, A. F. (1978): Treatment of hypercalcemia associated with malignancy. *Semin. Oncol.,* 5:141–153.
5. Besarab, A., and Caro, J. F. (1978): Mechanisms of hypercalcemia in malignancy. *Cancer,* 41:2276–2285.
6. Myers, W. P. L. (1977): Differential diagnosis of hypercalcemia and cancer. *CA,* 27:258–272.
7. Mundy, G. R., Raisz, L. G., Cooper, R. A., Schechter, G. P., and Salmon, S. E. (1974): Evidence for the secretion of an osteoclast stimulating factor in myeloma. *N. Engl. J. Med.,* 291:1041.
8. Faccini, J. (1974): The mode of growth of experimental metastases in rabbit femora. *Virchows Arch. [Pathol. Anat.],* 364:249–263.
9. Galasko, C. S. B. (1976): Mechanisms of bone destruction in the development of skeletal metastases. *Nature,* 263:507–508.
10. Singer, F. R., Sharp, C. F., Jr., and Rude, R. K. (1979): Pathogenesis of hypercalcemia in malignancy. *Mineral Electrolyte Metab.,* 2:161–178.
11. Case Records of the Massachusetts General Hospital (1941): Case 27461. *N. Engl. J. Med.,* 225:789–791.
12. Fry, L. (1962): Pseudohyperparathyroidism with carcinoma of bronchus. *Br. Med. J.,* 1:301–302.
13. Tashjian, A. H., Jr., Levine, L., and Munson, P. L. (1964): Immunochemical identification

of parathyroid hormone in nonparathyroid neoplasms associated with hypercalcemia. *J. Exp. Med.,* 119:467.

14. Benson, R. C., Jr., Riggs, B. L., Pickard, B. M., et al. (1974): Radioimmunoassay of parathyroid hormone in hypercalcemic patients with malignant disease. *Am. J. Med.,* 56:821–826.
15. Stephens, R. L., Hansen, H. H., and Muggia, F. M. (1973): Hypercalcemia in epidermoid tumors of the head and neck and esophagus. *Cancer,* 31:1487–1491.
16. Moses, A. M., and Spencer, H. (1963): Hypercalcemia in patients with malignant lymphoma. *Ann. Intern. Med.,* 59:531–536.
17. Zidar, B. L., Shadduck, R. K., Winkelstein, A., et al. (1976): Acute myeloblastic leukemia and hypercalcemia. *N. Engl. J. Med.,* 295:692–694.
18. Knill-Jones, R. P., Buckler, R. M., Parsons, V., et al. (1970): Hypercalcemia and increased parathyroid hormone activity in a primary hepatoma. *N. Engl. J. Med.,* 282:704–708.
19. Lafferty, F. W. (1966): Pseudohyperparathyroidism. *Medicine,* 45:247–260.
20. Hirshorn, J. E., Vrhovsek, E., and Posen, S. (1979): Carcinoma of the breast associated with hypercalcemia and the presence of parathyroid hormone-like substances in the tumor. *J. Clin. Endocrinol. Metab.,* 48:217–221.
21. Powell, D., Singer, F. R., Murray, T. M., et al. (1973): Nonparathyroid humoral hypercalcemia in patients with neoplastic diseases. *N. Engl. J. Med.,* 289:176–181.
22. Roof, B. S., Carpenter, B., Fink, D. J., et al. (1971): Some thoughts on the nature of ectopic parathyroid hormones. *Am. J. Med.,* 50:686–691.
23. Heath, D. A. (1976): Hypercalcemia and malignancy. *Ann. Clin. Biochem.,* 13:555.
24. Scholz, D. A., Riggs, L. A., Purnell, D. C., et al. (1973): Ectopic hyperparathyroidism with renal calculi and subperiosteal bone resorption. *Mayo Clin. Proc.,* 48:124–126.
25. Palmer, F. J., Nelson, J. C., and Bacchus, H. (1974): The chloride-phosphate ratio in hypercalcemia. *Ann. Intern. Med.,* 80:200–204.
26. Drezner, M. K., Neelon, F. A., Curtis, H. B., and Lebovitz, H. E. (1976): Renal cyclic adenosine monophosphate: An accurate index of parathyroid function. *Metab. Clin. Exp.,* 25:1103–1112.
27. Broadus, A. E., Mahaffey, J. E., Bartter, F. C., and Neer, R. M. (1977): Nephrogenous cyclic adenosine monophosphate as a parathyroid function test. *J. Clin. Invest.,* 60:771–783.
28. Riggs, B. L., Arnaud, O. D., Reynold, J. C., et al. (1971): Immunologic differentiation of primary hyperparathyroidism from hyperparathyroidism due to nonparathyroid cancer. *J. Clin. Invest.,* 50:2079.
29. Berson, S. A., and Yalow, R. S. (1966): Parathyroid hormone in plasma in adenomatous hyperparathyroidism, uremia and bronchogenic carcinoma. *Science,* 154:907–909.
29a. Raisz, L. G., Yajnik, C. H., Bockman, R. S., and Bower, B F. (1979): Comparison of commercially available parathyroid hormone immunoassays in the differential diagnosis of hypercalcemia due to primary hyperparathyroidism or malignancy. *Ann. Intern. Med.,* 91:739–740.
30. Klein, D. C., and Raisz, L. G. (1970): Prostaglandins: Stimulation of bone resorption in tissue culture. *Endocrinology,* 86:1436–1440.
31. Tashjian, A. H., Jr., Voelkel, E. F., Levine, L., and Goldhaber, P. (1972): Evidence that the bone resorption-stimulating factor produced by mouse fibrosarcoma cells is prostaglandin E_2: A new model for the hypercalcemia of cancer. *J. Exp. Med.,* 136:1329–1343.
32. Oates, J. A., Seyberth, H. W.,Frolich, J. C., Sweetman, B. J., and Watson, J. T. (1978): The role of prostaglandins in the pathogenesis of human disease: Elucidation with stable isotopic methods. In: *Stable Isotopes,* edited by T. A. Baillie, pp. 281–287. University Park Press, Baltimore.
33. Anggard, E., Green, K., and Samuelsson, B. (1965): Synthesis of tritium-labelled prostaglandin E_2 and studies on its metabolism in guinea pig lung. *J. Biol. Chem.,* 140:1932–1940.
34. Hamberg, M., and Samuelsson, B. (1971): On the metabolism of prostaglandin E_1 and E_2 in man. *J. Biol. Chem.,* 246:6713–6721.
35. Seyberth, H. W., Sweetman, B. J., Frolich, J. C., and Oates, J. A. (1976): Quantification of the major urinary metabolite of the E prostaglandins by mass spectrometry: Evaluation of the methods application to clinical studies. *Prostaglandins,* 11:381.
36. Tashjian, A. H., Jr. (1978): Role of prostaglandins in the production of hypercalcemia by tumors. *Cancer Res.,* 38:4138–4141.
37. Tashjian, A. H., Jr., Voelkel, E. F., Goldhaber, P., and Levine, L. (1973): Successful treatment of hypercalcemia by indomethacin in mice bearing a prostaglandin-producing fibrosarcoma. *Prostaglandins,* 3:515–524.

38. Seyberth, H. W., Segre, G. V., Morgan, J. L., Sweetman, B. J., Potts, J. T., and Oates, J. A. (1975): Prostaglandins as mediators of hypercalcemia associated with certain types of cancer. *N. Engl. J. Med.,* 293:1278–1283.
39. Santoro, M. G., Jaffe, B. M., and Simmons, D. J. (1977): Bone resorption in vitro and in vivo in PGE-treated mice. *Proc. Soc. Exp. Biol. Med.,* 156:373.
40. Vanderwiel, C. J., and Talmage, R. V. (1979): Comparison of the effects of prostaglandin E₂ and parathyroid hormone on plasma calcium concentration and osteoclast function. *Endocrinology,* 105:588–594.
41. Horton, J. E., Raisz, L. G., Simmons, H. A., Oppenheim, J. J., and Mergenhagen, S. E. (1972): Bone resorbing activity in supernatant fluid from cultured human peripheral blood leukocytes. *Science,* 177:793–795.
42. Mundy, G. R., Luben, R. A., Raisz, L. G., et al. (1974): Bone resorbing activity in supernatants from lymphoid cell lines. *N. Engl. J. Med.,* 290:869.
43. Mundy, G. R., Rick, M. E., Turcotte, R., and Kowalski, M. A. (1978): Pathogenesis of hypercalcemia in lymphosarcoma cell leukemia. *Am. J. Med.,* 65:600–606.
44. Mundy, G. R., and Raisz, L. G. (1977): Big and little forms of osteoclast activating factor. *J. Clin. Invest.,* 60:122.
45. Luben, R. A., Mohler, M. A., and Nedwin, G. E. (1979): Production of hibridomas secreting monoclonal antibodies against the lymphokine osteoclast activating factor. *J. Clin. Invest.,* 64:337–341.
46. Gordon, G. S., Fitzpatrick, M. E., and Lubich, W. P. (1967): Identification of osteolytic sterols in human breast cancer. *Trans. Assoc. Am. Physicians,* 80:183.
47. Gordon, G. S., Cantino, T. J., Erhardt, L., Hansen, J., and Lubich, W. (1966): Osteolytic sterol in human breast cancer. *Science,* 151:1226–1228.
48. Haddad, J. G., Jr., Couranz, S. J., and Avioli, L. V. (1970): Circulating phytosterols in normal females, lactating mothers and breast cancer patients. *J. Clin. Endocrinol. Metab.,* 30:174.
49. Verner, J. V., and Morrison, A. B. (1958): Islet cell tumor and a syndrome of refractory watery diarrhea and hypokalemia. *Am. J. Med.,* 25:374–380.
50. Clinical Pathologic Conference (1977): Metastatic pancreatic islet cell carcinoma with peptic ulcer disease and hypercalcemia (Washington School of Medicine). *Am. J. Med.,* 63:142–151.
51. Holdaway, I. M., Evans, M. C., and Clarke, E. D. (1977): Watery diarrhea syndrome with episodic hypercalcemia. *Aust. NZ J. Med.,* 7:63–65.
52. Inesi, G. (1978): Emergency management of hypercalcemia. *Drug Ther.,* 8:14–22.
53. Duarte, G. C., Winnacker, J. L., Becker, K. L., et al. (1971): Thiazide-induced hypercalcemia. *N. Engl. J. Med.,* 284:828–830.
54. Coburn, J. W., Brickman, A. S., and Massry, S. G. (1972): Medical treatment in primary and secondary hyperparathyroidism. *Semin. Drug Treat.,* 2:117–135.
55. Chakmakjian, Z. H., and Bethune, J. E. (1966): Sodium sulfate treatment of hypercalcemia. *N. Engl. J. Med.,* 275:862–869.
56. Dudley, H. R., Ritchie, A. C., Schillin, A., et al. (1955): Pathologic changes associated with the use of sodium ethylene diamine tetra-acetate in the treatment of hypercalcemia. *N. Engl. J. Med.,* 252:331–337.
57. Goldsmith, R. S., and Ingbar, S. H. (1966): Inorganic phosphate treatment of hypercalcemia of diverse etiologies. *N. Engl. J. Med.,* 274:1–7.
58. Rasmussen, H., and Bordier, P. (1974): *The Physiological and Cellular Basis of Metabolic Bone Disease.* Williams & Wilkins, Baltimore.
59. Raisz, L. G., and Niemann, I. (1969): Effect of phosphate, calcium and magnesium on bone resorption and hormonal response in tissue culture. *Endocrinology,* 85:446–452.
60. Carey, R. W., Schmitt, G. W., Kopald, H. H., et al. (1968): Massive extraskeletal calcification during phosphate treatment of hypercalcemia. *Arch. Intern. Med.,* 122:150–155.
61. Shackney, S., and Hasson, J. (1967): Precipitous fall in serum calcium, hypotension, and acute renal failure after intravenous phosphate therapy for hypercalcemia. *Ann Intern. Med.,* 66:906–916.
62. Yendt, E. R. (1972): Disorders of calcium, phosphorus and magnesium disorders. In: *Clinica. Disorders of Fluid and Electrolyte Metabolism,* edited by M. H. Maxwell and C. R. Kleeman pp. 416–417. McGraw-Hill, New York.
63. Deftos, L. J., and Potts, J. T., Jr. (1974): Parathyroid hormone, thyrocalcitonin, vitamin D

bone and mineral metabolism. In: *Duncan's Disease of Metabolism,* edited by P. L. Bondy, pp. 1225–1430. Saunders, Philadelphia.

64. Vaughn, C. B., and Vaitkevicius, K. (1974): The effects of calcitonin on hypercalcemia in patients with malignancy. *Cancer,* 34:1268–1271.
65. Brautbar, N., and Luboshitzky, R. (1977): Combined calcitonin and oral phosphate treatment for hypercalcemia in multiple myeloma. *Arch. Intern. Med.,* 137:914–916.
66. Au, W. Y. W. (1975): Calcitonin treatment of hypercalcemia due to parathyroid carcinoma— Synergistic effect of prednisone on long-term treatment of hypercalcemia. *Arch. Intern. Med.,* 135:1594–1597.
67. Kofman, S., and Eisenstein, R. (1963): Mithramycin in the treatment of disseminated cancer. *Cancer Chemother. Rep.,* 32:77–96.
68. Yarbro, J. W., Kennedy, B. J., and Barnum, C. P. (1966): Mithramycin inhibition of ribonucleic acid synthesis. *Cancer Res.,* 26:39.
69. Perlia, C. P., Gubisch, N. J., Wolter, J., et al. (1970): Mithramycin treatment of hypercalcemia. *Cancer,* 25:389–394.
70. Godfrey, T. E. (1971): Mithramycin for hypercalcemia of malignant disease. *Calif. Med.,* 115:1–4.
71. Margileth, D. A., Smith, F. E., and Lane, M. (1973): Sudden arterial occlusion associated with mithramycin therapy. *Cancer,* 31:708–712.
72. Eyster, F. E., Wilson, C. B., and Naibach, H. (1971): Mithramycin as a possible cause of toxic epidermal necrolysis (Lyell's syndrome). *Calif. Med.,* 114:42–43.
73. Caro, J. F., Besarab, A., and Glennon, J. A. (1978): Symptomatic hypocalcemia following combined calcitonin and mithramycin therapy for hypercalcemia due to malignancy. *Cancer Treat. Rep.,* 62:1561–1563.
74. Jee, W. S. S., Roberts, W. E., Park, H. Z., et al. (1972): Interrelated effects of glucocorticoid and parathyroid hormone upon bone remodelling. In: *Calcium, Parathyroid Hormone and the Calcitonins,* edited by R. V. Talmage and P. L. Munson, pp. 430–439. Excerpta Medica, Amsterdam.
75. Tashjian, A. H., Jr., Voelkel, E. F., McDonough, J., et al. (1975): Hydrocortisone inhibits prostaglandin production by mouse fibrosarcoma cells. *Nature,* 258:739–741.
76. Gryglewski, R. J., Panczenko, B., Korbut, R., et al. (1975): Corticosteroids inhibit prostaglandin release from perfused mesenteric blood vessels of rabbit and from perfused lungs of sensitized guinea pig. *Prostaglandins,* 10:345–355.
77. Seyberth, H., Segre, G., Morgon, J. L., et al. (1975): Prostaglandins as mediators of hypercalcemia associated with certain types of cancer. *N. Engl. J. Med.,* 293:1278–1283.

Medical Complications in Cancer Patients,
edited by J. Klastersky and M. J. Staquet.
Raven Press, New York © 1981.

Respiratory Complications During Cancer Therapy: Diagnosis and Management

*Franco M. Muggia, **James K. V. Willson, and
†Raymond B. Weiss

*Division of Oncology, New York University Medical Center, New York, New York 10016;
and **Medicine Branch, Clinical Onocology Program, and †Clinical Investigations Branch,
Cancer Therapy Evaluation Program, National Cancer Institute, National Institutes of
Health, Bethesda, Maryland 20205*

The increasingly aggressive diagnostic and supportive care that cancer patients receive has led to identification of previously undiagnosed pulmonary diseases, a number of which appear to be drug related. The importance of early recognition of these cytotoxic drug-induced diseases is emphasized by the necessity for early withdrawal of the drug in order to halt or reverse potentially lethal progression of pulmonary damage (79). At the same time, it is often difficult to differentiate drug-related toxicity from the toxicity of other potential insults in this group of patients (11). These insults include metastatic or primary malignancy, an opportunistic infection, pleural effusions, pulmonary edema, pulmonary emboli (including tumor emboli), and pulmonary reaction to therapeutic and diagnostic procedures. The nonspecific manifestations of all these potential insults mandate an analytic diagnostic approach once an interstitial pulmonary disease develops in the cancer patient.

In this chapter we review the tools available to the clinician for evaluating these patients and then discuss the findings associated with specific drugs. Finally, therapeutic recommendations are advanced. We also touch briefly on pleural effusions, as they represent another aspect of respiratory complications in the patient with cancer.

GENERAL DIAGNOSTIC FEATURES

Clinical Presentation

The clinical hallmark of the interstitial pneumonitis associated with cytotoxic drugs (e.g., bleomycin) is dyspnea. Pulmonary emboli, including those secondary to tumor embolization, and lymphangitic or hematogenous spread of carcinoma must be considered in the differential diagnosis of dyspnea in the absence of pneumothorax, effusions, or obvious cardiac decompensation. Unfortunately, once dyspnea is manifest, the interstitial pneumonitis is well established and may progress despite withdrawal of the offending agent (85). The early symptoms, usually a dry nonproductive cough, are insidious and may go unrecognized for weeks prior to the onset of exertional dyspnea. With some exceptions, fever is an infrequent sign of drug-induced pneumonitis, and its presence should alert the clinician to the possibility of an infectious process (74). However, the clinical pneumonitis which characteristically occurs 2 to 3 months following completion of irradiation usually includes dyspnea and fever to 102°F (35). In general, it is difficult to distinguish a drug-induced or radiation pneumonitis from an infection or neoplastic process on the basis of the symptomatic presentation.

Physical signs also provide little more than nonspecific findings which include tachypnea and diffuse rales, often out of proportion to the symptoms. Again, the presence of abnormal physical signs usually denotes established pneumonitis (68). The physical examination should be serially evaluated in patients receiving drugs which have been recognized to be associated with pneumonitis, but its limitation for diagnosing early disease must be recognized.

Roentgenographic and Radionuclide Evaluations

The various radiographic patterns of drug-induced lung disease were recently reviewed (58). Anticancer drugs are associated most prominently with two patterns: diffuse interstitial consolidation and diffuse air-space consolidation. They are not associated with pleural effusion, hilar enlargement, or localized consolidation.

Roentgenographic abnormalities in patients with drug-induced pneumonitis usually are not noted until the patient experiences respiratory symptoms. Serial monitoring of the chest X-ray in patients receiving drugs associated with interstitial pneumonitis has been advocated (40), but it must be recognized that such a practice fails to alert the physician to the early stage of pneumonitis in the asymptomatic patient (23). Characteristic radiographic changes have been described for many cytotoxic drugs. The chest X-ray in bleomycin-induced pneumonitis shows diffuse linear densities, predominantly in the lower lung zones (Figs. 1 and 2) (38). Pleural effusions have not been reported in bleomycin-induced pneumonitis. This is a helpful differential feature when considering alternative diagnoses, e.g., infection or pulmonary progression of the neoplasm. A more diffuse reticulonodular infiltrate than that seen with bleomycin is described in patients with a methotrexate-induced pneumonitis (26). The radiographic changes associated with methotrexate resolve more rapidly than those described for other cytotoxic drugs. Diffuse linear densities, usually reflecting extensive fibrosis, are characteristic of the radiographic changes described in the busulfan lung (13). Pleural effusions are rarely noted in busulfan- and methotrexate-induced pneumonitis (13,26).

The earliest radiographic evidence of *radiation* damage to the lung occurs at 2 to 3 months. A ground-glass opacification is described and, depending on

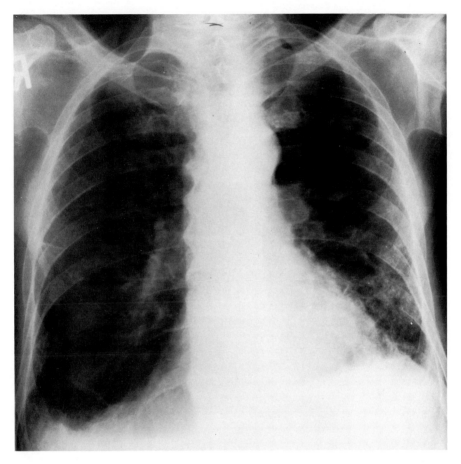

FIG. 1. Bilateral lower zone infiltrates in a patient with oropharyngeal carcinoma receiving bleomycin.

the severity of damage, may be alveolar, nodular, or dense, thus resembling a consolidation (51). The cardinal feature distinguishing radiation pneumonitis, however, is the sharp boundaries limited to the margins of the treatment port. This feature and the characteristic interval prior to the appearance of pneumonitis help to differentiate radiation pneumonitis from an alternative lung pathology (7). Depending on the degree of damage, volume loss with retraction of the hilum or mediastinum, local fibrosis, and pleural effusion may also be seen.

The gallium-67 lung scan may be a useful study for the early detection of drug-induced pneumonitis. In one report, gallium uptake was demonstrated in the lung at an early stage of bleomycin-induced pneumonitis in asymptomatic patients with normal chest X-rays (65). The specificity of the gallium-67 scan is limited, however, because it does not differentiate drug-induced pneumonitis

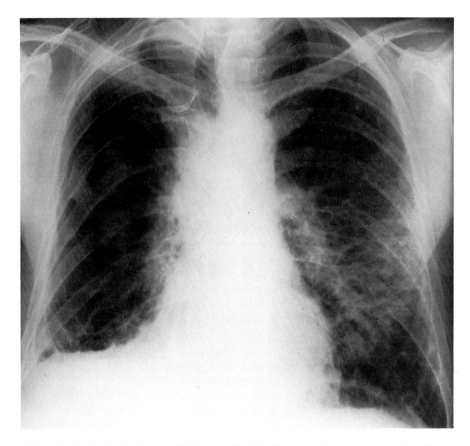

FIG. 2. Mediastinal and pulmonary infiltrates related to bleomycin for oropharyngeal carcinoma and prior irradiation.

from other inflammatory processes. In fact, it was recently advocated for the early detection of *Pneumocystis* in the immunosuppressed host. Increased uptake has also been seen by the Radiation Branch, National Cancer Institute, in association with radiation-induced reactions, even in radiographically normal areas. A prospective evaluation of the value of the gallium-67 scan in detecting early drug or radiation-induced pneumonitis in asymptomatic patients should be undertaken.

Pulmonary Function Tests

Readily available pulmonary function tests, including the diffusion capacity for carbon monoxide ($D_L CO$) and spirometry, are important for assessing established drug-induced pneumonitis and for monitoring asymptomatic patients. Interstitial pneumonitis results in decreased $D_L CO$, restrictive lung volumes, and hypoxia. Prospective studies of asymptomatic patients with normal chest X-rays receiving bleomycin show dramatic deterioration in the $D_L CO$ (20,61). These studies do not clearly delineate when drug therapy should be withdrawn in the asymptomatic patients with compromised pulmonary function. Future prospective studies should address the prognostic value of pulmonary function tests in the asymptomatic patient receiving a potential pulmonary toxin. At the present time, the $D_L CO$ and spirometry should be serially followed in these patients and significant changes carefully evaluated. In established drug-induced pneumonitis, the $D_L CO$ correlates with the course of pneumonitis, although abnormal pulmonary function may persist long after apparent clinical recovery (61). Hypoxia and hypocarbia are manifest in severe interstitial pneumonitis and reflect the clinical course.

Pulmonary Biopsy

The absence of specific diagnostic parameters which herald the onset of drug-induced pulmonary injury make it imperative that the clinician maintain a high index of suspicion for drug-associated pneumonitis. Significant symptoms, radiographic changes, or pulmonary function abnormalities should be evaluated by lung biopsy. It is imperative that treatable disorders, such as *Pneumocystis carinii,* or more common insults, such as viral pneumonitis, be excluded before withdrawing a therapeutic drug. Particular vigilance is urged when interpreting reports of drug-associated pneumonitis. Biopsy evidence, as well as a thorough evaluation for an infectious etiology, including viral cultures, should be required before a diagnosis of a drug-associated process is accepted.

The proper approach to obtaining a pulmonary biopsy is debated. A generous biopsy specimen is desired to provide the histologic detail required to make a diagnosis of a drug-induced pneumonitis. Transbronchial biopsy specimens are often inadequate, although drug-induced pneumonitis (3) as well as *Pneumocystis carinii* (57) have been diagnosed with a transbronchial biopsy. At this time, however, an open lung wedge biopsy is the preferred procedure for obtaining adequate tissue for diagnostic purposes (33).

The histopathology of drug-induced pneumonitis has been described for bleomycin (53), busulfan (45), cyclophosphamide (54), BCNU (25), and methotrexate (80). A common pathologic process has been postulated which culminates in a fibrosing alveolitis. Initially, a toxic insult to either the capillary endothelium (1) or alveolar epithelium (22) occurs; the site of this insult is debated. Inflammatory reaction to the initial injury results in a nonspecific interstitial pneumonitis with differing degrees of fibrosis. Cellular atypia, including atypia of the type II alveolar epithelium and bronchial epithelium, are characteristic of drug-induced pneumonitis. These atypical type II alveolar epithelial cells are exfoliated into the sputum, and examination of sputum cytology is recommended in the evaluation of suspected drug-induced pneumonitis. The severity of the fibrosis determines the degree of reversibility that might be expected.

The features of radiation-induced lung damage are not specific. Criteria for the diagnosis of radiation pneumonitis have been suggested and include atypical septal cell proliferation, vascular changes, and widespread hyaline membranes (10).

It must again be emphasized that the histopathology of a drug-induced or radiation-induced pneumonitis—like the clinical presentation—is characteristic but not specific. Proof of a drug-induced pneumonitis requires circumstantial evidence of drug therapy followed by a documented characteristic pneumonitis and the exclusion of other known causes of pneumonitis.

SPECIFIC TOXIC AGENTS

Bleomycin

Bleomycin is an active drug in lymphomas and is an essential component of the combination regimens which have proved curative for metastatic testicular cancer. The drug is a well-known cause of pulmonary fibrosis, which has been recognized in animal toxicologic as well as clinical tests in up to 40% of patients in one study (23). Factors associated with bleomycin pulmonary toxicity are dose, old age, and pre-existing pulmonary pathology (11,23,85). Bleomycin causes pulmonary fibrosis often enough for the relationship of dose to the pulmonary effect to have become well defined. When bleomycin is used as sole treatment, pulmonary toxicity is rare below 150 units and common (10 to 20%) when the cumulative dose exceeds 550 units (12).

In addition, the enhanced pulmonary toxicity from simultaneous administration of bleomycin and thoracic radiation was recently emphasized (15,44). A review of published clinical studies in which bleomycin and thoracic radiation were given concomitantly demonstrated that there was an increased incidence of pulmonary fibrosis over that seen from either treatment by itself, and that there was a 10% mortality from this toxicity (15). Moreover, the toxicity developed as a result of cumulative bleomycin doses which were considerably lower than those which usually produce lung toxicity. Thus the probability that severe pulmonary complications will occur with simultaneous irradiation appears to be extremely high.

Not only is there an enhanced pulmonary effect when bleomycin and radiation are used simultaneously, but also when they are used sequentially. In a study of patients with metastatic testicular carcinoma, prior thoracic irradiation (either whole lung or mediastinal) appeared to enhance the susceptibility to bleomycin-induced fibrosis (72). This complication developed in 5 of 12 patients receiving both treatments sequentially as opposed to only 4 of 89 who did not have prior irradiation. Careful consideration must therefore be given to the toxicity risk/benefit ratio whenever bleomycin is to be utilized in a patient who has received thoracic irradiation.

Combined chemotherapy regimens including bleomycin may also have an increased incidence of pulmonary toxicity as manifested by the experience of Schein et al. (73) with the BACOP regimen for lymphoma. With 15 units/m² twice monthly, 4 of 16 patients developed severe pulmonary toxicity. This was avoided when the dose was decreased to 5 units/m².

Another area of synergism for pulmonary toxicity is bleomycin and high oxygen concentrations in inspired air. Goldiner and colleagues (31) found that there was a 100% mortality after tumor bulk-reductive operations in five patients with testicular carcinoma who had previously received cumulative bleomycin doses of 200 to 400 units/m². All died of interstitial pneumonitis and fibrosis. A subsequent group of 12 patients treated similarly had their fluid balance carefully monitored and the FiO_2 kept at a low level during the anesthesia for their operations. None of these patients had pneumonitis (32). A similar phenomenon may have occurred in a series of patients who received bleomycin and radiation for esophageal cancer and were subsequently subjected to resection. Three of eight died of interstitial pneumonitis and fibrosis within 6 weeks of operation, whereas 10 patients not subjected to resection survived without toxicity.

Predisposition to oxygen toxicity is a phenomenon that may be shared by other chemotherapeutic agents. This suggests a common pathway of toxicity via superoxide formation. The importance of oxygen in bleomycin lipid peroxidation and DNA breakage has been demonstrated (82).

Furthermore, several quinone anticancer drugs have been shown to stimulate microsomal electron transport and are therefore likely to have free radical intermediates for their cytotoxicity. Hence the presence of molecular oxygen would lead to increased interaction with these free radicals and enhanced formation of superoxide (5). Further elucidation of such mechanisms may open the way for protection of toxicity (82).

A search has been initiated to find analogs of bleomycin which maintain antitumor activity but have less pulmonary toxicity. Umezawa and his colleagues in Japan (56), by fermentation, chemical modification, or partial synthesis, produced some 300 analogs of bleomycin which differ in their terminal amine moiety. Each of these compounds was tested in laboratory animals for antitumor activity and then, if active, was further tested for a tendency to cause pulmonary fibrosis using bleomycin as a control. The incidence and degree of fibrosis produced was quantitated using a value relative to bleomycin. The drug PEP-bleomycin [N-(3-aminopropyl)-α-phenethylamine bleomycin] (now designated pepleomycin) was selected for clinical trial in Japan based on high antitumor activity in experimental animals and a lower incidence of pulmonary toxicity (a ratio of 0.36 compared to the bleomycin control of 1.0 in mice). Studies in the United States in laboratory animals confirmed that pepleomycin has a lower pulmonary toxicity than bleomycin (78), and clinical trials are ongoing in Japan. These clinical studies will require careful comparison of pulmonary function abnormalities experienced in relation to bleomycin.

Nitrosoureas

The nitrosoureas are valuable drugs for treatment of gliomas, lymphomas, and myeloma. Some activity has also been present in small cell lung cancer, melanoma, and gastrointestinal cancer. Chloroethyl nitrosoureas which have been marketed in the United States include BCNU (carmustine) and CCNU (lomustine). Methyl CCNU and chlorozotocin are investigational drugs, the latter having been introduced more recently to modify myelotoxic manifestations. The naturally occurring methyl nitrosourea linked to glucosamine, streptozotocin, is mainly used for the treatment of islet cell tumors of the pancreas.

The preclinical toxicology studies of BCNU demonstrated pulmonary effects, but these were acute in nature (pleural effusion and pulmonary edema) and postmortem examination of experimental animals receiving the drug did not show pulmonary fibrosis (14). A report in 1966 (41) noted interstitial infiltrates during carmustine administration in four patients, but there was little evidence that carmustine was the cause of these infiltrates. Two patients had a benign course with clearing of the chest roentgenogram, and the other two had good explanations for the pulmonary abnormalities other than drug toxicity.

The first case of interstitial fibrosis attributable to carmustine was reported in 1976 (37). Since then there have been 12 additional patients receiving only carmustine who have been reported to have pulmonary fibrosis (6,9,21,25,43, 66,76,84). Most patients died from the pulmonary effect of the drug. In those patients who had biopsy or autopsy, the histologic changes in the lung induced by carmustine were similar to those seen as a result of bleomycin, busulfan, and the other lung-toxic drugs (79).

The cumulative carmustine doses that have produced fibrosis have varied from 1,380 to 3,300 mg (580 to 2,100 mg/m²). The duration of therapy has varied from 6 months to 3 years. Carmustine-induced fibrosis has so far been identified mostly in single case reports, and thus the probability of developing pulmonary fibrosis according to dose cannot be determined as has been done for bleomycin.

There is some evidence that there is a higher risk of interstitial pneumonitis and fibrosis when carmustine is used in combination with other drugs which are also known to cause the same problem, and it can occur at lower total doses. Durant and colleagues (25) had nine patients who developed pulmonary toxicity when carmustine and cyclophosphamide were given together. Since seven of the nine patients had total carmustine doses of less than 670 mg/m², a synergistic toxicity between these two drugs is suggested. Schreml et al. (75) reported two similar instances of patients receiving cyclophosphamide and carmustine.

Semustine was also reported to produce pulmonary fibrosis in one instance

(49). This patient received 4.1 g semustine over a 2-year period and incurred the typical pulmonary histologic changes seen with the other drugs under discussion. Since semustine is being widely used as part of long-term postoperative chemotherapy in patients with primary colon carcinoma, these patients should be closely observed for drug-induced pulmonary problems. Such toxic effects may have gone undetected in the past because of the relatively short survival of patients with metastatic tumor treated with the drug.

There have been no cases reported so far of pulmonary toxicity from streptozotocin with lomustine and chlorozotocin and other nitrosoureas that are closely related chemically; it is likely that similar toxicity will be observed in the future. In addition, one must be even more alert to these problems with high-dose nitrosourea regimens which are being utilized with autologous marrow rescue.

Mitomycin

Mitomycin is an antibiotic derived from *Streptomyces caespitosis,* which was first isolated in Japan in 1955. Studies with mitomycin began in the United States in 1958, and it was marketed there in 1974. It exhibits its greatest activity in gastrointestinal malignancies, but it is also used in breast, cervical, and esophageal carcinomas. However, in spite of this long history of clinical use, only recently was it recognized that this drug, too, may occasionally have pulmonary toxicity (4,28,46,55,60,71).

The first patient found to have pulmonary effect from mitomycin was only briefly reported, and the total dose was not recorded (71). The next three patients reported had cumulative mitomycin doses of 60, 102, and 156 mg, and the pulmonary lesions appeared 3 to 6 months after initiation of treatment (60). All three received only mitomycin. The histologic changes seen were similar to those noted with the other drugs under discussion, although interstitial fibrosis was not as prominent a feature.

Eleven other patients with fibrosis developing while on mitomycin have been studied in detail (4,28,46,55). All received 5-fluorouracil (5-FU) in addition, and two had cytosine arabinoside as well (4), but neither of these drugs is known to produce fibrosis. The cumulative doses were small in most cases, varying from 40 to 120 mg/m². Four patients (46,55) developed symptoms following only the second course of mitomycin. Again, the histologic appearance was similar to that previously described (4,28,55).

As with bleomycin, it appears that prior mitomycin therapy increases the risk of pulmonary toxicity when a patient is exposed to a high oxygen concentration from ventilatory support during and after surgery. Franklin and colleagues (29) had two patients with esophageal carcinoma in whom pulmonary infiltrates developed after receiving mitomycin, 5-FU and esophageal radiation followed by esophagectomy and postoperative ventilation with an FiO_2 of 50% or more. Other similarly treated patients who received an FiO_2 of less than 30% did not develop pulmonary problems. It is possible that a similar synergism exists for drugs other than bleomycin and mitomycin, and we reiterate that patients previously exposed to these pulmonary-toxic drugs should not be ventilated with high oxygen concentrations and incur a greater risk during surgery.

Methotrexate

Methotrexate seems to produce a more transient, treatable, and less fatal pulmonary reaction than any of the other cytotoxic agents, and its onset bears no relation to administered dose. A different mechanism of production of the pulmonary effect may be involved. Methotrexate causes a reversible drug hypersensitivity reaction rather than direct, alveolar epithelium toxicity with irreversible fibrosis (79).

Pneumonitis may occur from either oral or intravenous methotrexate administration, and even from intrathecal administration (36,48,86). Steroids may be helpful in methotrexate-induced pneumonitis. Fever may also be prominently associated with methotrexate administration (17).

Alkylating Agents

Busulfan has long been recognized to produce pulmonary toxicity, and the subject has been adequately reviewed (13,79). Atypical cytologic changes are also a hallmark of busulfan-induced abnormalities.

Cyclophosphamide is known occasionally to produce pneumonitis and fibrosis and was discussed in the review by Sostman et al. (79). Additional cases have been published (2,54,63) since 1977. Occurrence many years after cessation of the drug has been reported in children.

Two children received cyclophosphamide for 3 to 4 years in daily oral doses and were taken off the drug (2). At 4 and 6 years later, respectively, each developed hypoxemia and pulmonary fibrosis. Neither had received other cytotoxic drugs during the intervening period. Both had narrow anterior–posterior thoracic diameters. The authors surmised that this narrowing was due to a loss of lung volume from drug effect during the patients' adolescent growth spurt.

Chlorambucil was recently added to the list of drugs producing pulmonary fibrosis through three well-documented cases (19,47,64). Two brief publications cited six additional patients (67,70), with a fatal outcome in three.

Melphalan was also recently associated with pulmonary toxicity in two instances (18,81). In addition, an autopsy material review of patients with multiple myeloma disclosed one other case of pulmonary fibrosis and four cases in which alveolar epithelial cell dysplasia was present without progression to fibrosis. It is likely that instances of this toxicity have gone unrecognized.

Fibrosis is rare with these drugs, except for busulfan, and nonexistent with the parent nitrogen mustard or with thiotepa. When alkylating agents are combined with other drugs such as bleomycin and the nitrosoureas, an increased risk of pulmonary fibrosis is likely and may explain the toxicity associated with bleomycin, adriamycin, cyclophosphamide, vincristine, and prednisone (BACOP) combination chemotherapy (73).

Procarbazine

Procarbazine is known to occasionally produce pneumonitis. Its effect appears to have features of a hypersensitivity reaction (42,52). In four other patients reported to have developed pulmonary fibrosis, procarbazine had been given in combination, and it is difficult to assess the contribution of each individual drug (24,27,39). However, in two the lung histology was typical of hypersensitivity reaction, and procarbazine is thus the likely offender. Prednisone therapy has produced clinical improvement.

Miscellaneous Drugs

6-Mercaptopurine (6-MP) has been associated with interstitial pneumonitis, but this appears to be a rare phenomenon (79). However, the potential of a drug interaction leading to enhanced 6-MP toxicity as occurs in the liver must be borne in mind. The related azathioprine is similarly implicated (69).

Zinostatin is an investigational drug which is receiving clinical trial after studies in Japan. This agent was associated recently with development of pulmonary infiltrates. A hypersensitivity reaction is suspected to be responsible (34, 59,77).

THERAPEUTIC MEASURES—PULMONARY DISEASE

A high degree of suspicion of a drug-induced pulmonary process is probably the major safeguard against the inexorable progression toward a fatal syndrome of interstitial pneumonitis and pulmonary fibrosis. Recognition of milder forms of pulmonary impairment (e.g., mild dyspnea, cough, chest pain) and minimal physical findings which lead to interruption of the injurious agent's course, may be life-saving. In high-risk circumstances (e.g., a patient receiving bleomycin), serial pulmonary function studies including diffusion capacity may alert clinicians to abnormalities in the absence of other findings. It is very important to recognize that some situations lead to much greater risk of developing complications, as in patients who received prior thoracic irradiation. Follow-up at long intervals in those circumstances is inadequate.

Once the diagnosis appears probable and the drug has been withdrawn (a common circumstance upon hospital admission), efforts are made to exclude other (infectious) etiologies. In the presence of radiation-induced pneumonitis or suspicion of hypersensitivity reactions, glucocorticoids may be effective for reducing fever and respiratory symptoms. Exclusion of an infectious etiology is mandatory under these circumstances.

Clinical progression during the diagnostic work-up and antibiotic coverage (for neutropenic patients) becomes a requirement for biopsy. With biopsy, infectious etiologies such as fungi or *Pneumocystis carinii* can be excluded, but changes relating to fibrosis are of course nonspecific and fail to indicate the cause. Changes suggestive of hypersensitivity include eosinophilic cellular infiltration, vascular changes of endothelial cell hypertrophy, perivascular infiltration, edema of the vascular wall, and intra-alveolar or interstitial granulomatous lesions (17).

Glucocorticoids are the mainstay of treatment of hypersensitivity reactions leading to pulmonary manifestations. The experience with anticancer drug pneumonitis, however, is limited as described in individual case reports. Glucocorticoids have been most effective with reactions from methotrexate and procarbazine. It is of interest that daunorubicin was also cited as being capable of clearing methotrexate-induced infiltrates in leukemia (62). These cases may actually represent instances of leukemic leukostasis rather than methotrexate pulmonary toxicity. This entity must be included in the differential diagnosis in leukemia with pulmonary infiltrates (83).

There is extensive clinical experience with the treatment of radiation pneumonitis. The actual role of steroids, however, in the eventual outcome of pulmonary pathology has been the subject of much debate. Nevertheless, steroids are invaluable in attenuating the acute manifestations of pneumonitis, and they have been used commonly for these purposes.

A major aspect deserving investigation is the role of oxygen in promoting additional tissue damage from cytotoxic agents. Certainly, acute manifestations seem to be aggravated by its use during the postoperative period. Therefore, when providing assisted ventilation on any patient with cancer receiving or having received cytotoxic agents, this factor must be taken into consideration.

Finally, if a mechanism of pulmonary toxicity includes formation of the superoxide radical, then some preventive measure may be conceived by using agents which effectively prevent lipid peroxidation and act as free radical scavengers. Some attempts at testing such measures clinically have already been initiated.

PLEURAL EFFUSIONS: GENERAL THERAPEUTIC GUIDELINES

The management of neoplastic pleural effusion is a topic which has been discussed extensively, with an abundance of therapeutic measures being advocated (16,30,50). Unfortunately, no assessment of the survival benefit that these measures accrue is possible, since series include a heterogeneous group of disorders. Nevertheless, sclerosis of the pleural space by a variety of measures (e.g., surgical tube drainage, talc poudrage, nitrogen mustard, quinacrine, external radiation, radioactive colloids, and tetracycline) seems beneficial in over 50% of selected patients symptomatic with recurrent accumulation of fluid in one pleural space. One prospective randomized study indicates comparable control of fluid reaccumulation by tetracycline and quinacrine, but the latter was associated with considerably more toxicity (8). A study comparing tetracycline to tube drainage by itself would be of interest, particularly if confined to one disease entity for comparability. Bilateral sclerosis, if done simultaneously, invariably leads to marked deterioration in breathing from decreased compliance.

All these measures must, of course, ultimately be compared to application of effective systemic therapy. Such alternatives are often present for responsive tumors such as breast cancer, ovarian cancer, and lymphoma. Nevertheless, pleural effusions may represent an isolated area of disease progression in the absence of other manifestations, and local therapy represents an attractive alternative. On the other hand, respiratory failure may be present along with many other manifestations of disease progression, and it is doubtful under these circumstances that any local therapy would have much to offer. In particular, with advancing cachexia, hypoalbuminemia and recumbency become contributory factors to rather refractory effusions.

CONCLUSIONS

Respiratory complications of cancer or its treatment are common, particularly in late stages. Increased awareness of pulmonary complications of cytotoxic therapy has led to earlier diagnosis and prevention of severe pneumonitis. However, only recently has the deleterious interaction of radiation and chemotherapy become sufficiently emphasized. Similarly, it is surprising that the pathophysiology of pleural effusions secondary to cancer has not been well delineated and most therapeutic alternatives have not been properly evaluated. For example, prior radiation therapy to the chest wall may be a predisposing factor to effusions in breast cancer, but this has not been subjected to study. There is need for evaluation of treatments to be carried out with special consideration given to the overall disease status and pathophysiology of these complications.

REFERENCES

1. Adamson, I. R., and Bowden, D. H. (1974): The pathogenesis of bleomycin-induced pulmonary fibrosis in mice. *A. J. Pathol.*, 77:185–198.
2. Alvarado, C. S., Boat, T. F., and Newman, A. J. (1978): Late-onset pulmonary fibrosis and chest deformity in two children treated with cyclophosphamide. *J. Pediatr.*, 92:443.
3. Andersen, H. A. (1978): Transbronchoscopic lung biopsy for diffuse pulmonary diseases: Results in 939 patients. *Chest*, 73:734–736.
4. Andrews, A. T., Bowman, H. S., Patel, S. B., et al. (1979): Mitomycin and interstitial pneumonitis. *Ann. Intern. Med.*, 90:127.
5. Bachur, N. (1978): General mechanism for the biological activation of quinone anticancer agents to free radicals. *Curr. Chemother.*, 2:1124.
6. Bailey, C. C., Marsden, H. B., and Jones, P. H. M. (1978): Fatal pulmonary fibrosis following 1,3-bis(2-chloroethyl)-1-nitrosourea (BCNU) therapy. *Cancer*, 42:74.
7. Bate, D., and Guttman, R. J. (1957): Changes in lung and pleura following two-million-volt therapy for carcinoma of the breast. *Radiology*, 69:372–382.
8. Bayly, T. C., Kisner, D. L., Sybert, A., et al. (1978): Tetracycline and quinacrine in the control of pleural effusions: A randomized trial. *Cancer*, 41:1188–1192.
9. Bellot, P. A., and Valdiserri, R. O. (1979): Multiple pulmonary lesions in a patient treated

with BCNU (1,3-bis(2-chloroethyl)-1-nitrosourea) for glioblastoma multiforme. *Cancer,* 43:46.
10. Bennett, D. E., Million, R. R., and Ackerman, L. V. (1969): Bilateral radiation pneumonitis, a complication of the radiotherapy of bronchogenic carcinoma. *Cancer,* 23:1001–1018.
11. Blum, R. H., and Carter, S. K. (1973): Pulmonary complications of cancer chemotherapy. *N. Engl. J. Med.,* 288:266.
12. Blum, R. H., Carter, S. K., and Agre, K. (1973): A clinical review of bleomycin—A new antineoplastic agent. *Cancer,* 31:903.
13. Burns, W. A., McFarland, W., and Matthews, M. J. (1970): Busulfan-induced pulmonary disease. *Am. Rev. Respir. Dis.,* 101:408–413.
14. Carter, S. K., Schabel, F. M., Broder, L. E., et al. (1972): 1,3-bis(2-Chlorethyl)-1-nitrosourea (BCNU) and other nitrosoureas in cancer treatment: A review. *Adv. Cancer Res.,* 16:273.
15. Catane, R., Schwade, J. G., Turrisi, A. T., et al. (1979): Pulmonary toxicity after radiation and bleomycin—A review. *Int. J. Radiat. Oncol. Biol. Phys.,* 5:1513–1518.
16. Chernow, B., and Sahn, S. A. (1977): Carcinomatous involvement of the pleura. *Am. J. Med.,* 63:695–702.
17. Clarysse, M. M., Cathey, W. J., Cartwright, G. E., and Wintrobe, M. M. (1969): Pulmonary disease complicating intermittent therapy with methotrexate. *JAMA,* 209:1861–1864.
18. Codling, B. W., and Chakera, T. M. H. (1972): Pulmonary fibrosis following therapy with melphalan for multiple myeloma. *J. Clin. Pathol.,* 25:668.
19. Cole, S. R., Myers, T. J., and Klatsky, A. U. (1978): Pulmonary disease with chlorambucil therapy. *Cancer,* 41:455.
20. Comis, R. L., Ginsberg, S. J., Kuppinger, M., et al. (1977): Effects of bleomycin on carbon monoxide diffusion capacity in patients with testicular carcinomas. *Curr. Chemother.,* 2:1135–1137.
21. Crittenden, D., Tranum, B. L., and Haut, A. (1977): Pulmonary fibrosis after prolonged therapy with 1,3-bis-(2-chloro-ethyl)-1-nitrosourea. *Chest,* 72:372.
22. Daskal, Y., Gyorkey, F., Gyorkey, P., et al. (1976): Ultrastructural study of pulmonary bleomycin toxicity. *Cancer Res.,* 36:1267–1272.
23. DeLena, M., Guzzon, A., Monfardini, S., et al. (1972): Clinical, radiologic, and histopathologic studies on pulmonary toxicity induced by treatment with bleomycin (NSC-125066). *Cancer Chemother. Rep.,* 56:343.
24. Dohner, V. A., Ward, H. P., and Stanford, R. E. (1972): Alveolitis during procarbazine, vincristine and cyclophosphamide therapy. *Chest,* 62:636.
25. Durant, J. R., Norgard, M. J., Murad, T. M., et al. (1979): Pulmonary toxicity associated with bischloroethylnitrosourea (BCNU). *Ann. Intern. Med.,* 90:191.
26. Everts, C. S., Westcott, J. L., and Bragg, D. C. (1973): Methotrexate therapy and pulmonary disease. *Radiology,* 107:539–543.
27. Farney, R. J., Morris, A. H., and Armstrong, J. D. (1977): Diffuse pulmonary disease after therapy with nitrogen mustard, vincristine, procarbazine, and prednisone. *Am. Rev. Respir. Dis.,* 115:135.
28. Fielding, J. W. L., Stockley, R. A., and Brookes, V. S. (1978): Interstitial lung disease in a patient treated with 5-fluorouracil and mitomycin C. *Br. Med. J.,* 2:602.
29. Franklin, R., Buroker, T. R., Vaishampayan, G. V., et al. (1979): Combined therapies in esophageal squamous cell cancer. *Proc. Am. Assoc. Cancer Res.,* 20:223.
30. Friedman, M. S., and Slater, E. (1978): Malignant pleural effusions. *Cancer Treat. Rev.,* 5:49–66.
31. Goldiner, P. L., Carlon, G. C., Cvitkovic, E., et al. (1978): Factors influencing postoperative morbidity and mortality in patients treated with bleomycin. *Br. Med. J.,* 1:1664.
32. Goldiner, P. L., and Schweizer, O. (1979): The hazards of anesthesia and surgery in bleomycin-treated patients. *Semin. Oncol.,* 6:121–124.
33. Greenman, R. L., Goodall, P. T., and King, D. (1975): Lung biopsy in immunocompromised hosts. *Am. J. Med.,* 59:488–496.
34. Griffin, T. W., Comis, R. L., Lokich, J. J., et al. (1978): Phase I and preliminary phase II study of neocarzinostatin. *Cancer Treat. Rep.,* 62:2019.
35. Gross, N. J. (1977): Pulmonary effects of radiation therapy. *Ann. Intern. Med.,* 86:81–92.
36. Gutin, P. H., Green, M. R., Bleyer, W. A., et al. (1976): Methotrexate pneumonitis induced by intrathecal methotrexate therapy: A case report with pharmacokinetic data. *Cancer,* 38:1529.
37. Holoye, P. Y., Jenkins, D. E., and Greenberg, S. D. (1976): Pulmonary toxicity in long-term administration of BCNU. *Cancer Treat. Rep.,* 60:1691.

38. Horowitz, A. L., Friedman, M., Sikand, R. S., et al. (1973): The pulmonary changes of bleomycin toxicity. *Radiology,* 106:65–68.
39. Horton, L. W. L., Chappell, A. G., and Powell, D. E. B. (1977): Diffuse interstitial pulmonary fibrosis complicating Hodgkin's disease. *Br. J. Dis. Chest,* 71:44.
40. Iacovino, J. R., Leitner, J., Abbas, A. K., et al. (1976): Fatal pulmonary reaction from low doses of bleomycin. *JAMA,* 235:1253–1255.
41. Iriarte, P. V., Hananian, J., and Cortner, J. A. (1966): Central nervous system leukemia and solid tumors of childhood: Treatment with 1,3-bis-(2-chlorethyl)-1-nitrosourea (BCNU). *Cancer,* 19:1187.
42. Jones, S. E., Moore, M., Blank, N., et al. (1972): Hypersensitivity to procarbazine (Matulane ®) manifested by fever and pleuropulmonary reaction. *Cancer,* 29:498.
43. Kessinger, A., Lemon, H. M., and Foley, J. F. (1978): Sequential and adjuvant chemotherapy for malignant astrocytoma of the brain. *J. Surg. Oncol.,* 10:543.
44. Kodama, T., Shimosato, Y., Nishiwabi, Y., and Suzuki, A. (1976): Clinicopathologic study of pulmonary lesions induced by antitumor drugs. *Gan To Kazaku Ryoho,* 3:653–661.
45. Koss, L. G., Melamed, M. R., and Mayer, K. (1965): The effect of busulfan on human epithelia. *Am. J. Clin. Pathol.,* 44:385–397.
46. Krauss, S., Sonoda, T., and Solomon, A. (1979): Treatment of advanced gastrointestinal cancer with 5-fluorouracil and mitomycin C. *Cancer,* 43:1598.
47. Lane, S. D., Besa, E. C., Justh, G., et al. (1979): Fatal interstitial lung disease following high dose chlorambucil therapy. *Proc. Am. Soc. Clin. Oncol.,* 20:313.
48. Lascari, A. D., Strano, A. J., Johnson, W. W., et al. (1977): Methotrexate-induced sudden fatal pulmonary reaction. *Cancer,* 40:1393.
49. Lee, W., Moore, R. P., and Wampler, G. L. (1978): Interstitial pulmonary fibrosis as a complication of prolonged methyl-CCNU therapy. *Cancer Treat. Rep.,* 62:1355.
50. Leff, A., Hopewell, P. C., and Costello, J. (1978): Pleural effusions from malignancy. *Ann. Intern. Med.,* 88:532–537.
51. Libshitz, H. I., Brosof, A. B., and Southard, M. E. (1973): Radiographic appearance of the chest following extended field radiation therapy for Hodgkin's disease. *Cancer,* 32:206–215.
52. Lokich, J. J., and Maloney, W. C. (1972): Allergic reaction to procarbazine. *Clin. Pharmacol. Ther.,* 13:573.
53. Luna, M. A., Bedrossian, C. W., Lichtiger, B., et al. (1972): Interstitial pneumonitis associated with bleomycin therapy. *Am. J. Clin. Pathol.,* 58:501–510.
54. Mark, G. J., Lehimgar-Zadeh, A., and Ragsdale, B. D. (1978): Cyclophosphamide pneumonitis. *Thorax,* 33:89–93.
55. Martino, S., Baker, L. H., Pollard, R. J., et al. (1979): Pulmonary toxicity of mitomycin. In: *Mitomycin,* edited by S. K. Carter and S. T. Crooke, p. 233. Academic Press, New York.
56. Matsuda, A., Yoshioka, O., Yamashita, T., et al. (1978): Fundamental and clinical studies on new bleomycin analogs. *Recent Results Cancer Res.,* 63:191.
57. Matthay, R. A., Farmer, W. C., and Odero, D. (1977): Diagnostic fibreoptic bronchoscopy in the immunocompromised host with pulmonary infiltrates. *Thorax,* 32:539–545.
58. Morrison, A., and Goldman, A. (1979): Radiologic patterns of drug-induced lung disease. *Radiology,* 131:299–304.
59. Natale, R., and Yagoda, A. (1979): Phase II trial of neocarzinostatin (NCS) in bladder and prostatic cancer. *Proc. Am. Assoc. Cancer Res.,* 20:116.
60. Orwoll, E. S., Kiessling, P. J., and Patterson, J. R. (1978): Interstitial pneumonia from mitomycin. *Ann. Intern. Med.,* 89:352.
61. Pascual, R. S., Mosher, M. B., Sikand, R. S., et al. (1973): Effects of bleomycin on pulmonary function in man. *Am. Rev. Respir. Dis.,* 108:211–217.
62. Pasquinucci, G., Ferrara, P., and Castellari, R. (1971): Daunorubicin treatment of methotrexate pneumonia. (Letter). *JAMA,* 216:2017.
63. Patel, A. R., Shah, P. C., Rhee, H. L., et al. (1976): Cyclophosphamide therapy and interstitial pulmonary fibrosis. *Cancer,* 38:1542.
64. Refvem, O. (1977): Fatal intraalveolar and interstitial lung fibrosis in chlorambucil-treated chronic lymphocytic leukemia. *Mt. Sinai J. Med. NY,* 44:847.
65. Richman, S. D., Levenson, S. M., Bunn, P. A., et al. (1975): ^{67}Ga accumulation in pulmonary lesions associated with bleomycin therapy. *Cancer,* 36:1966–1972.
66. Richter, J. E., Hastedt, R., Dalton, J. F., et al. (1979): Pulmonary toxicity of bischloronitrosourea: Report of a case with transient response to corticosteroid therapy. *Cancer,* 43:1607.

67. Rose, M. S. (1975): Busulphan toxicity syndrome caused by chlorambucil. *Br. Med. J.,* 2:123.
68. Rosenow, E. C. (1972): The spectrum of drug-induced pulmonary disease. *Ann. Intern. Med.,* 77:977–991.
69. Rubin, G., Baume, P., and Vandenberg, R. (1972): Azathioprine and acute restrictive lung disease. *Aust. NZ J. Med.,* 3:272–274.
70. Rubio, F. A. (1972): Possible pulmonary effects of alkylating agents. *N. Engl. J. Med.,* 287:1150.
71. Samson, M. K., Comis, R. L., Baker, L. H., et al. (1978): Mitomycin C in advanced adenocarcinoma and large cell carcinoma of the lung. *Cancer Treat. Rep.,* 62:163.
72. Samuels, M. L., Johnson, D. E., Holoye, P. Y., et al. (1976): Large-dose bleomycin therapy and pulmonary toxicity: A possible role of prior radiotherapy. *JAMA,* 235:1117.
73. Schein, P. S., DeVita, V. T., Jr., Hubbard, S., et al. (1976): Bleomycin, adriamycin, cyclophosphamide, vincristine, and prednisone (BACOP) combination chemotherapy in the treatment of advanced histiocytic lymphoma. *Ann. Intern. Med.,* 85:417–422.
74. Schein, P. S., and Winokur, S. H. (1975): Immunosuppressive and cytotoxic chemotherapy: Long term complications. *Ann. Intern. Med.,* 82:84–95.
75. Schreml, W., Bargon, G., Anger, B., et al. (1978): Progressive pulmonary fibrosis during combination chemotherapy with BCNU. *Blut,* 36:353.
76. Selker, R. G., Jacobs, S. A., and Moore, P. (1978): Interstitial pulmonary fibrosis as a complication of 1,3-bis-(2-chloroethyl)-1-nitrosourea (BCNU) therapy. *Proc. Am. Soc. Clin. Oncol.,* 19:333.
77. Seltzer, S. E., Griffin, T., D'Orsi, C., et al. (1978): Pulmonary reaction associated with neocarzinostatin therapy. *Cancer Treat. Rep.,* 62:1271.
78. Sikic, B. I., Siddik, Z. H., and Gram, T. E. (1979): Relative pulmonary toxicity and antitumor effects of two new bleomycin analogs, pepleomycin and tallisomycin A. *Proc. Am. Assoc. Cancer Res.,* 20:182.
79. Sostman, H. D., Matthay, R. A., and Putman, C. E. (1977): Cytotoxic drug-induced lung disease. *Am. J. Med.,* 62:608.
80. Sostman, H. D., Matthay, R. A., Putman, C. E., et al. (1976): Methotrexate-induced pneumonitis. *Medicine,* 55:371–388.
81. Taetle, R., Dickman, P. S., and Feldman, P. S. (1978): Pulmonary histopathologic changes associated with melphalan therapy. *Cancer,* 42:1239.
82. Tamanaka, N., Fukushuma, M., Roizumi, K., Nishido, K., Kato, F., and Ota, K. (1978): Enhancement of DNA chain breakage by bleomycin and biological free radical producing systems. In: *Tocopherol, Oxygen, and Biomembranes,* edited by C. deDuve and O. Hayaishi, pp. 59–69. Elsevier/North-Holland, New York.
83. Vernant, J. P., Brun, B., Mannoni, P., and Dreyfus, B. (1979): Respiratory distress of hyperleukocytic granulocytic leukemias. *Cancer,* 44:264–268.
84. Weiss, R. B., Shah, S., and Shane, S. R. (1979): Pulmonary toxicity from carmustine (BCNU). *Med. Pediatr. Oncol.,* 6:255.
85. Yagoda, A., Mukherji, B., Young, C., et al. (1972): Bleomycin, an antitumor antibiotic: Clinical experience in 274 patients. *Ann. Intern. Med.,* 77:861–870.
86. Zusman, J., Frentz, J., and Waring, W. (1979): Rapid resolution of "methotrexate lung" (ML) with preoperative steroids. *Proc. Am. soc. Clin. Oncol.,* 20:412.

Medical Complications in Cancer Patients,
edited by J. Klastersky and M. J. Staquet.
Raven Press, New York © 1981.

Cutaneous Complications in Cancer Patients

J. Klastersky and R. De Jager

Medical Service and Henri Tagnon Laboratory of Clinical Investigation, Jules Bordet Institute, Free University of Brussels, 1000 Brussels, Belgium

In patients with cancer, dermatologic manifestations may present as primary or metastastic neoplastic involvement of the skin, distant effects associated with internal malignancies without malignant cells identified in the skin, infections secondary to the disease itself or its treatment, and cutaneous toxicity of radiation and chemotherapy (5,19). These four aspects are discussed in the present review.

NEOPLASTIC LESIONS OF THE SKIN

Primary skin cancers of epidermal origin (basal cell carcinoma, squamous cell carcinoma) may occur under the influence of known carcinogens [e.g., ionizing radiation, ultraviolet (UV) light, immunosuppressive drugs, arsenic] or genetic factors found in such diseases as xeroderma pigmentosum or basal cell nevus syndrome. They are often multicentric and recurrent. In contrast to these tumors, malignant melanomas, primary skin lymphomas (mycosis fungoïdes, Sézary syndrome), or sarcomas (Kaposi sarcoma) do metastasize widely to involve, at times, the entire body surface as well as internal organs. An analysis of primary skin cancers is beyond the scope of this review.

The true incidence of skin metastases from solid tumors is difficult to evaluate from published clinical or autopsy studies. Whereas metastases from malignant melanoma (63% of 164 patients in a clinical study) and breast carcinoma (35% of 71 autopsies) (33) are frequent, other primary tumors rarely metastasize to the skin (3.3% of 2,992 patients seen in a Department of Radiation Therapy). Among the primary cancers whose metastases were found in the skin were carcinomas of the kidney (6.3%), colon (3.5%), lung (3.1%), ovary (1.9%), bladder (1.8%), esophagus (1.6%), and cervix (0.6%) (3).

This was a highly selected sample, however, and probably does not reflect the true incidence of skin metastases, which is likely higher for lung cancer and intra-abdominal malignancies, especially ovarian carcinoma. Thoracotomy and laparotomy scars are frequently the site of metastases and represent iatrogenic dissemination of the neoplastic disease. Metastases to the skin occur through lymphatic or hematogenous spread. They present as single or multiple lesions often located in one area of the body. The scalp is often involved with metastases from breast cancer presenting as tumor nodules or circular areas of baldness mimicking alopecia areata or cicatrices; in this case, the carcinoma cells infiltrating the scalp are surrounded by a fibrotic reaction probably responsible for the disappearance of the hair follicles (30). The scalp is less frequently involved with metastases from lung, colon, bladder carcinomas, and lymphomas. The head and neck area may be the site of a solitary metastasis from renal carcinoma. The chest wall and back may be involved with metastases from breast, lung, and esophagus. More rarely, metastases from extrathoracic primary tumors are encountered (ovary, bladder, cervix). Their diagnosis offers little difficulty. The abdominal wall is mainly involved with metastases from intra-abdominal tumors (ovary, stomach, colon, pancreas). Worth emphasizing are umbilical metastases (Sister Joseph's sign) and those appearing at the site of puncture of malignant ascites (3). Skin metastases often do not raise diagnostic problems because of their appearance (malignant melanoma) or location (mastectomy scar). However, their aspect is not always characteristic when they are presenting as nonspecific papules, nodules, or plaques: They may occur at a distance from the primary site or be the first sign of the disease. In those circumstances, a needle or excision biopsy allows comparison of the pathology of the primary tumor and the skin metastasis or establishes the first diagnosis of malignant disease.

In the case of metastatic breast carcinoma determination of the hormone receptor level in the excised skin lesion can help establish the hormonal sensitivity of the tumor and orient further treatment selection.

Skin metastases are often easily measured or evaluated, and their size should be used and recorded as criteria of evaluation of treatment. Their presence reflects the advanced stage of the disease, but their impact on life expectancy is not as determinant as visceral lesions are. They may be a source of major discomfort to the patient however, because when they grow in size they tend to become exophytic, ulcerated, infected, and can bleed. These complications call for appropriate local palliative measures such as excision or radiation in addition to systemic treatment. Lymphatic spread through the dermis in breast cancer can result in a pseudocellulitis (inflammatory carcinoma) or, when associated with fibrosis, in a sclerosing cast on the chest wall (cancer en cuirasse). A similar pattern of spread can be observed in malignant melanoma. Lymphangiosarcoma of the arm is seen in 0.45% of women who undergo mastectomy; it is a late lethal complication of postmastectomy lymphedema.

DERMATOLOGIC EFFECTS OF CANCER

There are numerous cutaneous manifestations associated with internal malignancies (25). In most of these there is no real understanding of their pathogenesis. Some are very suggestive of the presence of an internal cancer, but most of the cutaneous changes can be seen in benign conditions as well. The relationship between the cutaneous manifestations and the malignant disease is based on the observation that they can regress when the cancer is adequately eradicated and recur when the neoplasia recurs. It should be mentioned also that the skin manifestations may also antedate or follow the diagnosis of malignancy. Some of these manifestations, of which the relationship to cancer is well recognized, are discussed briefly here.

Pruritus is a relatively common problem in patients with lymphoma, especially Hodgkin's disease. It is said to occur in 5% of these patients. It can be localized, but more often it is generalized; it is variably severe and not often constant; it can be increased by the absorption of alcohol. Usually, no skin lesions are detectable at the same time except for excoriations, but occasionally acquired ichthyosis is present, especially in Hodgkin's disease. Patients with Hodgkin's disease, in whom severe itching was a major clinical problem, when compared with similarly treated patients without pruritus appeared to have a more aggressive disease. Severe itching, alone or with B symptoms, needs further study as it may presage a poor prognosis in patients with Hodgkin's disease. Pruritus associated with cancer is often refractory to the usual symptomatic measures; it is often relieved by successful treatment of the underlying malignancy.

Acanthosis nigricans is often associated with adenocarcinoma arising in the abdomen or pelvis. It is a symmetrical hyperplasia of the skin with hyperpigmentation varying from brown to black; the lesions predominate in the body folds. Occasionally pruritus and hyperkeratosis of the palms and soles is present. Acanthosis nigricans can be a manifestation of many benign diseases, either idiopathic or associated with endocrine disease or drug ingestion.

Increased pigmentation (melanosis), either localized or generalized, is rarely observed in association with carcinoma or lymphoma; usually the mechanism remains obscure except when melanocyte-stimulating hormone or another hormone capable of stimulating melanocytes can be demonstrated. This is the case in some ACTH-producing tumors such as anaplastic small cell carcinoma of the lung.

Carcinoïd tumors can be responsible for erythema, or a red flushing, involving usually the face, neck, and upper trunk. After many episodes of flushing, permanent skin lesions may develop with cyanosis and telangectasia, giving the patient a plethoric appearance; a similar skin appearance can be seen in polycythemia.

Localized erythema, often associated with pain, can be indicative of thrombophlebitis. Migratory superficial thrombophlebitis, which is often refractory to therapy, can be an early manifestation of carcinoma of the lung, stomach, ovary, or pancreas. These tumors may be also associated with deep venous thromboses, sometimes in such atypical sites as the neck, chest, or pelvis.

Vasculitis may be the consequence of cryoglobulinemia or macroglobulinemia associated with lymphoma or myeloma. Immunoblastic lymphadenopathy, an immunoproliferative disorder of mixed-cell type has been reported in patients with hypocomplementemia and vasculitis, some of whom had cryoglobulinemia. As a manifestation of the vasculitis, cold urticaria, acral cyanosis, and gangrene may result. In those cases the vasculitis is the result of an immune-complex disease in which the complexes cause the vascular lesions. The pathogenic mechanism is probably similar to that of vasculitis resulting from infections such as hepatitis, subacute bacterial endocarditis, or infectious mononucleosis. That cancer can be responsible for immunologically mediated disease as exemplified by the occurrence of cancer-associated immune nephritis; in some cases antigens derived from the tumor have been found within the renal lesions.

Dermatomyositis is often (15 to 50%) associated with internal malignancy in patients over 40 years of age. It is a disorder of the skin, muscles, and blood vessels. Erythema and edema of the skin of the face are characteristic, as is painful and tender myositis; these lesions usually follow the course of the neoplasia as the skin changes often correlate with the results of therapy of the tumor, which is usually a carcinoma. The disease usually starts insidiously as a weakness in proximal muscles that progresses out of proportion to the loss of muscle bulk. Muscular pain and the skin rash may or may not be present at the onset of the disease. Dysphagia, secondary to the weakness of pharyngeal muscles, arthralgias, and Raynaud's phenomenon may be observed in some patients.

Amyloidosis can be associated with neoplastic diseases such as myeloma or lymphoma. It may cause macroglossia, purpura, and papular or/and nodular lesions of the skin. Bleeding occurs readily because amyloid is deposited in the vessel walls, as well as focally within the dermis. It was reported recently that skin biopsy, even in uninvolved areas, represents a valuable diagnostic approach for amyloidosis.

Plantar xanthomas are lesions seen in association with lipoprotein–paraprotein complexes principally in patients with multiple myeloma but also in those with lymphoma and leukemia (36).

A few specific dermatologic diseases are specifically associated with the presence of a malignant tumor. Among them are Bowen's disease and Paget's disease of the breast (pathognomonic of intraductal carcinoma of the breast).

Skin lesions and malignant diseases are also associated with various genetic disorders (20), the most important of which are summarized in Table 1. Another example of an association between skin lesions and cancer is the clubbing of digits, and osteoarthropathy, which can be associated with pachydermoperiostosis; these lesions are seen chiefly in patients with lung cancer.

SKIN INFECTIONS IN CANCER PATIENTS

Myelosuppression and immunosuppression are extremely frequent in cancer patients. They may be due to the malignant disease itself, especially in patients with leukemia, lymphoma, and myeloma. More often, alterations of the patient's natural defenses against infection are the consequence of myelotoxic or/and immunosuppressive chemotherapy.

Myelosuppression or immunosuppression predisposes to a quite different spec-

TABLE 1. Genetic disorders associated with skin manifestations and cancer

Disease	Type of inheritance[a]	Associated cancer	Clinical manifestation
Basal cell nevus syndrome	AD	Basal cell carcinoma, medulloblastoma, astrocytoma, ameloblastoma, ovarian cancer	Multiple basal cell carcinomas, multiple somatic abnormalities
Giant cell hairy nevus	AD	Malignant carcinoma	Congenital nevus
Hemochromatosis	AD	Hepatoma	Hyperpigmentation, cirrhosis, diabetes, cardiac failure
Kaposi's sarcoma	AD	Lymphoma, leukemia, multiple myeloma	
Palmar and plantar keratosis	AD	Esophageal cancer	
Neurofibromatosis (von Recklinghausen's disease)	AD	Neurofibrosarcoma, meningioma, pheochromocytoma	Café au lait spots
MEA-IIB	AD	Pheochromocytoma, medullary carcinoma of thyroid	Café au lait spots
Extramammary Paget's disease	AD	Rectal adenocarcinoma	Eczematous rash (genital region)
Intestinal polyposis (Peutz-Jeghers' syndrome)	AD	Malignant gastrointestinal polyps, granulosa cell tumor of ovaries	Perioral hyperpigmentation
Intestinal polyposis (Gardner's syndrome)	AD	Malignant degeneration of colon, adenomatous polyps	Osteomas
Neuroblastoma	AD	Ganglioneuroma, neuroblastoma, pheochromocytoma	Café au lait spots
Albinism	AR	Skin	Hyperpigmentation
Turcot's syndrome	AR	Malignant CNS tumors, malignant polyposis	Café au lait spots
Xeroderma pigmentosum	AR	Basal cell and squamous cell carcinomas	Photosensitivity, DNA repair deficiency to UV light

[a] AD, autosomal dominant; AR, autosomal recessive.

trum of infectious diseases; in myelosuppressed patients, neutropenia predisposes to bacterial infections, especially by Gram-negative rods, whereas in immunodepressed people fungal and viral infections are more frequent. Under both circumstances, skin infections are fairly common either as the source of sepsis or as a consequence of widespread seeding with blood-borne septic emboli originating from an extracutaneous focus. In patients with lymphoma or acute leukemia, especially when neutropenia is present, skin infections are frequent. In a group of patients with malignant lymphoma, skin infections represented 17% of the total number of serious infections. Half of these infections were of bacterial origin and half were viral, most often caused by herpes zoster (6). In neutropenic leukemia patients skin and soft tissues represented 14% of the infectious sites, and 39% of these infections were recognized as a source of bacteremia. In addition, 10% of these neutropenic patients had an infection of the perirectal region (30). Most of these skin infections in granulocytopenic patients are caused by bacteria, i.e., Gram-negative bacilli. Generally, these Gram-negative rods are *Pseudomonas aeruginosa, Klebsiella* sp., *Serratia* sp., *Enterobacter* sp., *Proteus* sp., and *Escherichia coli.* These microorganisms are acquired from the hospital environment; although these bacteria are relatively nonpathogenic in normal people, they can turn into aggressive pathogens in a compromised host.

A typical skin infection encountered in neutropenic patients is ecthyma gangrenosum, caused by *Ps. aeruginosa.* It is a necrotic lesion surrounded by an erythematous halo, and it is almost pathognomonic of *Ps. aeruginosa* septicemia. Differential diagnosis includes pyoderma gangrenosum, which can be seen in leukemics as well and which is the end result of a vasculitic process. Lesions similar to ecthyma gangrenosum can be observed in infections caused by Enterobacteriaceae; however, these skin infections are usually more extensive, progressing in a widening circle with the center becoming necrotic. From the therapeutic point of view, it should be stressed that bacterial cellulitis in neutropenic patients usually carries a poor prognosis. When neutropenia is severe, granulocyte transfusions are probably indicated in addition to broad-spectrum antibiotics if the lesions are progressing.

As already mentioned, perianal abscesses are particularly frequent in neutropenic patients; these abscesses are often less well characterized clinically than similar lesions in nonneutropenics; usually they present as an extensive and necrotic cellulitis. These lesions are a relatively common problem in neutropenic patients with acute monocytic and myelomonocytic leukemias. These infections usually occur during periods of pronounced granulocytopenia, and *Ps. aeruginosa* can often be cultured from the skin lesions. Septicemia is associated with perianal cellulitis in more than 50% of neutropenic patients. Thus the rectum should be considered as a possible site of infection in all febrile granulocytopenic patients with hematological malignancies, especially when rectal pain is present (29,31). There has been some suggestion that radiation therapy to these lesions might be helpful. Levi and co-workers (18) performed a double-blind randomized trial in which 17 of 35 episodes of localized inflammatory skin and perianal lesions received 400 rads of megavoltage irradiation in addition to intensive supportive care. Overall 65% of the irradiated infections and 44% of the nonirradiated lesions responded completely, a difference which was not statistically significant (18).

Fungal infections can be a problem in neutropenic patients: Aspergillosis, candidiasis, cryptococcosis, and mucormycosis can be associated with skin lesions during fungemia. These lesions are usually eroded, gangrenous, nonsuppurating ulcerations which are often deeply penetrating and sharply demarcated (2).

Disseminated cryptococcosis can present as palpable purpura due in fact to vasculitis (10). A similar presentation, as indurated skin nodules due to vasculitis, has been described in mucormycosis (23). Characteristic macronodular skin lesions develop in about 10% of the patients with disseminated candidiasis and *Candida* septicemia. *Aspergillus* skin lesions are not frequent; they can be primary inoculation sites or secondary foci that appear during disseminated disease. They present as cutaneous or subcutaneous abscesses and maculopapular lesions which progress to pustulation containing greenish-yellow purulent material. The hallmark of most *Aspergillus* infections is tissue and vascular invasion with thrombosis, infarction, and hemorrhage. In patients at high risk from fungal infections, the appearance of clinical manifestations of multiple thromboses should alert the physician to the possibility of aspergillosis (24,43). These fungal infections must be diagnosed specifically for the offending pathogen; usually demonstration of fungemia or evidence of fungal invasion on biopsy specimens from the lesion is needed. Therapy is best carried out with amphotericin B; the success rate is usually related to early antifungal therapy and to the remission of the underlying malignancy through adequate chemotherapy.

In immunosuppressed patients, mycotic infections present as more chronic disease; in cryptococcosis and chronic mucocutaneous candidiasis, skin involvement may occur. Once again, biopsy of the lesion rather than culture is diagnostic.

Also encountered in immunosuppressed patients are the opportunistic viral infections; cutaneous involvement is fairly common in herpes simplex and herpes zoster infections. Herpes simplex infections consist of vesicular lesions on an erythematous base which usually progress toward healing, even if they are fairly extensive. The cutaneous lesions in herpes zoster have a dermatomal distribution; they begin as crops of papulovesicles on a red base and progress to maculopapular plaques. Pain is often a presenting symptom and may persist after the cutaneous lesions heal. In severely immunosuppressed patients, herpes zoster lesions can coexist with varicella-type lesions. Although clinical herpes zoster is usually considered the result of a reactivation of latent viruses present in the host, there is some evidence that it may also, under special circumstances, be an acquired disease (9,27,28).

In immunosuppressed children who have not yet experienced varicella, prevention of the disease with hyperimmune globulins is indicated after contact with a person who has herpes zoster or varicella (7). Similarly, prevention might be indicated in some adult patients at high risk when exposed to active cases.

Therapy is rarely necessary; although not highly fatal, varicella–zoster infections are more severe in cancer patients than in the general population or in patients who have completed therapy. Human leukocyte interferon has been used recently for the treatment of herpes zoster and varicella in patients with cancer: Complications of varicella occurred more often in the placebo recipients, and patients with herpes zoster who were treated had a tendency toward less severe postherpetic neuralgia; visceral complications were six times less frequent in interferon recipients. Thus high-dosage interferon appears to be effective in limiting cutaneous dissemination, visceral complications, and progression of herpetic lesions within the primary dermatoma (1,22). Recent studies suggest that adenine arabinoside significantly shortens the course of herpes zoster infection in immunocompromised patients and lessens the morbidity associated with pain. It is most effective when administered during the first 6 days of disease and in patients who are less than 38 years old. Adenine arabinoside has also proved itself an effective therapy in herpes simplex encephalitis; there is a possibility that it might be useful in disseminated herpes simplex infections, although most of these have a spontaneously favorable course (21,40).

Other viral infections with cutaneous involvement appear not to occur more frequently in compromised patients than in a normal population.

CUTANEOUS COMPLICATIONS OF CANCER CHEMOTHERAPY

Tissues with replication rates comparable to those of malignant tumors (bone marrow, gastrointestinal mucosa, hair follicles) are particularly prone to damage by chemotherapeutic agents. (See Table 2 for an outline of these agents.) Buccal mucosa and to a lesser extent the skin are frequent targets for adverse effects of cytostatic drugs. In addition to the untoward effects related to interference of these compounds with cell proliferation, the skin also manifests a response to sensitization or direct toxic action of these aggressive medications. Finally, some cytostatic drugs (e.g., bleomycin) have very specific adverse effects on the skin. These various aspects are reviewed here.

The major cutaneous manifestations of toxicity from cancer chemotherapy are alopecia, cellulitis, hyperpigmentation, and hemorrhage.

Alopecia occurs with most chemotherapeutic agents currently in use except maybe procarbazine, the nitrosoureas, and L-asparaginase. The most frequent site of chemotherapy-caused hair loss is the scalp, although axillary, pubic, and facial hair may be lost as well with high-dose and prolonged therapy (26). Many cytostatic agents are extremely toxic for living cells by direct contact; extravasation of these products from vein into surrounding subcutaneous tissues can cause severe cellulitis and necrosis. Secondary superinfection is then a frequent complication. Therefore these drugs should be administered very carefully into the tubing of a running intravenous infusion set to avoid escape into the perivenous tissues. Hyperpigmentation with or without dermatitis has been re-

TABLE 2. *Summary of major cutaneous reactions associated with cancer chemotherapy*

Chemotherapy	Alopecia	Dermatitis, rash, or urticaria	Pigmentation	Local cellulitis	Other
Alkylating agents					
Busulfan	+		++		
Chlorambucil					
Cyclophosphamide	+++		+		Mucositis +
Nitrogen mustard	++		+	++	
Melphalan					
Triethylenethio- phosphoramide					
Antimetabolites					
Cytosine arabinoside	+				
5-Fluorouracil	+	+	+		Stomatitis
6-Mercaptopurine			+		
Methotrexate	+	+	+		Mucositis +++
6-Thioguanine					
Antibiotics					
Adriamycin	+++	+[a]	+	+	Mucositis
Daunomycin	++	+[a]	+	+	Mucositis
Bleomycin	+	+++	+		Mucositis
Dactinomycin		+[a]	+		Muscositis
Mithramycin					
Mitomycin C	+			+	
Plant alkaloids					
Vinblastine	+			+	
Vincristine	+			+	
VP 16-213					
VM 26					
Miscellaneous					
Nitrosoureas		+			
L-Asparaginase		+			
Dacarbazine	+			+	
Hydroxyurea		++			
Procarbazine		+	+		
Cis-platinum					
Methyl GAG					
Mitotane		++			
Neocarzinostatin					
Peptichemio					
Hormones					
Corticoids					Skin atrophy
Androgens	+				
Estrogens			+		
Progesterone					
Tamoxifen					

[a] Radiosensitizing.

ported with busulfan, cyclophosphamide, and adriamycin. The folic acid antagonists methotrexate and Baker's antifol can photosensitize the skin and cause
an exaggerated sunburn-like reaction followed by brownish pigmentation. Bleeding into the skin is usually associated with thrombocytopenia; petechiae and
ecchymoses are frequent manifestations in patients who have platelet counts
below 20,000/mm^3. Of course, bleeding into the skin is not specific for chemotherapy-induced thrombocytopenia; it may be a manifestation of other coagulation problems, e.g., disseminated intravascular coagulopathy, which is often
found in cancer patients. Thrombocytopenia that is not associated with intravascular coagulation is best treated by transfusions of fresh platelets; heparin may
be needed when intravascular coagulation is present, although in most cases
the phenomenon is self-limiting.

Alkylating Agents

Alkylating agents administered systemically have no major mucosal or cutaneous toxicity.

Cyclophosphamide administration frequently results in alopecia. In some series
it is reported as frequently as in 50% of the patients; its frequency increases
with increasing dosage. It is sometimes reversible despite continued treatment
with the drug, and it is usually reversible when cyclophosphamide therapy is
discontinued. Urticaria is occasionally reported; in such cases chlorambucil,
another alkylating agent, can be substituted without cross-sensitivity being noted.
Transverse ridging of nails or teeth and skin hyperpigmentation are rarely reported with cyclophosphamide. Stomatitis does not occur in more than 10%
of the patients and in some series does not occur at all (8).

Chlorambucil and melphalan are very rarely associated with skin toxicity.
A few cases of maculopapular rashes have been reported, sometimes requiring
discontinuation of therapy. Alopecia has not been a problem with those drugs,
especially with chlorambucil.

Cutaneous side effects of triethylene thiophosphoramide (thiotepa) are also
very rare. A few reactions characterized by fever, urticaria, and pruritus have
been reported; and several cases of depigmentation around the eyes after intraocu-
lar instillation of thiotepa have been observed, some of which progressed and
persisted after discontinuation of the chemotherapy.

Nitrogen mustard is a potent local irritant if injected subcutaneously, but
systemic administration of mechlorethamine has only rare skin effects. Topical
application of mechlorethamine, which is sometimes used in the treatment of
psoriasis or mycosis fungoides, often produces cutaneous side effects; primary
irritant dermatitis, which occurs within the first weeks of therapy, can disappear
despite continued drug use. Allergic contact dermatitis occurs in one-third to
one half of the patients treated with topical mechlorethamine; it is characterized
by pruritus with or without eczema; it can appear early or late during therapy.
These skin reactions, when present, manifest within 24 to 48 hr after a treatment.

Hyperpigmentation, which seems to be reversible after discontinuation of therapy, is more pronounced in patients with a higher degree of pigmentation.

Busulfan administration affects epithelia and especially the skin. Hyperpigmentation can be observed and may mimic a syndrome of adrenal insufficiency, although it is usually not accompanied by objective evidence of adrenal hypofunction (38). The exact incidence of this form of toxicity is difficult to evaluate since most reports are single case presentations. No correlation exists between the development of these side effects and age, sex, clinical condition, or total busulfan dose or duration of therapy. Rare hypersensitivity reactions have been reported with busulfan.

Antimetabolites

Folate antagonists cause redness and ulceration of mucosal tissue, chiefly buccal but also nasal and conjunctival. The adverse effects appear 2 to 7 days after administration of methotrexate. The degree of mucositis is a function of drug dose and duration of administration, and therapy should be discontinued at the first signs of it. Different dose schedules and route of administration are associated with a varying incidence and severity of mucositis. Patients treated with low-dose methotrexate therapy for psoriasis only rarely develop mouth ulcers, whereas patients receiving high-dose methotrexate therapy, even when given folinic acid rescue, have a high frequency of this complication (16,37).

Skin rash is observed in about 20% of patients treated with therapeutic methotrexate doses; its incidence increases with other signs of toxicity. The rash is usually maculopapular and most often involves the upper trunk and neck, although it can spread elsewhere. The severity of the rash is related to other signs and symptoms of toxicity. It appears usually after 1 to 3 days of treatment with methotrexate and is occasionally pruritic. Mucocutaneous toxicity of Baker's antifol (triazinate) is fairly common and consists of dermatitis and stomatitis; its incidence was found to be decreased by shortening the schedule of administration from 5 to 3 days. Hair loss occurs rarely with antifolate (5%) and is observed mainly in older patients and those receiving higher doses. Occasionally vasculitis or widespread herpetiform skin eruptions are observed, almost always in association with severe systemic toxicity.

Dermatologic manifestations are extremely rare after treatment with the *purine antagonists*. Although oral ulcerations have been reported in a small percentage (fewer than 5%) of patients given 6-mercaptopurine, true cutaneous toxicity seems exceptional and has not been reported for thioguanine or azathioprine. Among pyrimidine and pyrimidine nucleoside antimetabolities, 5-fluorouracil (5-FU) can cause severe stomatitis, an indication for discontinuing the therapy. The incidence of that complication in some earlier series was in the range of 50 to 70%. It increases with higher doses and with a more rapid intravenous infusion. Low-dose schedules, eliminating loading doses, are associated with severe stomatitis in less than 5% of the patients. Alopecia occurs rarely with low-dose schedules but has been reported in 20 to 50% of the patients with more intensive therapies (15,17). An interesting cutaneous side effect of systemic 5-FU is the response of actinic keratoses and other cutaneous neoplasms which react to systemic 5-FU. This response is characterized by erythema, scaling, and desquamation, often resulting in hyperpigmentation and atrophy. Sensitivity to sunlight, nail changes, dryness of the skin, and skin hyperpigmentation are also occasionally reported.

The major toxic effects observed with pyrazofurin are mucosal (erythema, erosion, and bullae). Toxic reactions are more pronounced in patients who previously received radiotherapy.

Efudex, a topical preparation of 5-FU is extremely effective in eradicating premalignant keratoses and multiple primary and superficial basal cell and squamous cell cancers. When applied to such lesions, 5-FU induces erythema, scaling, and crusting which spares the normal skin. Postinflammatory hyperpigmentation may persist for weeks or months. Irritation of the conjunctiva or lips may occur when topical 5-FU is applied in these areas. Topical administration is not associated with any serious systemic toxicity (41).

No serious cutaneous toxicity has been reported with cytosine arabinoside and 5-azacytidine except for oral inflammation or ulceration, which occurs in about 10% of the patients receiving cytosine arabinoside.

Antibiotics

Mitomycin C causes alopecia rarely. Stomatitis has been reported in about 10% of the patients but can be reduced to virtually 0% when lower individual doses are used. It is locally irritant if injected subcutaneously; it causes chronic ulcerations at the site of the perfusion.

Bleomycin is responsible for hypertrophic skin changes at sites of skin stress, e.g., elbows and hands. The lesions are slowly reversible and often result in residual pigmentation; they have no relation to pulmonary fibrosis and occur in 50 to 75% of patients. These scleroderma-like changes are dose-related and often represent dose-limiting side effects. Skin toxicity can occur as early as 5 days after the onset of bleomycin therapy, but more often a limiting toxicity is encountered with chronic biweekly administration of 15 mg/m² (32,42). Skin lesions caused by bleomycin administration consist of desquamation of hands, feet, and pressure areas; there is usually hardening and tenderness of the tips of the fingers, ridging of the nails, and occasionally bulla formation over pressure points. Hyperpigmentation may be generalized, but it more often involves skin folds, scars, and accompanying dermatoses. Occasionally a regression of this pigmentation is reported. Alopecia occurs in 10 to 75% of the patients, it usually involves the scalp and starts about 3 weeks after onset of therapy; alopecia associated with bleomycin is usually partial, and the hair grows back in most series. Mouth ulcerations occur during therapy with bleomycin in 15 to 40% of cases. Ulceration is preceded by erythema and pain, and usually occurs in patients with skin lesions. These ulcers heal fairly rapidly after discontinuation of the drug but recur when therapy is started again.

Daunomycin and adriamycin are often associated with stomatitis and alopecia. Alopecia usually develops between the third and fourth week after the initial dose. If affects almost all patients receiving adriamycin and may involve any hair-bearing area. Hair usually regrows completely within 2 to 5 months of cessation of therapy. Nail pigmentation, presumed to represent an effect of the chemotherapeutic agent in the growing nail bed, is another relatively common effect of adriamycin and daunomycin. Stomatitis is present in 3 to 30% of the patients receiving daunomycin and in 70 to 100% of those treated with adriamycin. Mucositis seems to be more frequent and more severe in patients who have liver disease and in those who are treated with doses in the range of 60 mg/M² every 3 weeks (35).

Adriamycin and daunomycin are vesicant if extravasated into subcutaneous tissues. Experimental necrosis caused by adriamycin heals more slowly than surgical wounds; the difference is due to a reduced rate of wound contraction, the cause of which is unknown. Urticaria above the site of injection with daunomycin (and occasionally a generalized urticaria) does not seem to represent a contraindication to further treatment with daunomycin provided the patient is closely observed. Increased pigmentation has been noted in patients on adriamycin therapy, especially on palms, soles, and nail beds.

Adriamycin can potentiate skin lesions induced by radiotherapy. Radiation therapy and chemotherapy that includes adriamycin can also produce severe esophageal reactions. Dermatitis in the form of a moist desquamation was observed in 5 of 10 patients receiving very low doses of supervoltage radiation therapy; radiosensitizing properties of adriamycin are probably involved in these adverse reactions, although precise mechanisms are unknown.

Actinomycin D, another anthracycline derivative, is also known as a radiosensitizing agent, causing erythema, desquamation, and hyperpigmentation of the skin at sites of concomitant or prior radiotherapy. The lesion starts usually within 3 months of the radiation therapy and resembles the usual radiation reaction of the skin. Acneform skin eruptions also occur with actinomycin D unrelated to radiotherapy; they are usually reversible after therapy. Alopecia is not common; it manifests 7 to 10 days after a course and continues over the next 2 to 4 weeks.

Actinomycin D causes oral ulcerations and redness of the tongue and buccal or oropharyngeal mucosa in about 40% of the patients. This type of toxicity can be delayed, maximal lesions being reached sometimes only 1 to 2 weeks after a course of therapy.

Plant Alkaloids

Vincristine and vinblastine have no major skin toxicity; hair loss has been reported in about 20% of the patients receiving vincristine, but it is uncommon with vinblastine. Regrowth may occur while maintenance therapy continues, and alopecia is rarely complete. Stomatitis has been seen in less than 10% of the patients receiving vinblastine and is not observed with vincristine. Both drugs are local irritants when injected subcutaneously. Vincristine can cause a cellulitis-like picture with erythema, edema, and vesiculation which usually resolves slowly (14).

The epidophyllotoxin derivatives VP 16–213 and VM 26 are not associated with great cutaneous untoward effects; alopecia occurs in about 10% of the patients treated with these agents.

Miscellaneous Agents

Skin reactions can be observed occasionally with most of the other cytostatic agents; however, they are not the major complications resulting from their use.

Mitotane (o,p'-DDD) produces cutaneous toxicity in 13 to 17% of the patients to whom it is administered. Generally the skin toxicity, manifesting as a skin rash, disappears while the patient is still on therapy, but usually the dose must be diminished or the drug discontinued. Toxicity is related to the dosage; 50% of patients in one study did not develop toxicity until higher doses were given. Urticaria, erythema multiforme, and drug rashes are observed occasionally, as is hyperpigmentation.

L-Asparaginase administration can produce hypersensitivity reactions in 5 to 20% of the patients; these manifestations may vary from mild allergic reactions (e.g., urticaria, which can usually be controlled by antihistamines without discontinuing chemotherapy) to anaphylactic shock (11,12,39).

Hydroxyurea is associated with relatively frequent skin reactions (30%), but none are really characteristic. Cutaneous vasculitis with or without flu-like symptoms have been reported, as have maculopapular rashes. Other skin side effects (alopecia, increased pigmentation) and mucositis are rare.

Nitrosoureas, including streptozotocin, have not been associated with severe dermatologic toxicity; occasionally local venous pain on administration has been reported, as well as a sensation of flushing of the skin, conjunctival injection, and burning pain in the extremity receiving an intravenous BCNU infusion. The incidence of this side effect can be reduced by slowing the infusion or reducing the volume of alcohol used as diluent.

Dacarbazine can also be a local irritant if injected subcutaneously and can cause phlebitis of the vein to which it is injected. Less frequently a flu-like syndrome of fever, myalgia, malaise, alopecia, facial flushing, and facial paresthesias has been observed. However, in some series no such toxicity has been found.

Procarbazine is often associated with skin reactions, but the incidence of these side effects is not very high (10%). Facial flushing is reported in patients who are on procarbazine therapy when they ingest small amounts of ethanol.

Hypersensitivity reactions (urticaria, exfoliative dermatitis, maculopapular eruptions) associated occasionally with a flu-like syndrome, eosinophilia, and pulmonary infiltration have been reported. Stomatitis and alopecia are rare (4,13,34).

Among the newer drugs, skin reactions have been reported with neocarzinostatin, manifesting as hypersensitivity reactions and skin rashes. Similarly methyl GAG can cause inflammatory skin lesions resembling erythema multiforme. These skin reactions have a tendency to be generally distributed and occur late in the course of drug administration. They subside rapidly when the drug is discontinued. Peptichemio has been associated with alopecia and dermatitis in a few patients. The exact frequency of these side effects is difficult to assess, but it is not very high.

Other chemotherapeutic agents have not been associated with cutaneous toxicity, although, as with any drug, occasional skin allergic reactions can be seen. Drugs which are essentially devoid of untoward cutaneous effects are hexamethylmelamine and cis-platinum. Alopecia has only rarely been reported with these agents.

Hormones

Hormones and hormone derivatives which are used in cancer chemotherapy can be associated with important actions on the skin. Corticosteroids induce skin changes which are well known and illustrated by the classical skin appearance in patients with Cushing's syndrome. Atrophy of the skin resulting in paper-thin skin and cutaneous striae due to loss of skin collagen are associated with capillary fragility. Androgen administration results in virilization, with well-known skin effects, e.g., increased hair growth and acneform eruptions.

Progesterone results in few skin reactions. Local soft tissue reactions due to sensitivity to the oil carrier are occasionally observed after intramuscular injection.

Estrogens increase capillary fragility, resulting in cutaneous purpuric areas at sites of minor trauma, especially on hands and forearms. Estrogenic stimulation may occur at target organs: Gynecomastia in males, hyperpigmentation of the areolae in both sexes, and vulvar pruritus in females are common side effects of estrogen administration.

Nafoxitine, an antiestrogen compound, causes dryness (ichthyosis) of the skin, photosensitivity skin reactions, and less commonly a partial loss of the hair in a substantial proportion of treated patients. These side effects are severe enough to make clinical use of nafoxitine very difficult. Tamoxifen, on the other hand, a newer antiestrogenic compound, is devoid of these adverse cutaneous reactions. Occasionally an estrogenic type of reaction is observed with tamoxifen, but in most patients the agent is extremely well tolerated.

CONCLUSIONS

Skin is easy to observe in any patient, and dermatologic diagnosis usually requires only clinical examination and skin biopsy.

Skin changes are frequent in cancer patients, and they may indicate progression of the neoplastic disease or complications of chemotherapy. In either case, they usually have an important influence on diagnosis and therapy. Attention to chemotherapy-induced cutaneous lesions, especially to skin infections in myelo-suppressed or immunosuppressed patients, may have a major role in reducing morbidity and mortality from these complications. Knowledge of the cutaneous complications in cancer patients and ability to treat them early and adequately is thus part of the supportive care in these patients.

REFERENCES

1. Arvin, A. M., Feldman, S., and Merigan, T. C. (1978): Human leukocyte interferon in the treatment of varicella in children with cancer: A preliminary controlled trial. *Antimicrob. Agents Chemother.,* 13:605–607.
2. Bodey, G. P., and Luna, M. (1974): Skin lesions associated with disseminated candidiasis. *JAMA,* 229:1466–1468.
3. Brady, L., O'Neill, E., and Farber, S. (1977): Unusual sites of metastases. *Semin. Oncol.,* 4:59–64.
4. Brunner, K. W., and Young, C. W. (1965): A methyldhydrazine derivative in Hodgkin's disease and other malignant neoplasms. *Ann. Intern. Med.,* 63:69–86.
5. Dreizen, S., Bodey, G. P., Rodriguez, V., and McCredie, K. B. (1975): Cutaneous complications of cancer chemotherapy. *Postgrad. Med.,* 58:150–158.
6. Feld, R., and Bodey, G. P. (1977): Infections in patients with malignant lymphoma treated with combination chemotherapy. *Cancer,* 39:1018–1025.
7. Feldman, S., Hughes, W. T., and Daniel, C. B. (1975): Varicella in children with cancers: Seventy-seven cases. *Pediatrics,* 56:388–397.
8. Fernbach, D. J., Griffith, K. M., Haggard, M. E., Holcomb, T. M., Schow, W. W., Vieth, I. J., and Windmiller, J. (1966): Chemotherapy of acute leukemia in childhood: Comparison of cyclophosphamide and mercaptopurine. *N. Engl. J. Med.,* 275:451–456.
9. Goffinet, D. R., Glatstein, E. J., and Merigan, T. C. (1972): Herpes zoster–varicella infections and lymphoma. *Ann. Intern. Med.,* 76:235–240.
10. Greene, M. H., Macher, A. M., Hernandez, A. D., Tomecki, K. J., and Chabner, B. (1978): Disseminated cryptococcosis presenting as palpable purpura. *Arch. Intern. Med.,* 138:1412–1413.
11. Haskell, C. M., Canellos, G. P., Leventhal, B. G., and Carbone, P. P. (1969): L-Asparaginase toxicity. *Cancer Res.,* 29:974–975.
12. Haskell, C. M., Canellos, G. P., Leventhal, B. G., Carbone, P. P., Block, J. B., Serpick, A. A., and Selawry, O. S. (1969): L-Asparaginase: Therapeutic and toxic effects in patients with neoplastic disease. *N. Engl. J. Med.,* 281:1028–1034.
13. Henry, M. C., and Marlow, M. (1973): Preclinical toxicology study of procarbazine (NSC-77213). *Cancer Chemother. Rep.,* 4:97–102.
14. Holland, J. F., Scharlau, C., Gailani, S., Krant, M. J., Olson, K. B., Horton, J., Shnider, B. I., Lynch, J. J., Owens, A., Carbone, P. P., Colsky, J., Grob, D., Miller, S. P., and Hall, T. C. (1973): Vincristine treatment of advanced cancer: a cooperative study of 392 cases. *Cancer Res.,* 1258–1264.
15. Horton, J., Olson, K. B., Sullivan, J., Reilly, C., Shnider, B., and The Eastern Cooperative Oncology Group (1970): 5-Fluorouracil in cancer: An improved regimen. *Ann. Intern. Med.,* 73:897–900.
16. Jaffe, N., Paed, D., Farber, S., Traggis, D., Geiser, C., Kim, B. S., Das, L., Frauenberger, G., Djerassi, I., and Cassady, J. R. (1973): Favourable response of metastatic osteogenic sarcoma to pulse high-dose methotrexate with citrovorum rescue and radiation therapy. *Cancer,* 31:1367–1373.
17. Kennedy, B. J., and Theologides, A. (1961): The role of 5-fluorouracil in malignant diseases. *Ann. Intern. Med.,* 55:719–730.
18. Levi, J. A., Schimpff, S. C., Slawson, R. G., and Wiernik, P. H. (1977): Evaluation of radiotherapy

for localized inflammatory skin and perianal lesions in adult leukemia: A prospectively randomized double-blind study. *Cancer Treat. Rep.,* 61:1301–1305.

19. Levine, N., and Greenwald, E. S. (1978): Mucocutaneous side effects of cancer chemotherapy. *Cancer Treat. Rev.,* 5:67–84.
20. Lynch, H. T., and Frichot, B. C. (1978): Skin, heredity and cancer. *Semin. Oncol.,* 4:67–84.
21. Merigan, T. C. (1976): Efficacy of adenine arabinoside in herpes zoster. *N. Engl. J. Med.,* 294:1233–1234.
22. Merigan, T. C., Rand, K. H., Pollard, R. B., Abdallah, P. S., Jordan, G. W., and Fried, R. P. (1978): Human leukocyte interferon for the treatment of herpes zoster in patients with cancer. *N. Engl. J. Med.,* 298:981–987.
23. Meyer, R. D., Kaplan, M. H., Ong, M., and Armstrong, D. (1973): Cutaneous lesions in disseminated mucormycosis. *JAMA,* 225:737–738.
24. Meyer, R. D., Young, L. S., Armstrong, D., and Yu, B. (1973): Aspergillosis complicating neoplastic disease. *Am. J. Med.,* 54:6–15.
25. Moschella, S. (1978): Cutaneous manifestations of internal malignancy. *Med. Clin. North Am.,* 59:471–479.
26. O'Brien, R., Zelson, J. H., Schwartz, A. D., and Pearson, H. A. (1970): Scalp tourniquet to lessen alopecia after vincristine. *N. Engl. J. Med.,* 283:1469.
27. Reboul, F., Donaldson, S. S., and Kaplan, H. S. (1978): Herpes zoster and varicella infections in children with Hodgkin's disease. *Cancer,* 41:95–99.
28. Schimpff, S. C., Serpick, A., Stoler, B., Rumack, B., Mellin, H., Joseph, J. M., and Block J. B. (1972): Varicella–zoster infection in patients with cancer. *Ann. Intern. Med.,* 76:241–254.
29. Schimpff, S. C., Wiernik, P. H., and Block, J. B. (1972): Rectal abscesses in cancer patients. *Lancet,* 2:844–847.
30. Schow, W., Swanson, P., Gomez, F., and Reyes, C. (1971): Alopecia neoplastica—Hair loss resembling alopecia areata caused by metastatic breast cancer. *JAMA,* 218:1335–1337.
31. Sehdev, M. K., Dowling, M. D., Jr., Seal, S. H., and Stearns, M. W., Jr. (1973): Perianal and anorectal complications in leukemia. *Cancer,* 31:149–152.
32. Shastri, S., Slayton, R. E., Wolter, J., Perlia, C. P., and Taylor, S. G., III (1971): Clinical study with bleomycin. *Cancer,* 28:1142–1146.
33. Smulders, J., and Smets, W. (1960): Les métastases des carcinomes mammaires—Fréquence des métastases hypophysaires. *Bull. Assoc. Fr. Cancer,* 47:434.
34. Stolinsky, D. C., Solomon, J., Pugh, R. P., Stevens, A. R., Jacobs, E. M., Irwin, L. E., Wood, D. A., Steinfield, J. L., and Bateman, J. R. (1970): Clinical experience with procarbazine in Hodgkin's disease, reticulum cell sarcoma, and lymphosarcoma. *Cancer,* 26:984–990.
35. Tan, C., Etcubanas, E., Wollner, N., Rosen, G., Gilladoga, A., Showel, J., Murphy, M. L., and Krakoff, I. H. (1973): Adriamycin—An antitumor antibiotic in the treatment of neoplastic disease. *Cancer,* 32:9–17.
36. Taylon, J., Lewis, L., Battle, J., Butkess, A., Robertson, A., Deoddher, S., and Roeneghk, H., Jr. (1979): Plane xanthoma and multiple myeloma with lipoprotein–paraprotein complexing. *Arch. Dermatol.,* 114:425–431.
37. Vogler, W. R., and Jacobs, J. (1971): Toxic and therapeutic effects of methotrexate–folinic acid (leucovorin) in advanced cancer and leukemia. *Cancer,* 28:894–901.
38. Ward, H. N., Konikov, N., and Reinhard, E. H. (1965): Cytologic dysplasia occurring after busulfan (Myleran) therapy: A syndrome resembling adrenocortical insufficiency and atrophic bronchitis. *Ann. Intern. Med.,* 63:654–660.
39. Whitecar, J. P., Jr., Bodey, G. P., Harris, J. E., and Freireich, E. J. (1970): L-Asparaginase. *N. Engl. J. Med.,* 282:732–734.
40. Whitley, R. J., Ch'ien, L. T., Dolin, R., Galasso, G. J., Alford, C. A., Jr., and The Collaborative Study Group (1976): Adenine arabinoside therapy of herpes zoster in the immunosuppressed NIAID collaborative viral study. *N. Engl. J. Med.,* 294:1193–1199.
41. Williams, A. C., and Klein, E. (1970): Experience with local chemotherapy and immunotherapy in premalignant and malignant skin lesions. *Cancer,* 25:450–462.
42. Yagoda, A., Mukherji, B., Young, C., Etcubanas, E., Lamonte, C., Smith, J. R., Tan, C. T. C., and Krakoff, I. H. (1972): Bleomycin, an antitumor antibiotic—Clinical experience in 274 patients. *Ann. Intern. Med.,* 77:861–870.
43. Young, R., Bennett, J. E., Vogel, C. L., Carbone, P. P., and DeVita, V. T. (1970): The spectrum of the disease in 98 patients. *Medicine,* 49:147–173.

Medical Complications in Cancer Patients,
edited by J. Klastersky and M. J. Staquet.
Raven Press, New York © 1981.

Gastrointestinal Complications of Neoplasms

Daniel D. Von Hoff and Esther Pollard

*Department of Medicine, University of Texas Health Science Center at San Antonio,
San Antonio, Texas 78284*

The purpose of this chapter is to review concisely the gastrointestinal problems associated with neoplastic diseases and the treatment of neoplastic diseases. The direct effects of cancer on the gastrointestinal system are covered first followed by a more detailed description of the effects of therapy of tumors on the gastrointestinal system.

DIRECT EFFECTS OF MALIGNANCY ON THE GASTROINTESTINAL SYSTEM

Most malignancies can have a direct effect on the gastrointestinal system. Cancers of the gastrointestinal tract itself, including head and neck, esophageal, stomach, small bowel, or colorectal cancer, obviously can cause problems of malnutrition, obstruction, ulceration, bleeding, or perforation. In addition to the gastrointestinal primary lesions, a number of tumors, including melanoma, breast cancer, ovarian cancer, lymphoma, and leukemia, can involve the gastrointestinal tract. Infiltration by these malignancies can cause the problems noted above and can also be responsible for protein-losing enteropathies (lymphoma or bowel, stomach, esophageal, and gastric cancer), malabsorption (lymphoma, leukemia), and secondary infections of the gastrointestinal tract (perirectal abscesses with leukemia) (12). By a destructive effect on normal pancreas, cancer of the pancreas may cause a deficiency of enzymes with resultant malabsorption. Chronic extrahepatic obstruction by tumor can cause decreased bile salt excretion into the bowel lumen, which also causes malabsorption (2).

The liver with its rich blood supply is the most common organ to be involved with metastatic disease. One-half to two-thirds of the patients who die of cancer of the gastrointestinal tract, and one-third of the patients who die of lung cancer, have liver metastases. Intrahepatic obstruction and cholestasis with decrease in bile acid secretion is another cause of malabsorption (10).

EFFECTS OF SURGERY

Radial excision of cancers of the oral cavity and pharynx can cause a number of nutritional consequences largely on a mechanical basis (19). Patients undergoing total or partial resection of the thoracic esophagus have varying degrees of steatorrhea and diarrhea following these procedures (30).

Gastrectomy, partial or total, for cancer can be responsible for malabsorption of fat, vitamin B_{12}, vitamin D, calcium, and iron. However, gastrectomy also limits caloric intake, which can cause difficulty in weight maintenance. The dumping syndrome—consisting of epigastric fullness, hyperperistalsis, borborygmi, and cramps with occasional nausea, vomiting, or diarrhea—may be seen after partial or total gastrectomy (30).

Resection of the small bowel can affect nutrient absorption. The jejunum is the area of major absorption of all nutrients except vitamin B_{12}. However, the ileum accomodates for any functional change produced by loss of the more proximal bowel (9,30). This adaptability to increase absorptive capabilities prevents major clinical problems after small bowel resection except for patients who have $\geq$ 75% of their total small bowel removed. Patients who have more than 2 feet of ileum and ileocecal valve removed can have vitamin B_{12} and fat malabsorption. Calcium and vitamin D supplements are also required (30).

Major resection of either the left or right colon usually does not cause major problems, but a subtotal resection of the colon may produce significant diarrhea if the ileum is anastomosed to the rectum. Similar problems with diarrhea occur after total colectomy with ileostomy (30).

Gastrointestinal problems after subtotal resection of the pancreas include pancreatic insufficiency with weight loss, malabsorption, and diarrhea (22).

EFFECTS OF RADIOTHERAPY

Radiation therapy can cause a number of problems for the gastrointestinal system. Radiotherapy to the head and neck may cause loss of appetite, altered taste, and mucositis (8,20). Growth of teeth may be retarded by radiotherapy; and several years after radiotherapy to the teeth, caries develop and teeth autoamputate at their neck (6). Exposure of the salivary glands to radiotherapy results in rapid thickening of saliva, a decrease in total amount of saliva, and acute siladenitis. These changes in saliva are probably important in the genesis of dental caries (17).

Radiotherapy delivered to areas of the esophagus can cause dysphagia secondary to inflammation and ulceration. Late effects can include fibrosis and obstruction (8). Enhancement of radiation effects on the esophagus can be noted with administration of adriamycin (11).

Gastric irradiation results in a temporary but often marked diminution of the mucous and acid content of the gastric secretions (14). Nausea, vomiting, and diarrhea are frequently acute side effects of irradiation to the small bowel (8). One may also see delayed transit time, increased intestinal secretions with dilated loops of small bowel, and malabsorption of glucose, fats, and protein. Late effects include ulceration and a reduction in intestinal caliber and elasticity

(1). Effects of radiation on the small bowel seem to be more profound in patients with pelvic adhesions (15).

The large bowel is considered less vulnerable to the effects of irradiation but can ulcerate and/or perforate with high-dose radium treatment of cervical cancer (26). Irradiation of the liver can result in hepatitis. This side effect can occur a few weeks to 6 months after high-dose radiotherapy to the liver (13).

EFFECT OF CHEMOTHERAPY

Nausea and vomiting are perhaps the most common manifestation of gastrointestinal toxicity of chemotherapeutic agents. This complication occurs with almost every major class of compounds including a majority of the alkylating agents (e.g., nitrogen mustard and cyclophosphamide), nitrosoureas, folate analogs (methotrexate, cytosine arabinoside), purine analogs (6MP 6TG), pyrimidine analogs (5-fluorouracil, 5-FU), anthracycline antibiotics (adriamycin and daunomycin), other antitumor antibiotics (actinomycin D, bleomycin, mitomycin C), and enzymes (e.g., asparaginase) (4,24). Violent and prolonged nausea and vomiting may occur after administration of *cis*-diamminedichloroplatinum, 5-azacytidine, streptozotocin, or DTIC. (3,4,24,28,29,32).

There is some evidence that certain of the alkylating agents may cause very little or less-severe nausea and vomiting (chlorambucil, busulfan, melphalan) (4), and that oral administration of some drugs (e.g., cyclophosphamide) may cause less nausea and vomiting than intravenous administration (4).

Stomatitis—which includes cheilosis, glossitis, pharyngitis, and other mucosal (3) toxicities of the alimentary canal—is seen with a number of chemotherapeutic agents. Severe and sometimes dose-limiting mucosal toxicities have been noted with actinomycin D, methotrexate, methyglyoxal-bis-guanylhydrazone (methyl GAG), azaserine, daunomycin, adriamycin, bleomycin, and during infusion with 5-FU. Mucosal ulcerations occur only rarely with alkylating agents but may be seen with phenylalanine mustard and cyclophosphamide (4,24). Ulceration of the stomach and/or duodenum is a well known complication of administration of corticosteroids (16).

Constipation and adynamic ileus are two of the major toxic effects of vincristine administration (24), and a number of patients have experienced paralytic ileus after vinblastine administration (4).

Diarrhea is particularly severe with actinomycin D, 5-FU, and methyl GAG administration. Diarrhea is also commonly seen after methotrexate, cyclophosphamide, 5-azacytidine, 6-mercaptopurine, procarbazine, or hydroxyurea administration (24).

Pancreatic dysfunction is induced by asparaginase with elevation of amylase and acute pancreatitis. Streptozotocin affects the islet cells of the pancreas, causing hyperglycemia, and methyl GAG can cause severe hypoglycemia (4, 5,24,27). New schedules of administration of the latter drug have not caused hypoglycemia (18).

Hepatic toxicity induced by chemotherapeutic agents can range from transient mild elevation in liver function tests to necrosis or permanent cirrhosis. 6-Mercaptopurine (6-MP) may induce jaundice with pronounced bile stasis (21). It also produces mild elevation in serum glutamic oxalate transaminase (SGOT) levels. Azathioprine, the active metabolite of which is 6-MP, has also been associated with elevations in SGOT and alkaline phosphatase (4).

It is well established that administrations of methotrexate may cause elevation of hepatic enzymes. The prolonged use of methotrexate may cause cirrhosis in a small but significant number of patients (4,24).

Mithramycin can be acutely hepatotoxic, with very high elevations of SGOT but only modest elevations in alkaline phosphatase. The pathology of this toxicity is acute liver necrosis (4).

Mild elevations of liver enzymes and bilirubin occur in patients who have received L-asparaginase. In addition, the synthetic capabilities of the liver are impaired (albumin and clotting factor production) (4,5,24).

Sporadic cases of hepatotoxicity secondary to alkylating agents (cyclophosphamide chlorambucil), anthracyclines (daunomycin and adriamycin, when used in combination regimens), and streptozotocin have also been reported (4,21, 24,25).

EFFECT OF IMMUNOTHERAPY

Nausea and vomiting have been reported with certain immunotherapeutic compounds, including *Corynebacterium parvum,* poly(IC) (polyriboinosinic, polyribocytidylic acid), and levamisole. Diarrhea has also been noted with levamisole therapy (7,23). Hepatic dysfunction, with alkaline phosphatase elevation, clinical jaundice, and hepatomegaly, has been noted to occur secondary to granulomatous hepatitis from BCG (31). As more immunotherapeutic agents are used, it is likely other gastrointestinal toxicities will be noted with that treatment modality.

SUMMARY

Gastrointestinal complications of the neoplastic process and of the treatment of the tumor are varied. The oncologist should be aware of these complications to correctly manage the patient with cancer.

REFERENCES

1. Brick, I. B. (1955): Effects of million volt irradiation on the gastrointestinal tract. *Arch. Intern. Med.,* 96:26–31.
2. Brooks, J. R., and Calebar, J. M. (1976): Cancer of the pancreas. *Am. J. Surg.,* 131:516–520.
3. Brunner, K. W., and Young, C. W. (1965): A methylhydrazine derivative in Hodgkin's disease and other malignant neoplasms: therapeutic and toxic effects studied in 51 patients. *Ann. Intern. Med.,* 63:69–86.

4. Cadman, E. (1977): *Toxicity of Chemotherapeutic Agents in Cancer—A Comprehensive Treatise,* edited by F. T. Becker, pp. 599–672. Plenum, New York.
5. Capizzi, R. L., Bertina, J. R., and Handschumacker, R. E. (1970): L-Asparaginase. *Annu. Rev. Med.,* 433–444.
6. Del Ragato, J. A. (1939): Dental lesions observed after roentgen therapy in cancer of the buccal cavity, pharynx and larynx. *Am. J. Roentgenol.,* 42:404–410.
7. DeVita, V. T., Canellos, G., Carbone, P. P., Baron, S., Levy, H., and Gralnick, H. (1970): Clinical trials with the interferon (InF) inducer polyinosinic-cytidylic acid. *Proc. Am. Assoc. Cancer Res.,* 11:21.
8. Donaldson, S. S. (1977): Nutritional consequences of radiotherapy. *Cancer Res.,* 37:2407–2413.
9. Dowling, R. H. (1967): Compensatory changes in Intestinal absorption. *Br. Med. Bull.,* 23:275–278.
10. Farmerly, K., Kirsner, J., and Joseph, F. (1969): Clinical observations on malabsorption. *Med. Clin. North Am.,* 53:1169–1190.
11. Greco, F. A., Brereton, H. D., Kent, H., Zimbler, H., Merrill, J., and Johnson, R. E. (1976): Adriamycin and enhanced radiation reaction on normal esophagus and skin. *Ann. Intern. Med.,* 85:294–298.
12. Holland, J. F., and Frei, E., III, editors (1973): *Cancer Medicine,* pp. 579 and 1140. Lea & Febiger, Philadelphia.
13. Ingold, J. A., Reed, G. B., Kaplan, H. S., and Bagshaw, M. A. (1965): Radiation hepatitis. *Am J. Roentgenol. Radium Ther. Nucl. Med.,* 93:200–208.
14. Ivy, A. C., Orndoff, B. H., Jacoby, A., and Whitlow, J. F. (1923): Studies on the effect of x-rays on glandular activity. *J. Radiol.,* 4:189–199.
15. Jackson, B. T. (1976): Bowel damage from radiation. *Proc. R. Soc. Med.,* 69:683–686.
16. Karnofsky, D. A. (1967): Late effects of immunosuppressive anticancer drugs. *Fed. Proc.,* 26:925–932.
17. Kashima, H. K., Kirkhan, W. R., and Andrews, J. R. (1965): Post irradiation siladenitis: a study of the clinical features, histopathologic changes and serum enzyme changes following irradiation of human salivary glands. *Am. J. Roentgenol. Radium Ther. Nucl. Med.,* 94:271–291.
18. Knight, W. A., III, Livingston, R. B., Fabian, C., and Costanzi, J. (1979): Methyl-glyoxal bis guanylhydrazine (methyl GAG, MGBG) in advanced human malignancy. *Proc. Am. Soc. Clin. Oncol.,* 20:319.
19. Laurence, W. J. (1977): Nutritional consequences of surgical resection of the gastrointestinal tract for cancer. *Cancer Res.,* 37:2179–2386.
20. MacCarthy-Leventhal, E. M. (1959): Post-radiation mouth dryness. *Lancet,* 2:1138–1139.
21. Minow, R. A., Stern, M. A., and Casey, J. H. (1976): Clinicopathologic correlations of liver damage in patients treated with 6-mercaptopurine and adriamycin. *Cancer,* 38:1524–1528.
22. Monge, J. J., Judd, E. S., and Gage, P. P. (1964): Radical pancreatico duodenectomy: A 22 year experience with the complications, mortality rate and survival rate. *Ann. Surg.,* 160:711–779.
23. Oettgen, J. F., Pinsky, C. M., and Delmonte, L. (1976): Treatment of cancer with immunomodulators *Corynebacterium parvum* and levamisole. *Med. Clin. North Am.,* 60:511–537.
24. Ohnuma, T., and Holland, J. F. (1977): Nutritional consequences of cancer chemotherapy and immunotherapy. *Cancer Res.,* 37:2395–2406.
25. Penta, J. S., Von Hoff, D. D., and Muggia, F. M. (1977): Hepatotoxicity of combination chemotherapy for acute myelocytic leukemia. *Ann. Intern. Med.,* 87:247–248.
26. Quam, S. H. (1968): Factitial proctitis due to irradiation for cancer of the cervix uteri. *Surg. Gynecol. Obstet.,* 126:70–74.
27. Regelson, W., and Holland, J. F. (1973): Clinical experience with methylglyoxal-bisguanyl-hydrazone dihydrochloride: A new agent with divided activity in acute myelogenous leukemia and the lymphomas. *Cancer Chemother. Rep.,* 27:15–26.
28. Rozencweig, M., Von Hoff, D. D., Slavik, M., and Muggia, F. M. (1975): *Cis*-diammine dichloroplatinum. II. A new anticancer drug. *Ann. Intern. Med.,* 86:803–812.
29. Schein, P. S., O'Connell, J. J., Blom, J., Hubbard, S., Magrath, I. T., Bergevin, P., Wiernik, P. H., Ziegler, J. L., and DeVita, V. T. (1974): Clinical antitumor activity and toxicity of streptozotocin (NSC85998). *Cancer,* 34:993–1000.

30. Shils, M. F., and Gilot, T. (1966): The effect of esophagectomy on absorption in man: Clinical and metabolic observations. *Gastroenterology,* 50:347–357.
31. Sparks, F. C., Silverstein, M. J., Hùnt, J. S., Haskell, C. M., Pilch, Y. H., and Morton, D. L. (1973): Complications of BCG immunotherapy in patients with cancer. *N. Engl. J. Med.,* 289:827–830.
32. Von Hoff, D. D., Slavik, M., and Muggia, F. M. (1976): 5-Azacytidine: A new anticancer drug with effectiveness in acute myelogenous leukemia. *Ann. Intern. Med.,* 85:237–245.

Medical Complications in Cancer Patients,
edited by J. Klastersky and M. J. Staquet.
Raven Press, New York © 1981.

Cardiac Disorders in Cancer Patients

*Marcel Rozencweig, *Martine Piccart, and **Daniel D. Von Hoff

*Medical Service and Henri Tagnon Laboratory of Clinical Investigation, Jules Bordet
Institute, Tumor Center, Free University of Brussels, 1000 Brussels, Belgium; and
**University of Texas Health Science Center, San Antonio, Texas 78284*

Cardiac signs and symptoms are often encountered in cancer patients, particularly in the advanced stage of the disease. In addition to preexisting cardiac problems, these manifestations may be accounted for by a large variety of cardiac and extracardiac abnormalities. Overwhelming disease in other organs as well as the simultaneous occurrence of anemia, electrolyte disturbances, and hypoalbuminemia frequently contribute to the difficulty in assessing cardiac function in these patients. Hemorrhagic disorders and systemic infections may also involve the heart. Thus, cardiac candidiasis may be found in 20% of cancer patients with disseminated *Candida* infection studied at necropsy (61). In patients with far-advanced malignancies, nonbacterial thrombotic endocarditis is increasingly recognized as a significant cause of morbidity and mortality (26,70,100).

Case reports have also described the development of pulmonic stenosis by extrinsic pressure from mediastinal masses (31,116). Arrhythmia has been noted with vagal stimulation by intrathoracic tumor growth (38), and with severe tumor-induced hypoglycemia (79). Hyperdynamic heart failure has been associated with the development of arteriovenous fistula (95,107). Cardiac signs may also be produced by carcinoid tumors (124) and pheochromocytoma (110).

Because of this myriad of cardiac complications associated with neoplastic diseases, it may become difficult to identify disorders related to metastatic involvement of the heart and toxic effects of anticancer treatments. This chapter focuses on these latter aspects, with particular emphasis on the cardiotoxic potential of commonly used anticancer agents. Primary malignancies of the heart are extremely rare and will not be considered here.

CARDIAC METASTASES

The prevalence of cardiac metastases and their clinical manifestations have been studied in a large number of autopsy series (40). The available information generally does not lend itself to accurate interpretation of the data. The extent of investigation devoted to the cardiac status and methods of data reporting vary widely from one series to another. True embolic metastases are not always clearly separated from continuous overgrowth to the heart and pericardial invasion is not consistently analyzed. Clinical findings are usually restricted to patients with cardiac metastases at postmortem examination, whereas no data are given for the others. The retrospective nature of the correlation between clinical and pathologic findings further underlines the limitations of these studies.

Metastases to the heart and pericardium are usually associated with the presence of additional intrathoracic malignant tumors (50). They are more likely to develop with extensive dissemination but may occasionally represent the only site of metastasis. Cardiac invasion may be seen with almost all types of primary tumors and is particularly common in melanoma, leukemia, and lymphoma. It has been noted in 30 to 64% of patients dying of metastatic melanoma (50,53). In this disease, tumor invasion is usually nodular rather than interstitial and areas of tumor necrosis are frequently observed. Among necropsy cases of acute or chronic leukemia, malignant cardiac infiltrates have been found in 34 to 53% of the patients (97). These infiltrates appear to be focal, usually few in number, and located most frequently in the pericardium with only occasional extension through the entire cardiac wall. In non-Hodgkin's lymphoma, cumulative data in 1,177 patients indicate that cardiac involvement may occur in 22% (98). This figure seems even higher in autopsy cases of mycosis fungoides but is definitely lower in Hodgkin's disease. The vast majority of lymphoma patients with cardiac involvement have pericardial invasion.

Clinical manifestations of cardiac metatases are related to the extent and site of involvement. Pericardial and myocardial metastases are most frequently encountered whereas endocardial invasion is unusual (50,115,122). Rare cases of massive angioinvasion with extension of tumor thrombus to the heart have been observed with a variety of tumor types including renal cell carcinoma (48,87), Wilms' tumor (127,128), hepatoma (43), follicular carcinoma of the thyroid (123), and pheochromocytoma (102).

Cardiac metastases are rarely diagnosed while the patient is still alive although heart disorders may be the initial manifestation of a malignant disease. These metastases appear to develop at a late stage and produce signs and symptoms that often may be attributable to many other sources. Thus, in an autopsy series of 420 children and adult patients with acute lymphocytic or myelocytic leukemia (97), pathologic examination of the heart revealed the presence of thrombocytopenia-related hemorrhages (54%), pericardial abnormalities not attributable to local metastases (13%), myocardial infection that was almost always associated with systemic infection (7%), chronic cardiac valvular lesions (6%), congenital malformation of heart or great vessels (2%), and noninfective thrombotic endocarditis (0.7%). These findings and the frequent occurrence of anemia and hypoalbuminemia explained why the incidence of dyspnea, chest pain, effusion into body cavities, precordial murmurs, ventricular gallops, edema, and electrocardiographic disturbances might be similar in patients with or without cardiac metastases (97).

Generally, in patients with malignant tumors and no prior heart disease, the most suggestive findings of cardiac metastases include acute pericarditis, cardiac tamponade or constriction, rapid increase in the size of the heart as shown by roentgenogram, onset of ectopic tachycardia, development of second or third degree atrioventricular block, and onset of unequivocal cardiac failure (53).

Little information has been published on the treatment of metastatic cardiac disorders. Most available data concern the therapeutic approach to pericardial effusions.

Pericardiocentesis should be performed at the first sign of tamponade. This procedure can demonstrate the presence of pericardial effusion and its malignant origin may be confirmed by cytologic examination. After fluid aspiration, injection of CO_2 into the pericardium allows the assessment of the extent of tumor infiltration as well as the monitoring of fluid reappearance.

Pericardiocentesis may provide immediate relief but is rarely followed by long-term complete remissions without additional measures (59). Local conservative and adjunctive therapy includes radiation therapy and intracavitary chemotherapy (114). Firm therapeutic recommendations can hardly be made because reported series are small and heterogenous and a possible contribution of systemic chemotherapy generally cannot be ruled out. Radiation therapy has proved useful in radiosensitive tumors and in patients with no prior radiotherapy to the mediastinum. In lymphomas and leukemias, 1,500 to 2,000 rads in 1.5 to 2 weeks may be sufficient to control the effusions effectively (121). Intrapericardial administration of mechlorethamine hydrochloride, 5-fluorouracil, radioactive chromic phosphate, and radioactive colloidal gold have been used with inconclusive results (74,99,114). More recently, instillation of tetracycline hydrochloride into the pericardial sac has been advocated by Davis et al. (39). This treatment produces nonspecific irritative sclerosis with permanent concrescence of the pericardium to the epicardium. Its successful use in a series of six consecutive patients and the apparent lack of serious complications make this procedure attractive for further investigation. Rapid and life-threatening reaccumulation of fluid may require surgical management consisting of pericardiectomy or the creation of a pleuropericardial window.

RADIATION-INDUCED HEART DISEASE

Radiotherapy may produce progressive cardiac fibrosis, especially when megavoltage treatments are administered. The process leading to this complication has not yet been clearly elucidated. Experimental studies suggest that this phenomenon might result from radiation damages to capillary endothelial cells and subsequent ischemia (46). Pericardial lesions are most frequently seen and pathologic findings primarily consist of organizing pericarditis and extensive fibrosis (45). Myocarditis with diffuse interstitial fibrosis is common (23,45, 105,117) and may occasionally involve the conduction system (4,105,117). Coronary artery disease and/or myocardial infarction may be encountered

(4,76,117,125). Valvulopathies are rare (81,117). Limited and focal endocardial fibrosis or fibroelastosis of questionable clinical significance have also been noted (45).

The reported incidence of radiation-induced heart disease ranges between 5 and 30% (89,106,117). This wide variation may be at least partially ascribed to the retrospective nature of these analyses, the selection of different endpoints, and perhaps differences in radiation technics, e.g., anteriorly weighted mantle field (89,106) versus equally weighted opposed fields (117) in patients with Hodgkin's disease. Occurrence of heart disease seems related to dose, fractionation, and the volume of heart that is irradiated (118). Limits of pericardial tolerance have been defined as 1,500 rets in large-volume treatments and 1,850 rets in small-volume treatments (118). However, a dose-response relationship has not been consistently found above 1,500 rets (106,118).

Clinical problems generated by radiation damages are most commonly related to pericardial lesions. Detectable disease develops after a delay of several months and in the majority of patients it occurs within 1 year after completion of radiation therapy. Pericarditis may be seen during irradiation, possibly in relation to necrosis of pericardial metastases and secondary inflammatory reactions (117).

Acute and chronic pericarditis have been described in a series of 25 patients reported at Stanford University (117). The acute form is clinically indistinguishable from other varieties of acute pericarditis and is characterized by fever, chest pain, pericardial friction rubs, electrocardiographic changes, and often pericardial effusion and tamponade. After apparent complete recovery, acute pericarditis may be followed by clinically silent but progressive pancarditis.

Chronic pericarditis develops with an insidious onset and is generally first suggested by the discovery of an enlarging cardiac silhouette on routine chest roentgenograms. Of 15 patients with chronic pericarditis in the Stanford series (117), 12 had pericardial effusion, 10 had constrictive pericarditis, and 7 had both. Among the 12 patients with pericardial effusion, the disease progressed to tamponade and constriction in 8.

The effusions are usually serofibrinous exudates and may be bloody. Simultaneous cardiac catheterization and pericardiocentesis as well as injection of sterile CO_2 into the pericardial cavity may help evaluate the relative effect of cardiac tamponade and pericardial constriction.

Acute radiation injury to the heart may be successfully treated with salicylates (117) or high-dose corticosteroids (64). The latter treatment requires some caution since rapid tapering of corticosteroid dosage may apparently exacerbate radiation injuries (32).

Subtotal pericardiectomy has been advocated at the National Cancer Institute in patients who have diseases highly responsive to anticancer treatments and who present with chronic pericardial effusion leading to symptomatic tamponade or persisting with no symptoms for more than 6 months (81). This surgical approach effectively relieves the cardiac tamponade and may prevent the subsequent development of constrictive pericarditis. Pericardiectomy may be very difficult and seems much less effective in this latter complication. The procedure may occasionally reveal a recurrent malignancy that is undetected at cytologic examination of the pericardial fluid and that may be of favorable prognosis if appropriate therapy is initiated.

CARDIOTOXICITY OF ANTHRACYCLINES

The anthracyclines include some of the most useful antitumor agents in current cancer chemotherapy but cardiotoxicity remains their most disturbing dose-limiting effect. Much experience has been gained, particularly with adriamycin (18) but also with daunomycin (133). Clinical trials of new derivatives have been recently initiated with hopes of decreasing cardiotoxicity.

Adriamycin

The cardiotoxic effects of adriamycin may be categorized into two distinct groups of abnormalities, i.e., early or immediate nonspecific electrocardiographic abnormalities and cumulative dose-dependent cardiomyopathies.

When patients are closely monitored, electrocardiographic changes are found in approximately 30% (90). These changes are more likely to develop in the presence of electrocardiographic alterations prior to adriamycin treatment (21,42,80).

A large variety of single or combined electrocardiographic abnormalities may be encountered, particularly ST–T wave changes, sinus tachycardia, premature ventricular contractions, atrial tachyarrhythmia, low voltage of the QRS complex, and ectopic atrial contractions (90,130). Similar electrocardiographic alterations have been noted in children and in adults (52).

A reduction in voltage of the QRS complex might be an early expression of myocardial damage (67). This alteration appears to be irreversible and related to the total cumulative dose of adriamycin (5,35,67). However, its lack of specificity lessens its potential usefulness for predicting the development of cardiomyopathy.

Other electrocardiographic changes are usually reversible but spontaneous resumption to original electrocardiographic patterns may require up to 2 months (80,120). They may occur at any cumulative dose levels, apparently irrespective of schedule (80). They are rarely of clinical significance, although antiarrhythmic medication or electroconversion may be required occasionally (35).

Adriamycin induces progressive cardiac damages that may result in congestive heart failure with significant morbidity and mortality. The clinical presentation of cardiomyopathies secondary to adriamycin is indistinguishable from other cardiomyopathies. They may develop with a sudden or an insidious onset. Signs and symptoms of adriamycin-induced congestive heart failure primarily include tachycardia, shortness of breath, neck vein distension, gallop rhythms, ankle edema, hepatomegaly, cardiomegaly, and pleural effusions. Serum enzyme elevations (CPK, SGOT) have been noted in serial determinations but no correlations with total doses have been observed (78).

This congestive heart failure is diagnosed at median intervals of 3 to 4 weeks (range: 0–33 weeks) after the last drug administration and reportedly related death occurs in 38 to 43% of these patients (90,130). In the series of Minow et al. (80), the median time from the last dose of adriamycin to diagnosis of cardiomyopathy was 25 days in fatal cases and 54 days in nonfatal cases, suggesting that the patients who died had more fulminating congestive heart failure.

The incidence of adriamycin-induced congestive heart failure varies with the cumulative dose of drug administered (35,67). There is a continuum of increasing risk, especially above a total dose of 550 mg/m^2 (90,130). Schedule of drug administration (33,135) and age of the patient (24,91) significantly modulate this risk. Prolonged treatments are safer with a weekly schedule than with the administration of single doses every 3 weeks. There is apparently no clear difference in risk between children and adults but among adults there is an increasing probability of developing drug-induced cardiac failure in older patients. At the cumulative dose of 550 mg/m^2, the risk may be estimated as 0.8% in young adults (15–35 years) treated at a weekly schedule and 13.9% in patients more than 60 years of age treated with single doses repeated at 3-week intervals (130). The corresponding figures for cumulative doses of 400 and 700 mg/m^2 are 0.3 versus 4.4% and 3.0 versus 43.5%, respectively (130).

There is a strong suggestion that adriamycin-induced cardiomyopathy may be more severe in patients with prior heart disease or hypertension (14,24,35, 75,77,80,130). Other anticancer treatments have also been reported to potentiate the cardiac effect of adriamycin, i.e., mediastinal radiation therapy (15,35,52, 77,80,92), cyclophosphamide (80), actinomycin D, mithramycin (65), mitomycin C (29), dacarbazine (113), vincristine (90), and bleomycin (90). The potential role of these additional risk factors cannot yet be properly evaluated.

The pathogenesis of adriamycin-induced cardiotoxicity remains poorly understood (69). It has been related to progressive damage to DNA and inhibition of DNA repair (109), to an inhibitory effect on coenzyme Q_{10}-dependent enzymes of the electron transfer reactions in mitochondria and Golgi apparatus (11,12,63), to intracellular increase of calcium concentration (85), and to peroxidation of cardiac lipids (82) resulting from the activation of anthracyclines to free radical forms by microsomal enzymes (7,57). Lipid peroxidation could be inhibited by α-tocopherol (82,83) and by coenzyme Q_{10} (141). A drug-conditioned autoimmune antiheart reaction is another mechanism that has been proposed to explain the cardiac effects of anthracyclines (51).

Light microscopic studies of chronic cardiac toxicity show interstitial edema and fibrosis as well as myocyte degeneration characterized by myofibrillar loss and cytoplasmic vacuolization (18,47). These lesions are initially focal and tend to become diffuse with larger doses. Serial myocardial biopsy specimens have demonstrated ongoing degenerative changes months after cessation of therapy

(18). Extensive documentation of cardiac damage by electron microscopy is also available (47).

At present, the usefulness of conventional medical management in the therapy of adriamycin-induced cardiomyopathy is controversial (8,35,52,67,80). It would appear that early detection of congestive heart failure could notably improve the therapeutic efficacy of standard measures such as rest, digitalis, diuretics, and salt restrictions. In addition, discontinuation of adriamycin is an absolute must (35).

A prophylactic regimen to prevent drug-induced cardiomyopathy is highly desirable. Clinical studies with digitalis preparations (139) and coenzyme Q_{10} (34) have been reported with inconclusive results.

Daunomycin

The cardiotoxic effects of daunomycin can also be divided into two distinct categories, i.e., early electrocardiographic alterations and a cumulative dose-dependent cardiomyopathy. In a large collected series of patients, children had a 0.49% and adults a 1.13% incidence of electrocardiographic changes (132). Most common electrocardiographic findings consisted of nonspecific ST-T wave modifications, low voltage of QRS complex, low voltage of the T wave, tachycardia, and abnormal T axis. Electrocardiographic changes were essentially reversible. Of note, fatal acute arrhythmia occurred in one patient and myocardial infarction was found at postmortem examination. Electrocardiographic abnormalities do not seem to presage the development of congestive heart failure with the possible exception of lowered voltage of QRS, but this remains controversial (13,55,132). In one report, none of the 45 patients who had electrocardiographic abnormalities developed congestive heart failure but lack of serial electrocardiographic examinations precluded any conclusions (132).

Drug-induced cardiomyopathy has been reported in up to 10% of the patients treated with daunomycin (55). It may occur within 2 to 40 weeks after the last drug administration (131). Its clinical presentation is characterized by a rather sudden onset of severe congestive heart failure. It usually seems unresponsive to therapy with digitalis and diuretics (132), although favorable results with standard treatments have been reported (52).

Daunomycin-related cardiomyopathy is fatal in 79% of the cases, with death usually occurring within 24 hr. At postmortem examination, light microscopy may reveal interstitial edema and scattered foci of myocardial fiber degeneration (28,55,96). Damage to intrinsic cardiac neurons (112) and endomyocardial fibrosis (138) have also been described.

In an analysis of 5,613 patients receiving daunomycin, the incidence of congestive failure was definitely related to the total dose of drug administered, with higher risk as the total dose of drug was increased (132). There was a 1.5% incidence of development of congestive heart failure at a total dose of

600 mg/m^2. This figure reached 12% at $1,000 \text{ mg/m}^2$ and sharply increased thereafter. Cumulative dose dependence was observed in children and adults but age-related differences in the susceptibility to the induction of daunomycin cardiomyopathy has been noted with a risk of 17% in children versus 6% in adults at a total dose of $1,100 \text{ mg/m}^2$. Opposite observations have been reported by others (20).

There is a paucity of information available for correlating cardiomyopathy secondary to daunomycin and dose schedule of drug administration. Whether the risk for a same cumulative dose could be reduced by administering this dose over longer periods of time is uncertain (52,137). An intermittent schedule has been reported to possibly affect the heart to a lesser extent than daily treatments (20,71). These observations remain to be confirmed. The role of preexisting cardiovascular disease in the development of drug-induced cardiomyopathy is not established.

Investigational Anthracyclines

Efforts to develop anthracycline derivatives are primarily directed to the detection of compounds endowed with significantly lesser cardiotoxicity relative to conventional anthracyclines. However, a clinical comparison of these derivatives focusing on the occurrence of congestive heart failure can hardly be undertaken. This complication is observed essentially with prolonged treatments. It is frequently irreversible and lethal, although it would appear that its severity might be noticeably reduced with the serial use of reliable predictive tests of sufficient accuracy.

A number of anthracycline analogs have been clinically investigated to various extents but, to date, a clear advantage over conventional anthracyclines in terms of cardiotoxicity remains to be demonstrated. These new anthracycline derivatives include daunorubicin-DNA and adriamycin-DNA complexes (10,104,126), carminomycin (1,88), 4'-epiadriamycin (22), N-trifluoroacetyladriamycin-14-valerate (19), rubidazone (9,10), quelamycin (25,36), and aclacinomycin A (84).

Cardiac Monitoring for Anthracycline-Induced Cardiomyopathy

Various tests have been developed to monitor anthracycline-induced cardiac toxicity. Noninvasive methods are used to assess left ventricular function directly (radionuclide angiogram and echocardiogram) or indirectly (systolic time intervals and pulse wave delay). These procedures have elicited results that correlate to some extent with the cumulative dose of adriamycin and might help evaluate cardiotoxicity in groups of patients treated with new anthracycline derivatives or with potentially protective measures. There is currently no evidence that these tests might accurately predict individual tolerance to further treatment at any cumulative dose level of adriamycin. However, the radionuclide angiogram is presently emerging as a promising predictive test. Endomyocardial biopsies have also been advocated but a relationship between anatomic findings and the development of clinically significant heart failure has not yet been established.

Radionuclide Angiography

First-pass quantitative radionuclide angiocardiograms appear to allow rapid and reproducible determination of left ventricular ejection fraction (LVEF). This procedure was used sequentially by Alexander et al. (3) in a series of 55 patients. Five of these exhibited a decline in ejection fraction of at least 15% to a final value of ≤ 45% and developed congestive heart failure with additional adriamycin. The drug was withdrawn in six subsequent patients showing such a decline and none of these presented with congestive heart failure. This toxic effect was not encountered with smaller reduction of the ejection fraction. In this study, criteria for congestive heart failure were not given. Both the absolute decline in LVEF from initial to lowest value and the lowest level recorded during therapy correlated weakly but significantly with cumulative drug dose. However, the significance of this correlation was based on all patients and a statistical analysis excluding patients who developed congestive heart failure was not performed.

Echocardiography

Various parameters of left ventricular function may be calculated from echocardiograms and minimal changes can be accurately monitored and consistently reproduced. A significant decrease of myocardial contractility has been reported with increasing cumulative dose of adriamycin (17,44,58,75,93). However, evidence is still lacking that echocardiogram findings could adequately replace the rule of stopping adriamycin at the cumulative dose of 550 mg/m² (58).

Systolic Time Intervals

Systolic time intervals (STI) are measured from simultaneous recordings of electrocardiogram, phonocardiogram, and carotid pulse (136). Total electromechanical systole (QS2) is measured from the onset of the QRS complex to the first high-frequency vibration of the aortic component of the second heart sound. Left ventricular ejection time (LVET) is measured from the rapid upstroke of the carotid pulse to the through of the carotid incisura. The systolic preejection period (PEP) is defined as the difference between QS2 and LEVT. In the failing left ventricle, PEP is prolonged, LEVT is diminished, and total electromechanical systole remains relatively unchanged.

STI were serially determined in a series of 48 patients receiving adriamycin (8). There was no clear relationship between cumulative doses of the drug and STI abnormalities. All patients who presented with congestive heart failure had significant and persistent or progressive increase of the PEP:LVET ratio but this finding was followed by congestive heart failure in 50% of the cases, apparently including patients with no further adriamycin treatment.

The limited predictive value of STI has also been reported in other series (3,60), although a significant change in the PEP:LVET ratio may be observed with high cumulative doses of adriamycin (44,58). Mason et al. (75) could not find any correlation between STI and cardiac dysfunction defined by catheterization and clinical findings.

Pulse Wave Delay

The pulse wave delay or QKd time interval is the time interval between the start of the QRS complex (Q) and the start of the Korotkoff arterial sound (K) over the brachial artery at diastolic pressure (d). QKd is the sum of the cardiac PEP and the pulse transmission time to the brachial artery. Significant and usually transient prolongations of QKd are seen after administration of adriamycin. Failure of QKd to return to pretreatment levels may herald the development of congestive heart failure but this may also occur in patients with normal QKd (54).

Endomyocardial Biopsy

Percutaneous transvenous endomyocardial biopsies have shown that virtually all patients present with cardiac damages after doses of 240 mg/m² of adriamycin (15). A pathologic grading of toxicity was proposed by Billingham et al. and appeared to correlate much better than total cumulative dose with cardiac dysfunction based on catheterization and clinical findings (75). However, cardiac dysfunction was also noted with no or with minor anatomic alterations.

CARDIOTOXICITY OF OTHER ANTICANCER AGENTS

Many anticancer drugs have been implicated in the development of cardiac manifestations. Generally, clear evidence of a direct relationship between heart damage and drug treatment is often difficult to establish. Drug-related cardiotoxicity seems to be very rare with currently available conventional agents given at common dose schedules. Cardiac effects have been more frequently encountered with high-dose chemotherapy and with some investigational agents.

Cyclophosphamide

Hemorrhagic cardiac necrosis has been observed in patients receiving massive dosages of cyclophosphamide (120–240 mg/kg) (27,111). Clinical manifestations of this complication may occur as late as 2 weeks after the last dose has been administered. Electrocardiographic changes include sinus tachycardia, low voltage of the QRS complex, and ST-T wave modifications. About one-half of the patients have significant rises in LDH and CPK levels, suggesting myocardial damage. Chest X-ray films may show transient increases in the size of the heart. Cardiac necrosis is generally fatal within 11 to 14 days after drug administration. At postmortem examination, histologic changes include noninflammatory toxic vasculitis in small coronary vessels, myocardial necrosis as well as interstitial hemorrhages, edema, and fibrin deposition in the myocardium and the pericardium.

An acute lethal myopericarditis has also been described in four of 15 patients treated with high dose-combination chemotherapy consisting of cyclophosphamide, 6-thioguanine, cytosine arabinoside, and BCNU (6).

Methotrexate

Transient nonspecific ST-T alterations have been encountered after methotrexate infusions in patients receiving high doses of the drug alternated with adriamycin (101).

5-Fluorouracil

A few case reports have suggested that 5-fluorouracil has cardiotoxic potential (41,66,103). These patients had chest pain and occasionally ischemic electrocardiographic changes that usually developed 2 to 4 hr after drug administration.

Mitomycin C

Histologic myocardial changes similar to radiation-induced heart injury have been found in five of 15 patients treated with mitomycin C (94).

Busulfan

An apparently drug-related cardiopathy has been described in one patient treated for 9 years with busulfan. This patient died with signs of acute respiratory failure and autopsy disclosed interstitial pulmonary fibrosis and endocardial fibrosis in the absence of myocardial fibrosis (134).

Vincristine

Myocardial infarction developed in one patient after large weekly doses of vincristine (72). However, one episode of myocardial infarction had already been noted in this patient 2 years earlier.

Diethylstilbestrol

The Veterans' Administration Cooperative Urological Research Group has demonstrated that daily doses of 1 or 5 mg of diethylstilbestrol are similarly effective in controlling prostatic carcinoma. However, the higher dose is associated with higher incidence of cardiovascular deaths (16).

Investigational agents

Thalicarpine (37), emetine (86), and dehydroemetin (62) are plant alkaloid derivatives that may produce a variety of electrocardiographic changes.

Cytembena is structurally related to norepinephrine. This compound may produce a dose-limiting syndrome characterized by hypertension, tachycardia, tachypnea, hyperperistaltis, frequent explosive defecation, facial flushing, paresthesias, and chest pain with accompanying ischemic electrocardiographic changes (49).

8-Azaguanine administration may result in conduction defects, atrial fibrillation, ventricular tachycardia, and a syndrome suggestive of myocardial infarction. The cardiac effect of this purine derivative has been related to the absence of guanase in the heart and the subsequent inability to deaminate the drug (56).

Isolated cases of cardiotoxicity have also been reported with VP-16123 (108), cis-platinum (119, 140), 4'-(9-acridinylamino)methanesulfon-m-anisidide (68, 129), and guanazol (30). Mithramycin has been associated with multiple arterial occlusive episodes in one young patient with testicular cancer (73). No details are available to substantiate a possible cardiac effect of anhydro-ara-5-fluorocytidine (2).

CONCLUSIONS

When cardiac disorders occur in cancer patients, several diagnostic possibilities arise including preexisting cardiac disease, metastatic involvement of the heart, invasion of the pericardium with effusion, pulmonary emboli, and nonbacterial thrombotic endocarditis. It is important to realize that cardiac dysfunction may also be iatrogenic and result from radiotherapy, chemotherapy, or both.

A number of potent antineoplastic drugs may induce cardiotoxic complications. As the use of antineoplastic drugs expands, particularly in high-dose regimens, and as newer drugs are introduced into clinical trials, cardiac manifestations of cancer chemotherapy may be expected to become increasingly important in the differential diagnosis of cardiac dysfunction in patients with cancer.

ACKNOWLEDGMENTS

This work was supported by grant 3–4535–70 from the "Fonds de la Recherche Scientifique Médicale" (FRSM, Belgium) and contract NIH N01/CM 53840 from the National Cancer Institute (NCI, Bethesda, Maryland).

The authors greatly acknowledge the assistance of Ms. G. Decoster and Ms. N. Giet in the preparation of this manuscript.

REFERENCES

1. Abele, R., Rozencweig, M., Body, J.-J., Bedogni, P., Reich, S. D., Crooke, S. T., Lenaz, L., and Kenis, Y. (1980): Carminomycin (NSC-180024): A phase I study. *Eur. J. Cancer (in press).*
2. Alberto, P., Medenica, R., Germano, G., and Bollag, W. (1976): Phase I study of weekly administration of anhydro-ara-5-fluorocytidine (NSC-166641). *Cancer Treat. Rep.,* 60:281–283.
3. Alexander, J., Dainiak, N., Berger, H. J., Goldman, L., Johnstone, D., Reduto, L., Duffy, T., Schwartz, P., Gottschalk, A., and Zaret, B. L. (1979): Serial assessment of doxorubicin cardiotoxicity with quantitative radionuclide angiocardiography. *N. Engl. J. Med.,* 300:278–283.
4. Ali, M. K., Khalil, K. G., Fuller, L. M., Leachman, R. D., Sullivan, M. P., Loh, K. K., Gamble, J. F., and Shullenberger, C. C. (1976): Radiation-related myocardial injury. Management of two cases. *Cancer,* 38:1941–1946.
5. Ali, M. K., Soto, P. A., Maroongroge, D., Bekheit-Saad, S., Buzdar, A. U., Blumenschein, G. R., Hortobagyi, G. N., Tashima, C. K., Wiseman, C. L., and Shullenberger, C. C. (1979): Electrocardiographic changes after adriamycin chemotherapy. *Cancer,* 43:465–471.
6. Appelbaum, F. R., Strauchen, J. A., Graw, R. G., Jr., Savage, D. D., Kent, K. M., Ferrans, V. J., and Herzig, G. P. (1976): Acute lethal carditis caused by high-dose combination chemotherapy. A unique clinical and pathological entity. *Lancet,* 1:58–62.
7. Bachur, N. R. (1979): Anthracycline antibiotic pharmacology and metabolism. *Cancer Treat. Rep.,* 63:817–820.
8. Balcerzak, S. P., Christakis, J., Lewis, R. P., Olson, H. M. and Malspeis, L. (1978): Systolic time intervals in monitoring adriamycin-induced cardiotoxicity. *Cancer Treat. Rep.,* 62:893–899.
9. Benjamin, R. S., Keating, M. J., Swenerton, K. D., Legha, S., and McCredie, K. B. (1979): Clinical studies with rubidazone. *Cancer Treat. Rep.,* 63:925–929.
10. Benjamin, R. S., Mason, J. W., and Billingham, M. E. (1978): Cardiac toxicity of adriamycin-DNA complex and rubidazone: Evaluation by electrocardiogram and endomyocardial biopsy. *Cancer Treat. Rep.,* 62:935–939.
11. Bertazzoli, C., Sala, L., Solcia, E., and Ghione, M. (1975): Experimental adriamycin cardiotoxicity prevented by ubiquinone *in vivo* in rabbits. *Int. Res. Commun. Sys. Med. Sci.,* 3:468.
12. Bertazzoli, C., Sala, L., and Tosana, M. G. (1975): Antagonistic action of ubiquinone on the experimental cardiotoxicity of adriamycin in the isolated rabbit heart. *Int. Res. Commun. Sys. Med. Sci.,* 3:367.
13. Bezwoda, W. R., Lynch, S. R., Sacks, P., Gale, D., Bothwell, T. H., and Stevens, K. (1974): Local experience in the treatment of acute non-lymphoblastic leukaemia. *S. Afr. Med. J.,* 48:963–967.
14. Billingham, M. E., Bristow, M. R., Glatstein, E., Mason, J. W., Masek, M. A., and Daniels, J. R. (1977): Adriamycin cardiotoxicity: Endomyocardial biopsy evidence of enhancement by irradiation. *Am. J. Surg. Pathol.,* 1:17–23.
15. Billingham, M. E., Mason, J. W., Bristow, M. R., and Daniels, J. R. (1978): Anthracycline cardiomyopathy monitored by morphologic changes. *Cancer Treat. Rep.,* 62:865–872.
16. Blackard, C. E. (1975): The Veterans' Administration Cooperative Urological Research Group studies of carcinoma of the prostate: A review. *Cancer Chemother. Rep.,* 59:225–227.
17. Bloom, K. R., Bini, R. M., Williams, C. M., Sonley, M. J., and Gribbin, M. A. (1978): Echocardiography in adriamycin cardiotoxicity. *Cancer,* 41:1265–1269.
18. Blum, R. H., and Carter, S. K. (1974): Adriamycin: A new anticancer drug with significant clinical activity. *Ann. Intern. Med.,* 80:249–259.
19. Blum, R. H., Garnick, M. B., Israel, M., Canellos, G. P., Henderson, I. C., and Frei, E. III (1979): Initial clinical evaluation of N-trifluoroacetyladriamycin-14-valerate (AD-32), an adriamycin analog. *Cancer Treat. Rep.,* 63:919–923.
20. Bonadonna, G., and Monfardini, S. (1969): Cardiac toxicity of daunorubicin. *Lancet,* 1:837.
21. Bonadonna, G., Monfardini, S., De Lena, M., Fossati-Bellani, F., and Beretta, G. (1972): Clinical trials with adriamycin. Results of three-years study. In: *International Symposium on Adriamycin,* edited by S. K. Carter, A. Di Marco, M. Ghione, I. H. Krakoff, and G Mathé, pp. 139–152. Springer-Verlag, Berlin.

22. Bonfante, V., Bonadonna, G., Villani, F., Di Fronzo, G., Martini, A., and Casazza, A. M. (1979): Preliminary phase I study of 4'-epi-adriamycin. *Cancer Treat. Rep.*, 63:915–918.
23. Botti, R. E., Driscol, T. E., Pearson, O. H., and Smith, J. C. (1968): Radiation myocardial fibrosis simulating constrictive pericarditis. A review of the literature and a case report. *Cancer*, 22:1254–1261.
24. Bristow, M. R., Mason, J. W., Billingham, M. E., and Daniels, J. R. (1978): Doxorubicin cardiomyopathy: Evaluation by phonocardiography, endomyocardial biopsy, and cardiac catheterization. *Ann. Intern. Med.*, 88:168–175.
25. Brugarolas, A., Pachon, N., Gosalvez, M., Perez Llanderal, A., Lacave, A. J., Buesa, J. M., and Garcia Marco, M. (1978): Phase I clinical study of quelamycin. *Cancer Treat. Rep.*, 62:1527–1534.
26. Bryan, C. S. (1969): Nonbacterial thrombotic endocarditis with malignant tumors. *Am. J. Med.*, 46:787–793.
27. Buckner, C. D., Rudolph, R. H., Fefer, A., Clift, R. A., Epstein, R. B., Funk, D. D., Neiman, P. E., Slichter, S. J., Storb, R., and Thomas, E. D. (1972): High-dose cyclophosphamide therapy for malignant disease. Toxicity, tumor response, and the effects of stored autologous marrow. *Cancer*, 29:357–365.
28. Buja, L. M., Ferrans, V. J., Mayer, R. J., Roberts, W. C., and Henderson, E. S. (1973): Cardiac ultrastructural changes induced by daunorubicin therapy. *Cancer*, 32:771–788.
29. Buzdar, A. U., Legha, S. S., Tashima, C. K., Hortobagyi, G. N., Yong Yap, H., Krutchik, A. N., Luna, M. A., and Blumenschein, G. R. (1978): Adriamycin and mitomycin C: Possible synergistic cardiotoxicity. *Cancer Treat. Rep.*, 62:1005–1008.
30. Caoili, E. M., Talley, R. W., Smith, F., Salem, P., and Vaitkevicius, V. K. (1975): Guanazole (NSC-1895)—A phase I clinical study. *Cancer Chemother. Rep.*, 59:1117–1121.
31. Carney, E. K., Oppelt, W. W., Gleason, W. L., and Brindley, C. O. (1962): Cardiac Hodgkin's disease. A clinical, hemodynamic, and angiocardiographic evaluation of a case. *Am. Heart J.*, 64:106–110.
32. Castellino, R. A., Glatstein, E., Turbow, M. M., Rosenberg, S., and Kaplan, H. S. (1974): Latent radiation injury of lungs or heart activated by steroid withdrawal. *Ann. Intern. Med.*, 80:593–599.
33. Chlebowski, R., Pugh, R., Paroly, W., Heuser, J., Pajak, T., Jacobs, E., and Bateman, J. R. (1979): Adriamycin on a weekly schedule: Clinically effective with low incidence of cardiotoxicity. *Clin. Res.*, 27:53A.
34. Cortes, E. P., Gupta, M., Chou, C., Amin, V. C., and Folkers, K. (1978): Adriamycin cardiotoxicity: Early detection by systolic time interval and possible prevention by coenzyme Q10. *Cancer Treat. Rep.*, 62:887–891.
35. Cortes, E. P., Lutman, G., Wanka, J., Wang, J. J., Pickren, J., Wallace, J., and Holland, J. F. (1975): Adriamycin (NSC-123127) cardiotoxicity: A clinicopathologic correlation. *Cancer Chemother. Rep., Part 3*, 6:215–225.
36. Cortès-Funes, H., Gosalvez, M., Moyano, A., Manas, A., and Mendiola, C. (1979): Early clinical trial with quelamycin. *Cancer Treat. Rep.*, 63:903–908.
37. Creaven, P. J., Cohen, M. H., Selawry, O. S., Tejada, F., and Broder, L. E. (1975): Phase I study of thalicarpine (NSC-68075), a plant alkaloid of novel structure. *Cancer Chemother. Rep.*, 59:1001–1006.
38. Davies, P. (1957): Sino-auricular block associated with intrathoracic new growths. *Br. Heart J.*, 19:431–434.
39. Davis, S., Sharma, S. M., Blumberg, E. D., and Kim, C. S. (1978): Intrapericardial tetracycline for the management of cardiac tamponade secondary to malignant pericardial effusion. *N. Engl. J. Med.*, 299:1113–1114.
40. DeLoach, J. F., and Haynes, J. W. (1953): Secondary tumors of heart and pericardium. Review of the subject and report of one hundred thirty-seven cases. *Arch. Intern. Med.*, 91:224–249.
41. Dent, R. G., and McColl, I. (1975): 5-Fluorouracil and angina. *Lancet*, 1:347–348.
42. Dindogru, A., Barcos, M., Henderson, E. S., and Wallace, H. J., Jr. (1978): Electrocardiographic changes following adriamycin treatment. *Med. Pediatr. Oncol.*, 5:65–71.
43. Ehrich, D. A., Widmann, J. J., Berger, R. L., and Abelmann, W. H. (1975): Intracavitary cardiac extension of hepatoma. *Ann. Thorac. Surg.*, 19:206–211.
44. Ewy, G. A., Jones, S. E., Friedman, M. J., Gaines, J., and Cruze, D. (1978): Noninvasive cardiac evaluation of patients receiving adriamycin. *Cancer Treat. Rep.*, 62:915–922.

45. Fajardo, L. F., Stewart, J. R., and Cohn, K. E. (1968): Morphology of radiation-induced heart disease. *Arch. Pathol.,* 86:512–519.
46. Fajardo, L. F., and Stewart, J. R. (1973): Pathogenesis of radiation-induced myocardial fibrosis. *Lab. Invest.,* 29:244–257.
47. Ferrans, V. J. (1978): Overview of cardiac pathology in relation to anthracycline cardiotoxicity. *Cancer Treat. Rep.,* 62:955–961.
48. Freed, S. Z., and Gliedman, M. L. (1975): The removal of renal carcinoma thrombus extending into the right atrium. *J. Urol.,* 113:163–165.
49. Frytak, S., Moertel, C. G., Schutt, A. J., Ahmann, D. L., Donadio, J. V., and Weinshilboum, R. M. (1976): A phase I study of cytembena. *Cancer,* 37:1248–1255.
50. Gassman, H. S., Meadows, R., Jr., and Baker, L. A. (1955): Metastatic tumors of the heart. *Am. J. Med.,* 19:357–365.
51. Ghione, M. (1978): Cardiotoxic effects of antitumor agents. *Cancer Chemother. Pharmacol.,* 1:25–34.
52. Gilladoga, A. C., Manuel, C., Tan, C. T. C., Wollner, N., Sternberg, S. S., and Murphy, M. L. (1976): The cardiotoxicity of adriamycin and daunomycin in children. *Cancer,* 37:1070–1078.
53. Glancy, D. L., and Roberts, W. C. (1968): The heart in malignant melanoma. A study of 70 autopsy cases. *Am. J. Cardiol.,* 21:555–571.
54. Greco, F. A. (1978): Subclinical adriamycin cardiotoxicity: Detection by timing the arterial sounds. *Cancer Treat. Rep.,* 62:901–905.
55. Halazun, J. F., Wagner, H. R., Gaeta, J. F., and Sinks, L. F. (1974): Daunorubicin cardiac toxicity in children with acute lymphocytic leukemia. *Cancer,* 33:545–554.
56. Hall, T. C., Lovina, T. O., and McCombs, H. L. (1966): Cardiotoxicity of 8 azaguanine. *Proc. Am. Assoc. Cancer Res.,* 17:28.
57. Handa, K., and Sato, S. (1975): Generation of free radicals of quinone group-containing anticancer chemicals in NADPH-microsome system as evidenced by initiation of sulfite oxidation. *Gann,* 66:43–47.
58. Henderson, I. C., Sloss, L. J., Jaffe, N., Blum, R. H., and Frei, E., III (1978): Serial studies of cardiac function in patients receiving adriamycin. *Cancer Treat. Rep.,* 62:923–929.
59. Hirsch, D. M., Jr., Nydick, I., and Farrow, J. H. (1966): Malignant pericardial effusion secondary to metastatic breast carcinoma. A case of long-term remission. *Cancer,* 19:1269–1272.
60. Hutchinson, R. J., Bailey, C., Wood, D., and Donaldson, M. H. (1978): Systolic time intervals in monitoring for anthracycline cardiomyopathy in pediatric patients. *Cancer Treat. Rep.,* 62:907–910.
61. Ihde, D. C., Roberts, W. C., Marr, K. C., Brereton, H. D., McGuire, W. P., Levine, A. S., and Young, R. C. (1978): Cardiac candidiasis in cancer patients. *Cancer,* 41:2364–2371.
62. Israel, L., Depierre, A., and Chahinian, P. (1974): Dehydroemetin in 50 disseminated carcinomas unresponsive to other drugs. *Proc. Am. Assoc. Cancer Res.,* 15:11.
63. Iwamoto, Y., Hansen, I. L., Porter, T. H., and Folkers, K. (1974): Inhibition of coenzyme Q_{10}-enzymes, succinoxidase and NADH-oxidase by adriamycin and other quinones having antitumor activity. *Biochem. Biophys. Res. Commun.,* 58:633–638.
64. Keelan, M. H., Jr., and Rudders, R. A. (1974): Successful treatment of radiation pericarditis with corticosteroids. *Arch. Intern. Med.,* 134:145–147.
65. Kushner, J. P., Hansen, V. L., and Hammar, S. P. (1975): Cardiomyopathy after widely separated courses of adriamycin exacerbated by actinomycin-D and mithramycin. *Cancer,* 36:1577–1584.
66. Lang Stevenson, D., Mikhailidis, D. P., and Gillett, D. S. (1977): Cardiotoxicity of 5-fluorouracil. *Lancet,* 2:406–407.
67. Lefrak, E. A., Pitha, J., Rosenheim, S., and Gottlieb, J. A. (1973): A clinicopathologic analysis of adriamycin cardiotoxicity. *Cancer,* 32:302–314.
68. Legha, S. S., Latreille, J., McCredie, K. B., and Bodey, G. P. (1979): Neurologic and cardiac rhythm abnormalities associated with 4'-(9-acridinylamino)methanesulfon-*m*-anisidide (AMSA) therapy. *Cancer Treat. Rep.,* 63:2001–2003.
69. Lenaz, L., and Page, J. A. (1976): Cardiotoxicity of adriamycin and related anthracyclines. *Cancer Treat. Rev.,* 3:111–120.
70. MacDonald, R. A., and Robbins, S. L. (1957): The significance of nonbacterial thrombotic endocarditis: An autopsy and clinical study of 78 cases. *Ann. Intern. Med.,* 46:255–273.

71. Malpas, J. S., and Bodley Scott, R. (1969): Daunorubicin in acute myelocytic leukaemia. *Lancet,* 1:469–470.
72. Mandel, E. M., Lewinski, U., and Djaldetti, M. (1975): Vincristine-induced myocardial infarction. *Cancer,* 36:1979–1982.
73. Margileth, D. A., Smith, F. E., and Lane, M. (1973): Sudden arterial occlusion associated with mithramycin therapy. *Cancer,* 31:708–712.
74. Martini, N., Freiman, A. H., Watson, R. C., and Hilaris, B. S. (1977): Intrapericardial instillation of radioactive chromic phosphate in malignant pericardial effusion. *Am. J. Roentgenol.,* 128:639–641.
75. Mason, J. W., Bristow, M. R., Billingham, M. E., and Daniels, J. R. (1978): Invasive and noninvasive methods of assessing adriamycin cardiotoxic effects in man: Superiority of histopathologic assessment using endomyocardial biopsy. *Cancer Treat. Rep.,* 62:857–864.
76. McReynolds, R. A., Gold, G. L., and Roberts, W. C. (1976): Coronary heart disease after mediastinal irradiation for Hodgkin's disease. *Am. J. Med.,* 60:39–45.
77. Merrill, J., Greco, F. A., Zimbler, H., Brereton, H. D., Lamberg, J. D., and Pomeroy, T. C. (1975): Adriamycin and radiation: Synergistic cardiotoxicity. *Ann. Intern. Med.,* 82:122–123.
78. Middleman, E., Luce, J., and Frei, E., III (1971): Clinical trials with adriamycin. *Cancer,* 28:844–850.
79. Miley, G. B., Binnick, S. A., and Block, P. J. (1975): Hypoglycemia and ventricular tachycardia due to adenocarcinoma of the stomach. *Am. J. Med. Sci.,* 269:403–408.
80. Minow, R. A., Benjamin, R. S., and Gottlieb, J. A. (1975): Adriamycin (NSC-123127) cardiomyopathy. An overview with determination of risk factors. *Cancer Chemother. Rep.,* 6:195–201.
81. Morton, D. L., Glancy, D. L., Joseph, W. L., and Adkins, P. C. (1973): Management of patients with radiation-induced pericarditis with effusion: A note on the development of aortic regurgitation in two of them. *Chest,* 291–297.
82. Myers, C. E., McGuire, W. P., Liss, R. H., Ifrim, I., Grotzinger, K., and Young, R. C. (1977): Adriamycin: The role of lipid peroxidation in cardiac toxicity and tumor response. *Science,* 197:165–167.
83. Myers, C. E., McGuire, W., and Young, R. (1976): Adriamycin: Amelioration of toxicity by α-tocopherol. *Cancer Treat. Rep.,* 60:961–962.
84. Ogawa, M., Inagaki, J., Horikoshi, N., Inoue, K., Chinen, T., Ueoka, H., and Nagura, E. (1979): Clinical study of aclacinomycin A. *Cancer Treat. Rep.,* 63:931–934.
85. Olson, H. M., Young, D. M., Prieur, D. J., LeRoy, A. F., and Reagan, R. L. (1974): Electrolyte and morphologic alterations of myocardium in adriamycin-treated rabbits. *Am. J. Pathol.,* 77:439–450.
86. Panettiere, F., and Coltman, C. A., Jr. (1971): Phase I experience with emetine hydrochloride (NSC-33669) as an antitumor agent. *Cancer,* 27:835–841.
87. Paul, J. G., Rhodes, D. B., and Skow, J. R. (1975): Renal cell carcinoma presenting as right atrial tumor with successful removal using cardiopulmonary bypass. *Ann. Surg.,* 181:471–473.
88. Perevodchikova, N. I., Lichinitser, M. R., and Gorbunova, V. A. (1977): Phase I clinical study of carminomycin: Its activity against soft tissue sarcomas. *Cancer Treat. Rep.,* 61:1705–1707.
89. Pierce, R. H., Hafermann, M. D., and Kagan, A. R. (1969): Changes in the transverse cardiac diameter following mediastinal irradiation for Hodgkin's disease. *Radiology,* 93:619–624.
90. Praga, C., Beretta, G., Vigo, P. L., Lenaz, G. R., Pollini, C., Bonadonna, G., Canetta, R., Castellani, R., Villa, E., Gallagher, C. G., von Melchner, H., Hayat, M., Ribaud, P., De Wash, G., Mattsson, W., Heinz, R., Waldner, R., Kolaric, K., Buehner, R., Ten Bokkel-Huyninck, W., Perevodchikova, N. I., Manziuk, L. A., Senn, H. J., and Mayr, A. C. (1979): Adriamycin cardiotoxicity: A survey of 1273 patients. *Cancer Treat. Rep.,* 63:827–834.
91. Pratt, C. B., Ransom, J. L., and Evans, W. E. (1978): Age-related adriamycin cardiotoxicity in children. *Cancer Treat. Rep.,* 62:1381–1385.
92. Prout, M. N., Richards, M. J. S., Chung, K. J., Joo, P., and Davis, H. L., Jr. (1977): Adriamycin cardiotoxicity in children. Case reports, literature review, and risk factors. *Cancer,* 39:62–65.
93. Ramos, A., Meyer, R. A., Korfhagen, J., Yuen Wong, K., and Kaplan, S. (1976): Echocardio-

graphic evaluation of adriamycin cardiotoxicity in children. *Cancer Treat. Rep.,* 60:1281-1284.
94. Ravry, M. J. R. (1979): Cardiotoxicity of mitomycin C in man and animals. *Cancer Treat. Rep.,* 63:555.
95. Reybet-Degat, O., and Jeannin, L. (1975): Insuffisance cardiaque par fistule artério-veineuse, révélatrice d'un cancer du rein. A propos d'un cas. *Lyon Med.,* 233:385-390.
96. Ripault, J., Weil, M., and Jacquillat, C. (1967): Etude nécropsique de quatre malades traités par la rubidomycine. *Pathol. Biol.,* 15:955-957.
97. Roberts, W. C., Bodey, G. P., and Wertlake, P. T. (1968): The heart in acute leukemia. A study of 420 autopsy cases. *Am. J. Cardiol.,* 21:388-412.
98. Roberts, W. C., Glancy, D. L., and DeVita, V. T. (1968): Heart in malignant lymphoma (Hodgkin's disease, lymphosarcoma, reticulum cell sarcoma and mycosis fungoides). A study of 196 autopsy cases. *Am. J. Cardiol.,* 22:85-107.
99. Rose, R. G. (1962): Intracavitary radioactive colloidal gold: Results in 257 cancer patients. *J. Nucl. Med.,* 3:323-331.
100. Rosen, P., and Armstrong, D. (1973): Nonbacterial thrombotic endocarditis in patients with malignant neoplastic diseases. *Am. J. Med.,* 54:23-29.
101. Rosen, G., Suwansirikul, S., Kwon, C., Tan, C., Wu, S. J., Beattie, E. J., Jr., and Murphy, M. L. (1974): High-dose methotrexate with citrovorum factor rescue and adriamycin in childhood osteogenic sarcoma. *Cancer,* 33:1151-1163.
102. Rote, A. R., Flint, L. D., and Ellis, F. H., Jr. (1977): Intracaval recurrence of pheochromocytoma extending into right atrium. Surgical management using extracorporeal circulation. *N. Engl. J. Med.,* 296:1269-1271.
103. Roth, A., Kolaric, K., and Popovic, S. (1975): Cardiotoxicity of 5-fluorouracil (NSC-19893). *Cancer Chemother. Rep.,* 59:1051-1052.
104. Rozencweig, M., Kenis, Y., Atassi, G., Duarte-Karim, M., and Staquet, M. (1975): DNA-adriamycin. Preliminary results in animals and man. *Cancer Chemother. Rep.,* 6:131-136.
105. Rubin, E., Camara, J., Grayzel, D. M., and Zak, F. G. (1963): Radiation-induced cardiac fibrosis. *Am. J. Med.,* 34:71-75.
106. Ruckdeschel, J. C., Chang, P., Martin, R. G., Byhardt, R. W. O'Connell, M. J., Sutherland, J. C., and Wiernik, P. H. (1975): Radiation-related pericardial effusions in patients with Hodgkin's disease. *Medicine,* 54:245-259.
107. Sanyal, S. K., Saldivar, V., Coburn, T. P., Wrenn, E. L., Jr., and Kumar, M. (1976): Hyperdynamic heart failure due to A-V fistula associated with Wilms' tumor. *Pediatrics,* 57:564-568.
108. Schechter, J. P., and Jones, S. E. (1975): Myocardial infarction in a 27-year-old woman: Possible complication of treatment with VP-16-213 (NSC-141540), mediastinal irradiation, or both. *Cancer Chemother. Rep.,* 59:887-888.
109. Schwartz, H. S., and Kanter, P. M. (1975): Cell interactions: Determinants of selective toxicity of adriamycin (NSC-123127) and daunorubicin (NSC-82151). *Cancer Chemother. Rep. Part 3,* 6:107-114.
110. Short, I. A., and Padfield, P. L. (1976): Malignant phaeochromocytoma with severe constipation and myocardial necrosis. *Br. Med. J.,* 2:793-794.
111. Slavin, R. E., Millan, J. C., and Mullins, G. M. (1975): Pathology of high dose intermittent cyclophosphamide therapy. *Hum. Pathol.,* 6:693-709.
112. Smith, B. (1969): Damage to the intrinsic cardiac neurones by rubidomycin (daunorubicin). *Br. Heart J.,* 31:607-609.
113. Smith, P. J., Ekert, H., Waters, K. D., and Matthews, R. N. (1977): High incidence of cardiomyopathy in children treated with adriamycin and DTIC in combination chemotherapy. *Cancer Treat. Rep.,* 61:1736-1738.
114. Smith, F. E., Lane, M., and Hudgins, P. T. (1974): Conservative management of malignant pericardial effusion. *Cancer,* 33:47-57.
115. Spindola-Franco, H., Björk, L., and Berger, M. (1975): Intracavitary metastasis to the left ventricle: An angiocardiographic diagnosis. *Br. J. Radiol.,* 48:649-651.
116. Steinberg, I. (1968): Angiocardiography in diagnosis of pericardial effusion and pulmonary stenosis in Hodgkin's disease. *Am. J. Roentgenol.,* 102:619-626.
117. Stewart, J. R., Cohn, K. E., Fajardo, L. F., Hancock, E. W., and Kaplan, H. S. (1967): Radiation-induced heart disease. A study of twenty-five patients. *Radiology,* 89:302-310.
118. Stewart, J. R., and Fajardo, L. F. (1971): Dose response in human and experimental radiation-

induced heart disease. Application of the nominal standard dose (NSD) concept. *Radiology,* 99:403–408.
119. Talley, R. W., O'Bryan, R. M., Gutterman, J. U., Brownlee, R. W., and McCredie, K. B.: Clinical evaluation of toxic effects of *cis*-diamminedichloroplatinum (NSC-119875). Phase I clinical study. *Cancer Chemother. Rep.,* 57:465–471.
120. Tan, C., Etcubanas, E., Wollner, N., Rosen, G., Gilladoga, A., Showel, J., Murphy, M. L., and Krakoff, I. H. (1973): Adriamycin. An antitumor antibiotic in the treatment of neoplastic diseases. *Cancer,* 32:9–17.
121. Terry, L. N., and Kligerman, M. M. (1970): Pericardial and myocardial involvement by lymphomas and leukemias. The role of radiotherapy. *Cancer,* 25:1003–1008.
122. Thomas, J. H., Panoussopoulos, D. G., Jewell, W. R., and Pierce, G. E. (1977): Tricuspid stenosis secondary to metastatic melanoma. *Cancer,* 39:1732–1737.
123. Thompson, N. W., Brown, J., Orringer, M., Sisson, J., and Nishiyama, R. (1978): Follicular carcinoma of the thyroid with massive angioinvasion: Extension of tumor thrombus to the heart. *Surgery,* 83:451–457.
124. Thorson, A., Björck, G., Björkman, G., and Waldenström, J. (1954): Malignant carcinoid of the small intestine with metastases to the liver, valvular disease of the right side of the heart (pulmonary stenosis and tricuspid regurgitation without septal defects), peripheral vasomotor symptoms, bronchoconstriction, and an unusual type of cyanosis. *Am. Heart J.,* 47:795–817.
125. Tracy, G. P., Brown, D. E., Johnson, L. W., and Gottlieb, A. J. (1974): Radiation-induced coronary artery disease. *JAMA,* 228:1660–1662.
126. Trouet, A., and Sokal, G. (1979): Clinical studies with daunorubicin-DNA and adriamycin-DNA complexes: A review. *Cancer Treat. Rep.,* 63:895–898.
127. Utley, J. R., Mobin-Uddin, K., Segnitz, R. H., Belin, R. P., and Utley, J. F. (1973): Acute obstruction of tricuspid valve by Wilms' tumor. *J. Thorac. Vasc. Surg.,* 66:626–628.
128. Vaughan, E. D., Jr., Crosby, I. K., and Tegtmeyer, C. J. (1977): Nephroblastoma with right atrial extension: Preoperative diagnosis and management. *J. Urology,* 117:530–533.
129. Von Hoff, D. D., Elson, D., Pollard, G., and Coltman, C. A., Jr. (1980): Acute ventricular fibrillation and death during infusion of *m*-AMSA. *Cancer Treat. Rep. (in press).*
130. Von Hoff, D. D., Layard, M. W., Basa, P., Davis, H. L., Jr., Von Hoff, A. L., Rozencweig, M., and Muggia, F. M. (1979): Risk factors of doxorubicin-induced congestive heart failure. *Ann. Intern. Med.,* 91:710–717.
131. Von Hoff, D. D., Layard, M., Rozencweig, M., and Muggia, F. M. (1977): Time relationship between last dose of daunorubicin and congestive heart failure. *Cancer Treat. Rep.,* 61:1411–1413.
132. Von Hoff, D. D., Rozencweig, M., Layard, M., Slavik, M., and Muggia, F. M. (1977): Daunomycin-induced cardiotoxicity in children and adults. A review of 110 cases. *Am. J. Med.,* 62:200–208.
133. Von Hoff, D. D., Rozencweig, M., and Slavik, M. (1978): Daunomycin: An anthracycline antibiotic effective in acute leukemia. *Adv. Pharmacol. Chemother.,* 15:1–50.
134. Weinberger, A., Pinkhas, J., Sandbank, U., Shaklai, M., and de Vries, A. (1975): Endocardial fibrosis following busulfan treatment. *JAMA,* 231:495.
135. Weiss, A. J., Metter, G. E., Fletcher, W. S., Wilson, W. L., Grage, T. B., and Ramirez, G. (1976): Studies on adriamycin using a weekly regimen demonstrating its clinical effectiveness and lack of cardiac toxicity. *Cancer Treat. Rep.,* 60:813–822.
136. Weissler, A. M., Harris, W. S., and Schoenfeld, C. D. (1968): Systolic time intervals in heart failure in man. *Circulation,* 37:149–159.
137. Wiernik, P. H., Schimpff, S. C., Schiffer, C. A., Lichtenfeld, J. L., Aisner, J., O'Connell, M. J., and Fortner, C. (1976): Randomized clinical comparison of daunorubicin (NSC-82151) alone with a combination of daunorubicin, cytosine arabinoside (NSC-63878), 6-thioguanine (NSC-752), and pyrimethamine (NSC-3061) for the treatment of acute nonlymphocytic leukemia. *Cancer Treat. Rep.,* 60:41–53.
138. Wilcox, R. G., James, P. D., and Toghill, P. J. (1976): Endomyocardial fibrosis associated with daunorubicin therapy. *Br. Heart J.,* 38:860–863.
139. Williams, C. J. (1978): Doxorubicin cardiotoxicity: Role of digoxin in prevention. *Br. Med. J.,* 1:176.
140. Wiltshaw, E., and Carr, B. (1974): *Cis*-platinum (II) diammine-dichloride. Clinical experience of the Royal Marsden Hospital and Institute of Cancer Research, London. In: *Platinum Coordi-*

nation Complexes in Cancer Chemotherapy. Recent Results in Cancer Research, Vol. 48, edited by T. A. Connors and J. J. Roberts, pp. 178–182. Springer-Verlag, Berlin.

141. Yamanaka, N., Kato, T., Nishida, K., Fujikawa, T., Fukushima, M., and Ota, K. (1979): Elevation of serum lipid peroxide level associated with doxorubicin toxicity and its amelioration by [dl]-α-tocopheryl acetate or coenzyme Q_{10} in mouse (doxorubicin, toxicity, lipid peroxide, tocopherol, coenzyme Q_{10}). *Cancer Chemother. Pharmacol.,* 3:223–227.

Medical Complications in Cancer Patients,
edited by J. Klastersky and M. J. Staquet.
Raven Press, New York © 1981.

Malnutrition and Artificial Nutrition in Cancer Patients

Yvon Algrain Carpentier

Surgical Metabolism Unit, Department of Surgery, Saint-Pierre Hospital, Free University of Brussels, 1000 Brussels, Belgium

Malnutrition and cachexia have long been considered initial and common manifestations of cancer. It is difficult to determine among the clinical and metabolic consequences of cancer those that are due to the tumor itself and those that are the result of malnutrition. Moreover, carcinolytic treatments (surgery, radiotherapy, immunotherapy, and chemotherapy) severely affect the host and increase the complexity of the general picture.

During the past 10 years, the development of clinical and laboratory methods for assessing nutritional status led to the observation that malnutrition was a widespread and often unrecognized problem in hospitalized patients. New techniques of alimentation—i.e., total parenteral nutrition (TPN)—have become available. Their usefulness and efficacy in the treatment of various diseases associated with impaired oral feeding is now well established. Recent reports suggest that they could be a useful adjunct to the treatment of cancer (17). These nutritional techniques could not only correct the nutritional depletion of cancer patients but also allow adequate identification of the nonnutritional effects of cancer.

However, there is at the present time no general consensus on the benefit of improving the nutritional status of cancer patients. Although it seems that the fear of feeding the tumor rather than the host (55) is not justified (17), some oncologists still feel that anorexia could be a defense of the host against the tumor growth (9).

CACHEXIA

Cachexia is the result of the metabolic alterations induced by tumor growth. The manifestations of cachexia are weakness, fatigue, anorexia, and weight loss with depletion and redistribution of host components leading to an altered anatomic picture of the patient as well as to the inability to conserve normal regulatory functions. These symptoms are not clearly correlated to the caloric intake or to the amount, type, and anatomical site of neoplastic tissues. It is amazing

231

to observe that some patients bearing widespread tumors with disseminated metastases are not cachectic whereas others with limited tumors exhibit a severe degree of cachexia. The fact that tumor mass in cancer patients, even at the time of death, infrequently represents more than 5% of the host weight and that the effects of cancer cannot be entirely explained by the impaired food intake and absorption, led to the concept of "systemic effects of cancer" induced by chemical mediators released from neoplastic tissues (20). Various endocrine effects of some tumors induce well-recognized paraneoplastic hormonal syndromes. Several nonhormonal mediators have been isolated, and the subject has been reviewed extensively (20).

CLINICAL AND LABORATORY PARAMETERS OF NUTRITIONAL ASSESSMENT

General clinical examination of the patient provides an overall indication of the nutritional state and detects some abnormalities due to deficiencies in vitamins or trace elements. Weight loss is a common finding and is known to occur at some time in the history of cancer patients. When it does occur, if there is no intervention against the cancer, the evolution is progressive inanition and ultimate death. In two recent surveys (11,40), weight loss exceeding 6% of previous body weight was found in 40 to 75% of cancer patients. There was no significant difference in weight loss between a group of patients with limited bronchogenic cancers and another group with extensive diseases, but the median survival times in the depleted patients were less than half those observed in better nourished patients (40). Weight loss can represent either a depletion of the various compartments of the host or the selective depletion of one compartment. Selective deficits in visceral proteins and skeletal muscle with no detectable change in fat stores were observed in patients with colorectal neoplasms (48). Children with the diencephalic syndrome exhibit selective depletion of the fat compartment (4). Body weight measurements do not indicate specific depletion in one compartment, and their significance is dubious in case of fluid accumulation. However, body weight changes over rather long periods of time correlate well with changes in the nutritional status.

Measurement of skinfold thickness provides an estimation of the body fat stores (27). However, the range of normality is wide, and the correlation of this determination to total body fat is both age and sex dependent.

Skeletal muscle represents about 75% and visceral compartment the remaining 25% of the body cell mass (46), which cannot be measured directly. A method for an indirect determination of total exchangeable potassium was developed by Shizgal (53) which he claimed to be an accurate quantitative assessment of total body cell mass. An estimation of the whole body skeletal muscle mass can be given by anthropometric measurement of muscle circumference of the nondominant arm (37). Another estimation of skeletal muscle mass can be obtained by determining the creatinine height index (5).

The visceral protein compartment is responsible for maintaining tissue function, protein synthesis, and the immune response (6). Proteins from this compartment have different half-lives (34). However, nutritional assessment in most patients is generally limited to the determination of albumin and transferrin concentrations in the plasma. Each of these proteins has a long half-life, and their concentrations are affected by factors other than malnutrition.

That malnutrition—and hypoproteinemia—induces an increased susceptibility to infection is suggested by many clinical and epidemiologic data. However, the heterogeneity of the patient population, the presence of coexisting infections, and the difficulty of accurately assessing the nutritional status make it difficult to study the association between nutrition and immune competence so that an exact relationship remains unclear (3). Very severe and prolonged protein–calorie malnutrition is known to alter T-lymphocyte and polymorphonuclear cell functions, whereas B-lymphocyte function is better maintained. Therefore, lymphocyte functions do not indicate an early or mild alteration in nutritional status, but might be appropriate for detection of vitamin or trace element deficiencies (45). The delayed cutaneous hypersensitivity skin tests, widely used as an index of immune competence, require the participation of not only T-cells, but also B-cells and other leukocytes (45). They can be impaired in several pathological conditions (38). Anergy is therefore not specific of immune deficiency, and in a recent review Miller (45) proposed measurements of leukocyte sensitivity to migration inhibitory factor, chemotaxis, and bactericidal activity as the best possible immunologic tests for indicating early nutritional depletion.

Further studies are needed to define more adequate parameters for assessing nutritional status of the patient. Besides specific protein–calorie malnutrition, increased attention should be paid—particularly in patients with cancer—to the diagnosis of vitamin and mineral deficiencies (11).

CAUSES OF NUTRITIONAL DEPLETION IN CANCER PATIENTS

Effects of Cancer on Nutritional Status

The classic causes of nutritional depletion in cancer are decreased food intake, altered intestinal absorption, loss of nutrients, and altered metabolic adaptations. Whether other factors are involved in malnutrition associated with cancer, as suggested by some authors (20), is still a matter of controversy.

Decreased Food Intake and Anorexia

Estimating the quantitative decrease of food intake in cancer patients is problematic, due to the difficulty of defining appropriate control groups. Mechanical difficulties for normal oral feeding are encountered in patients bearing head or neck cancer, or they can be due to an extrinsic or intraluminal compression of the gastrointestinal tract. Besides these mechanical alterations, anorexia is a frequent problem in cancer patients. Indeed, impaired food consumption has been demonstrated in studies of patients with a variety of neoplastic diseases (56). Decreased taste was correlated with an elevated taste threshold for sweet and was associated with extensive neoplastic process, low calorie intake, and massive weight loss (21). Recently the correction of such taste abnormality after protein repletion with TPN (49) led to the hypothesis that deficiency in vitamins, minerals, and structural proteins could be responsible for altered taste sensation. Aversion for meat is correlated with a lowered taste threshold for bitter (21).

Psychological factors frequently observed in cancer patients—anxiety, discomfort, pain, nausea—may contribute to anorexia. Other factors (22) have been suggested as well, e.g., a high lactate production by the tumor, an altered amino acid pattern or hormonal profile, and by-products released by the neoplasm. Prolonged stimulation of gastrointestinal receptors due to impaired intestinal absorption could increase the feeling of satiety and account for the symptom of decreased eating later in the day observed in cancer patients. Heat generated by tumor metabolism could stimulate thermostatic sensors and have a regulatory effect on food intake.

Altered Function of the Gastrointestinal Tract

Malabsorption can occur regardless of whether the cancer is related to the gastrointestinal tract. When the tumor growth does not directly affect the digestive tract, alterations in the gastrointestinal system are secondary to decreased food consumption. Because the digestive tract is one of the most metabolically active systems in the body, decreased food intake induces a marked nitrogen loss from the small intestine, liver, and pancreas, as shown by experimental studies in rats (39). Decreased protein synthesis results in villous atrophy of the intestinal mucosa and impaired activity of the enzymes involved in digestive processes. Ovarian tumors, because of their propensity for seeding the peritoneal cavity, can cause intestinal obstruction or induce the development of ascites (52). Cancers unrelated to the digestive system can affect hepatic function by spreading metastases in the liver.

Involvement of the gastrointestinal tract by the tumoral process usually induces marked alterations in nutritional status. Partial or complete, progressive or acute obstruction of the alimentary tract is commonly caused by neoplasms and is associated with dysphagia, anorexia, pain, nausea, vomiting, diarrhea, or anemia (52). Besides the previously mentioned alterations in the small bowel mucosa, impaired absorption of food can result from lymphatic compression or node invasion by tumoral process, pancreatic exocrine deficiency caused by carcinoma, excess gastric acid production as observed with Zollinger-Ellison syndrome, bypass of portions of the small bowel due to neoplastic fistulas, blind loop syndrome, achylia, and vitamin B_{12} deficiency caused by tumoral gastric invasion. Diarrhea is commonly observed in these situations. It is a symptom characteristic of the presence of a neoplasm in the ascending colon or a villous tumor of the rectum. It can also result from biologically active substances formed by tumors of the alimentary tract (42). Malignant gastrocolic, enteroenteric, enterocolic, or external enterocutaneous fistulas of the alimentary tract can cause very severe nutrient losses.

Primary or secondary neoplastic invasion of the liver frequently results in ascites and impaired liver function, leading occasionally to renal failure.

Metabolic Alterations in Cancer Patients

Nonmalignant starvation is characterized by a shift of the host to fat fuel economy with glucose and protein sparing. Basal metabolic rate, O_2 consumption, CO_2 production, and respiratory quotient are decreased (10). Brain acquires the ability to consume ketone bodies so that glucose consumption accounts for less than 15% of the oxidative metabolism.

These adaptations do not take place during cancer starvation, where the metabolic picture looks more like the one observed after major injury or during sepsis (8). Measurements of resting metabolic rate in cancer patients have generally but not unequivocally provided supranormal values (61), together with high O_2 consumption and CO_2 production.

Fasting glucose and insulin concentrations of tumor-bearing patients are generally in the normal range, whereas hypoglycemia occurs in rare cases (7). Glucose tolerance is decreased in a large proportion of patients irrespective of the type of the cancer, but in association with cachexia and hypoalbuminemia (36). Impaired insulin release was recently reported (36).

Experimental studies showed markedly increased glucose transport and consumption in tumor cells resulting in glucose depletion in the interstitial fluid with intracellular glucose enrichment (32). At the interface between tumor and host, ability to survive and grow in a locally glucose-depleted environment could represent a selective advantage for tumoral tissue, allowing its expansion at the expense of normal tissue (8). Although various neoplastic tissues are able to use glucose aerobically (59), high glucose consumption and lactate production in tumoral tissue were demonstrated by Cori and Cori (18). Cori cycle activity is increased in cancer patients, especially in those who have lost weight (58). It seems unlikely that this glucose–lactate recycling alone could account for the elevated energy expenditure observed in cancer patients, but other gluconeogenic and/or futile cycles could be involved in this phenomenon (61). Administration of an exogenous glucose load to the tumor-bearing host does not turn off either gluconeogenesis or fatty acid mobilization and oxidation (57). This metabolic behavior is strikingly similar to the one observed in injured and septic patients (13,28). Endogenous lipid metabolism has not been widely investigated in cancer patients; increased peripheral lipolysis was reported, maybe due to the effect of substances released by the tumor. Since the correlation observed in normal subjects between glycerol plasma concentration and turnover was no longer found in injured patients (13), kinetic studies should be encouraged rather than determinations of plasma concentration.

Nitrogen balance does not separate host and tumor metabolism and does not take into account N_2 production. Measurements of this parameter in cancer patients have not been very revealing and have led to controversial results. The wasting of lean body mass, which is frequently observed in association with cancer, results from decreased protein synthesis (30)—and possibly increased breakdown—in muscle cells. These alterations could be specific to cancer disease, but they can be overcome by supplying large amounts of amino acids to muscle (43). Hypoalbuminemia is probably the result of decreased synthesis, but consumption of albumin by the tumor or distribution of albumin into abnormal spaces has been suggested (20). No data are available to clearly separate the specific effect of decreased protein intake from the consequence of cancer disease on lowering albumin level. It was shown, however, that parenteral nutrition could restore normal albumin levels in cancer patients, even in the absence of change in the tumor (25).

Protein synthesis in the tumor appears to be maintained irrespective of the nutritional intake. Indeed, an experimental study on tumor-bearing rats showed that during starvation DNA synthesis in the liver of the host is markedly reduced, whereas it is unaffected or even increased in the tumor (8). Other experimental work led to the concept of the tumor behaving as a nitrogen trap (44), but these findings were not confirmed by studies using various animal models (19). It is unlikely that this concept should be strictly applied in man, especially since tumor growth is more limited in human subjects than in animal models. Imbalances in the pattern of plasma amino acids have been observed in cancer patients. Amino acids seem to behave differently in tumor than in normal tissue (50). In injured and septic patients, alterations in amino acid composition within muscle were shown to be larger than and to precede modifications in plasma (1). Similar investigations performed in cancer patients could provide interesting information on protein metabolism.

Effects of Cancer Therapy on Nutritional Status

The various oncological treatments—surgery, radiotherapy, and chemotherapy—affect major organ systems more or less severely. They can induce or aggravate profound nutritional depletion. It can become critical in some debilitated patients to weigh the risks of treatment versus the possible benefits.

Surgery

Radical surgical treatment of cancer often causes severe injury. The resulting metabolic alterations are similar to the ones observed in traumatized patients. Besides these significant metabolic consequences, surgery of the digestive tract can alter food intake and absorption (41). Mechanical problems after surgery for cancer of the head or neck can compromise oral feeding and necessitate the use of a feeding tube. Resection of the esophagus and/or the stomach leads to decreased food intake and impaired absorption of various nutrients, i.e., fat and vitamins. Extensive resection of the small intestine (which is not frequently performed in cancer surgery) results in the well-known "short bowel syndrome" and its extreme nutritional consequences. Occasionally, moderately extensive resection of irradiated small bowel leads to severe malabsorption. Surgical removal of all or part of the colon can induce disturbances in water and electrolyte balance, but does not seriously impair food intake and absorption.

Radical resection for carcinoma of the pancreas induces endocrine and exocrine insufficiency with impaired fat absorption. Major hepatic resection, ligation of the common hepatic artery, and infusion of chemotherapeutic agents in the hepatic arterial system are frequently associated with liver dysfunction. The incidence of hepatic decompensation and encephalopathy is higher in nutritionally deprived patients.

Anastomotic leakage represents the major complication in abdominal surgery. Septic contamination and nutrient losses used to lead to catastrophic rates of morbidity and mortality, but the prognosis of these complications has dramatically improved since TPN has been available (12).

Radiation Therapy

Because the gastrointestinal tract is one of the most metabolically active tissues of the body, radiotherapy directed to any of its organs impairs digestive function and has serious nutritional consequences. The alterations depend on the dose, time, fractionation of radiation, and the volume included in the treatment field; these changes are more severe if other carcinolytic treatment, surgery or chemotherapy, is associated (23). Radiotherapy for head and neck cancer induces temporary local inflammation of the oral cavity or the pharynx, decreased taste sensation, impaired saliva secretion, and dental caries. Weight loss is observed in 90% of the patients. Radiotherapy directed to the thorax can produce esophageal irritation with dysphagia; fibrosis and stenosis can occur later. Involvement of the stomach in the irradiation field can decrease the acidity of gastric secretions; high doses can cause ulcer and alter appetite. Abdominal radiotherapy directed on the small bowel and colon is frequently associated with nausea, vomiting, and diarrhea. Decreased cell proliferation and atrophy of intestinal villi together with impaired enzyme activity lead to malabsorption. Chronic diarrhea and partial or complete obstruction are the classical symptoms of delayed radiation-induced enteritis; they are associated with mucosal ulceration, vascular thrombosis, submucosal fibrosis, altered enteric flora, and perforation or fistula. As for most iatrogenic diseases, the incidence of these complications is not precisely known, but weight loss is found in almost 90% of the patients who undergo total abdominal irradiation.

Chemotherapy and Immunotherapy

Because of its lack of specificity, aggressive neoplastic drug therapy severely affects host cells. The specific effect on various organs of the most commonly used agents was recently reviewed (47) and so is not detailed here. Nausea and vomiting resulting in anorexia and decreased food intake are almost constant symptoms induced by most compounds. The toxicity of many agents on the mucosa of the alimentary tract and on the major secreting organs causes stomatitis, malabsorption, diarrhea, abdominal pain, rectitis, and proctitis. Mucosal ulceration, bleeding, and perforation can occur in the most severe cases. Ileus is a frequent side effect of vincristine. Leukopenia, thrombocytopenia, and/or anemia resulting from the toxicity on the hematopoietic system are dose-limiting for many chemotherapeutic compounds. Fever and chills are frequent side effects of immunotherapy or chemotherapy but can be the manifestations of sepsis; these specific symptoms are associated with anorexia and increased energy expenditure. Impaired food intake is the more common consequence of dysfunction of the central nervous system induced by chemotherapy agents or tranquilizers. Liver function is often altered by chemotherapy and immunotherapy. Steroids and methotrexate can induce muscle atrophy and osteoporosis. Some agents can cause electrolyte imbalance, e.g., decreased sodium or calcium plasma levels. It seems established that the chances of response to oncological treatment are better in patients whose nutritional status has not been seriously altered (17). New types of treatment are, or could be, based on the qualitative and quantitative difference in substrate requirements between tumor and normal cells.

ARTIFICIAL NUTRITION IN CANCER PATIENTS

Enteral feeding with an elemental diet and parenteral alimentation (TPN) are the two types of artificial nutrition that have preferentially been used for the nutritional support of cancer patients during the past 10 years. Enteral nutrition by tube was recently reviewed by Shils (51). The discussion here is limited to the use of TPN in cancer patients.

Technical and Metabolic Aspects of TPN

After more than 10 years of widespread experience with TPN, septic contamination and metabolic alterations remain the major complications of this technique. Although these problems are even more acute in cancer disease, they should not prevent the depleted patient from receiving nutritional support.

The effects of TPN on the metabolism of cancer patients have not been widely studied. The analogies between cancer-bearing and severely injured patients suggest that recent findings on the metabolic consequences of TPN in trauma patients should be taken into account. However, the application of these data to the treatment of cancer patients is speculative. Rates of mobilization and oxidation of endogenous fat are elevated in surgical patients and persist even when large amounts of glucose are administered (13). Carbohydrate intake exceeding the energy expenditure induces an increase in metabolic rate, oxygen consumption, and CO_2 production (28). Excessive liver storage of glycogen and fat is associated with impaired hepatic function. These alterations are minimized when fat is included as part of the energy intake (2). Moreover, injured patients exhibit higher rates of removal and oxidation of exogenous lipids when compared to normal controls and depleted patients without malignancy (14). It seems therefore reasonable to avoid excessive calorie intake and to include fat in the intravenous diet of cancer patients. However, two fundamental questions are still unanswered: What is the energy requirement of the cancer patient? What is the optimal proportion of lipid in the energy intake? Without strong data to provide clear answers, we suggest that the calorie intake would not exceed 150% of the energy expenditure estimated for each patient [i.e., following the tables provided by Wilmore (60)], and that fat would account for 30 to 45% of the infused calories. Crystalline amino acids should be administered to provide 1 g nitrogen per 150 cal; specially adapted solutions should be used in case of renal or hepatic insufficiency. The need for electrolytes, minerals, and oligo and trace elements, as well as folate and vitamins, should be covered (25). Despite the increased susceptibility of cancer patients to infection, the risk of TPN-related sepsis is minimal if a careful nursing of the infusion system is provided by a specialized team (15). We recently described a safe system for infusing TPN without mixing exogenous fat with the water-soluble nutrients (29). The application of special methods for ambulatory and home parenteral alimentation presents a special interest in cancer patients (25,54). The aim of nutritional repletion is to replenish lean body mass rather than fat. Since physical exercise is essential for regeneration of skeletal muscle, a program of physical rehabilitation should accompany TPN (25).

First Results of TPN as an Adjunct to Cancer Therapy

The controversy about the role of TPN as an adjunct to cancer therapy is due to the lack of large randomized studies providing objective evaluation. The available data show that the fear of feeding the tumor rather than the host, thereby accelerating cancer growth, is not justified (17). No harmful effect due to feeding was observed in a series of 2,000 cancer patients (25). The major established effect of TPN is to rehabilitate some patients who would otherwise have been poor or noncandidates to cancer treatment. Weight gain, improved anthropometric measurements, increased albumin level, and restoration of immune defenses were observed in most depleted patients after about 2 weeks of therapy (26).

Preoperative TPN, while improving the nutritional status, allows optimal bowel preparation. The availability of postoperative TPN permits more extensive resections and slower and more progressive reutilization of the digestive tract.

Faster recovery eventually allows early initiation of other oncological therapies. Finally, the efficacy of TPN in the treatment of such complications as digestive fistulas has been clearly demonstrated.

Protection against toxic intestinal effects during radiation therapy of the abdomen was demonstrated by using an elemental diet in rats (33) and TPN in dogs (24). This protection could be due to a reduction in pancreatic secretion. Increased tolerance to abdominal irradiation associated with weight gain and no apparent intestinal damage, nausea, or vomiting was reported in previously debilitated patients (23). No data are available to demonstrate a protection against bone marrow alterations during radiation therapy.

Weight gain and restoration of immune defenses obtained with TPN (16,17) can provide some previously debilitated patients a chance for chemotherapy that would otherwise have been denied to them (26). It seems well established that the nutritional status can affect the impact of chemotherapeutic drugs. TPN during the course of chemotherapy and/or immunotherapy has been shown to reduce nausea and vomiting in most instances as well as other symptoms of intestinal toxicity (17). There was no deterioration of nutritional status, and a feeling of well-being was generally observed. Regeneration of neutrophilic granulopoiesis after chemotherapy was accelerated by TPN (31,35). These data suggest that more aggressive chemotherapy could be administered to intravenously fed patients. However, the response rate or the survival has not significantly increased after using TPN in well-nourished patients receiving chemotherapy.

CONCLUSION

Malnutrition is commonly associated with cancer and can result from the disease and/or therapy. It is difficult to separate the specific effects of malnutrition from the consequences of bearing a tumor. This would be possible if the patients were nutritionally repleted. Tumor cells tolerate food deprivation better than normal tissues and live at the expense of the host. Thus starvation is not good for the cancer patient. TPN can adequately replenish debilitated patients and can provide new candidates for oncological therapy. However, TPN should not be given to patients who will not receive further treatment. The interest of TPN in cancer surgery is well established. Better tolerance and protection against toxicity of radiation therapy, chemotherapy, and immunotherapy have been demonstrated, but large prospective studies are needed to assess the role of TPN as an adjunct of these treatments. It is obvious that ideally cancer therapy should selectively affect tumoral tissue and artificial nutrition should selectively replenish normal tissues of the host and deprive neoplastic cells.

In this review, we have emphasized the need for further research in order to provide definition of better parameters for nutritional assessment, better knowledge of the factors involved in the development of cachexia, and better understanding of the metabolism of tumor and its host as well as the metabolic consequences of nutritional repletion.

REFERENCES

1. Askanazi, J., Elwyn, D. H., Kinney, J. H., Gump, F. E., Michelsen, C. B., and Stinchfield, F. E. (1978): Muscle and plasma aminoacids after injury: The role of inactivity. *Ann. Surg.,* 188:797–803.
2. Askanazi, J., Carpentier, Y. A., Elwyn, D. H., Nordenstrom, J., Jeevanandam, M., Rosenbaum, S. H., Gump, F. E., and Kinney, J. M. (1980): Influence of total parenteral nutrition on fuel utilization in injury and sepsis. *Ann. Surg.,* 191:40–46.
3. Awdeh, Z. L., Bengoa, J., Demayer, E. M., et al. (1972): A survey of nutritional–immunological interactions. *Bull. WHO,* 46:537–546.
4. Bain, H. W., Darte, J. M., Keith, W. S., and Kruyff, E. (1966): The diencephalic syndrome of early infancy due to silent brain tumor: With special reference to treatment. *Pediatrics,* 38:473–482.
5. Bistrian, B. R., Blackburn, G. L., Sherman, M., and Scrimshaw, N. S. (1975): Therapeutic index of nutritional depletion in hospitalized patients. *Surg. Gynecol. Obstet.,* 141:512–516.
6. Blackburn, G. L., Bistrian, B. R., Maini, B. S., Schlamm, H. J., and Smith, M. F. (1977): Nutritional and metabolic assessment of the hospitalized patient. *J. Parent. Ent. Nutr.,* 1:11–22.
7. Brennan, M. F. (1977): Uncomplicated starvation versus cancer cachexia. *Cancer Res.,* 37:2359–2364.
8. Brennan, M. F., and Goodgame, J. T. (1977): Nutrition and cancer: host tumour interaction during varying conditions of substrate availability. In: *Nutritional Aspects of Care in the Critically Ill,* edited by J. R. Richards and J. M. Kinney, pp. 523–540. Churchill Livingstone, Edinburgh.
9. Burke, M., and Kark, A. E. (1977): Parenteral feeding and cancer. *Lancet,* 2:999.
10. Cahill, G. F., Jr. (1970): Starvation in man. *N. Engl. J. Med.,* 282:668–675.
11. Calman, K. C. (1978): Nutritional support in malignant disease. *Proc. Nutr. Soc.,* 37:87–93.
12. Carpentier, Y., and Janne, P. (1978): Artificial nutrition and the gastrointestinal tract: Some clinical and experimental data. In: *Advances in Parenteral Nutrition,* edited by I. D. A. Johnston, pp. 501–508. MTP Press, Lancaster, England.
13. Carpentier, Y. A., Askanazi, J., Elwyn, D. H., Jeevanandam, M., Gump, F. E., Hyman, A. I., Burr, R., and Kinney, J. M. (1979): Effects of hypercaloric glucose infusion on lipid metabolism in injury and sepsis. *J. Trauma,* 19:649–654.
14. Carpentier, Y. A., Nordenstrom, J., Askanazi, J., Elwyn, D. H., Gump, F. E., and Kinney, J. M. (1979): Relationship between rates of clearance and oxidation of ^{14}C-intralipid in surgical patients. *Surg. Forum,* 30:72–74.
15. Copeland, E. M., III, MacFadyen, B. V., and Dudrick, S. J. (1974): The risk of hyperalimentation in patients with potential sepsis. *Surg. Gynecol. Obstet.,* 138:377–380.
16. Copeland, E. M., MacFadyen, B. V., and Dudrick, S. J. (1976): Effect of intravenous hyperalimentation on established delay hypersensitivity in the cancer patient. *Ann. Surg.,* 184:60–64.
17. Copeland, E. M., III, Daly, J. M., and Dudrick, S. J. (1977): Nutrition as an adjunct to cancer treatment in the adult. *Cancer Res.,* 37:2351–2456.
18. Cori, C. F., and Cori, G. T. (1925): Carbohydrate metabolism of tumors; changes in sugar, lactic acid, and CO_2-combining power of blood passing through tumor. *J. Biol. Chem.,* 63:397–405.
19. Costa, G., and Holland, J. F. (1962): Effects of Krebs-2 carcinoma on the lipid metabolism of male swiss mice. *Cancer Res.,* 22:1081–1083.
20. Costa, G. (1977): Cachexia, the metabolic component of neoplastic diseases. *Cancer Res.,* 37:2325–2327.
21. Dewys, W. D., and Walters, K. (1975): Abnormalities of taste sensation in cancer patients. *Cancer,* 36:1888–1896.
22. Dewys, W. D. (1977): Anorexia in cancer patients. *Cancer Res.,* 37:2354–2358.
23. Donaldson, S. S. (1977): Nutritional consequences of radiotherapy. *Cancer Res.,* 37:2407–2413.
24. Dubois, J. B., Joyeux, H., Yakoun, M., Pourquier, H., and Solassol, C. (1976): Total abdominal

irradiation and parenteral nutrition: an experimental study in the dog. *Biomedicine,* 25:123–125.

25. Dudrick, S. J., MacFadyen, B. V., Jr., Souchon, E. A., Englert, D. M., and Copeland, E. M., III (1977): Parenteral nutrition techniques in cancer patients. *Cancer Res.,* 37:2440–2450.

26. Dudrick, S. J. (1977): Summary of the informal discussion of nutritional management. *Cancer Res.,* 37:2462–2468.

27. Durnin, J. V., and Womersley, J. (1974): Body fat assessed from total body density and its estimation on 481 men and women aged from 16 to 72 years. *Br. J. Nutr.,* 32:77–97.

28. Elwyn, D. H., Kinney, J. M., Jeevanandam, M., Gump, F. E., and Broell, J. R. (1979): Influence of increasing carbohydrate intake on glucose kinetics in injured patients. *Ann. Surg.,* 190:117–127.

29. Francois, N., Vanderveken, L., and Carpentier, Y. A. (1979): A safe and inexpensive system for infusion of TPN with lipids. *J. Parent. Ent. Nutr.,* 3:314.

30. Goodlad, G. A. J., and Raymond, M. J. (1973): The action of the Walker 256 carcinoma and toxohormone on amino acid incorporation into diaphragm protein. *Eur. J. Cancer,* 9:139–145.

31. Hartlapp, J. H., Drebber, G., Noack, D., Walbert, G., Illiger, J., and Labedzki, L. (1979): Parenteral nutrition during aggressive chemotherapy accelerates neutrophilic granulopoietic recovery. In: *Abstracts (IV) of the Fifth Meeting of International Society of Hematology* (European and African Division), p. 51.

32. Hatanaka, M. (1974): Transport of sugars in tumor cell membranes. *Biochim. Biophys. Acta,* 355:77–104.

33. Hugon, J. S. (1976): Intestinal ultrastructure after prolonged use of an elemental diet. *Strahlentherapie,* 151:541–548.

34. Ingenbleek, Y., Van Den Schrieck, H. G., and De Nayer, P. (1975): Albumin, transferrin and the thyroxine-binding prealbumin/retinol-binding protein (TBPA-RBP) complex in assessment of malnutrition. *Clin. Chim. Acta,* 63:61–67.

35. Issell, B. F., Valdivieso, M., Zaren, H. A., Dudrick, S. J., Freireich, E. J., Copeland, E. M., and Bodey, G. P. (1978): Protection against chemotherapy toxicity by IV hyperalimentation. *Cancer Treat. Rep.,* 62:1139–1143.

36. Jasani, B., Donaldson, L. T., Ratcliffe, J. G., and Sokhi, G. S. (1978): Mechanism of impaired glucose tolerance in patients with neoplasia. *Br. J. Cancer,* 38:287–292.

37. Jelliffe, D. B. (1966): *Assessment of the Nutritional Status of the Community.* World Health Organization, Geneva.

38. Johnson, M. W., Maibach, H. I., and Salmon, N. E. (1971): Skin reactivity in patients with cancer: Impaired delayed hypersensitivity or faulty inflammatory response? *N. Engl. J. Med.,* 284:1255–1257.

39. Ju, J. S., and Nasset, E. S. (1959): Changes in total nitrogen content of some abdominal viscera in fasting and realimentation. *J. Nutr.,* 68:633–645.

40. Lanzotti, V. J., Thomas, D. R., Boyle, L. D., et al. (1977): Survival with inoperable lung cancer: An integration of prognostic variables based on simple clinical criteria. *Cancer,* 39:303–313.

41. Lawrence, W., Jr. (1977): Nutritional consequences of surgical resection of the gastrointestinal tract for cancer. *Cancer Res.,* 37:2379–2386.

42. Lipsett, M. B. (1977): Effects of cancers of the endocrine and central nervous systems on nutritional status. *Cancer Res.,* 37:2373–2376.

43. Lundholm, K., Bylund, A. C., Holm, J., and Schersten, T. (1976): Skeletal muscle metabolism in patients with malignant tumor. *Eur. J. Cancer,* 12:465–473.

44. Mider, G. B., Tesluk, J., and Morton, J. J. (1948): Effects of Walker carcinoma 256 on food intake, body weight and nitrogen metabolism of growing rats. *Acta Un. Intern. Contra Cancrum,* 6:409–420.

45. Miller, C. L. (1978): Immunological assays as measurements of nutritional status: a review. *J. Parent. Ent. Nutr.,* 2:554–566.

46. Moore, F. D., Olson, K. H., McMurray, J. E., Parker, H. V., Ball, N. R., and Boyden, C. M. (1963): In: *Body Cell Mass and Its Supporting Environment.* Saunders, Philadelphia.

47. Ohnuma, T., and Holland, J. F. (1977): Nutritional consequences of cancer chemotherapy and immunotherapy. *Cancer Res.,* 37:2395–2406.

48. Rombeau, J. L., Goldman, S. L., Apelgren, K. N., Sanford, I., and Frey, C. F. (1978): Protein–calorie malnutrition in patients with colorectal cancers. *Dis. Colon Rectum,* 21:587–589.
49. Russ, J. E., and Dewys, W. D. (1978): Correction of taste abnormality of malignancy with intravenous hyperalimentation. *Arch. Intern. Med.,* 138:799–800.
50. Shils, M. E. (1973): Nutrition and neoplasia. In: *Modern Nutrition in Health and Disease,* 5th ed., edited by R. S. Goodhart and M. E. Shils, pp. 981–996. Lea & Febiger, Philadelphia.
51. Shils, M. E. (1977): Enteral nutrition by tube. *Cancer Res.,* 37:2432–2439.
52. Shils, M. E. (1977): Nutritional problems associated with gastrointestinal and genitourinary cancer. *Cancer Res.,* 37:2366–2372.
53. Shizgal, H. M. (1976): Total body potassium and nutritional status. *Surg. Clin. North Am.,* 56:1185–1194.
54. Solassol, C., and Joyeux, H. (1976): Ambulatory parenteral nutrition. In: *Parenteral Alimentation,* edited by C. Manni, S. I. Magalini, and E. Sorascia, p. 143. Elsevier, New York.
55. Terepka, A. R., and Waterhouse, C. (1956): Metabolic observations during the forced feeding of patients with cancer. *Am. J. Med.,* 20:225–238.
56. Theologides, A., Ehlert, J., and Kennedy, B. J. (1976): The calorie intake of patients with advanced cancer. *Minn. Med.,* 59:526–529.
57. Waterhouse, C., and Kemperman, J. H. (1971): Carbohydrate metabolism in subjects with cancer. *Cancer Res.,* 31:1273–1278.
58. Waterhouse, C. (1974): Lactate metabolism in patients with cancer. *Cancer,* 33:66–71.
59. Weinhouse, S. (1955): Newer pathways of carbohydrate metabolism. *Diabetes,* 4:173–177.
60. Wilmore, D. H. (1977): *The Metabolic Management of the Critically Ill.* Plenum, New York.
61. Young, V. R. (1977): Energy metabolism and requirements in the cancer patient. *Cancer Res.,* 37:2336–2347.

Medical Complications in Cancer Patients,
edited by J. Klastersky and M. J. Staquet.
Raven Press, New York © 1981.

Prevention and Therapy of Infection in Myelosuppressed Patients

Jean Klastersky

Medical Service and Henri Tagnon Laboratory of Clinical Investigation, Jules Bordet Institute, Tumor Center, Free University of Brussels, 1000 Brussels, Belgium

Infection has long been recognized as a major cause of disease and death in patients with cancer. Infectious morbidity and mortality have been particularly important in patients with acute leukemia who undergo prolonged periods of severe granulopenia. Patients with fewer than 1,000 granulocytes/mm³ have an increased risk of serious infection, and this is magnified considerably as the granulocyte count decreases further (1).

Most infections in patients with acute nonlymphocytic leukemia (ANLL) are caused by microorganisms acquired in the hospital which colonize these high-risk patients (2). Since bacterial infections play an overwhelming role in myelosuppressed patients, most of this discussion is devoted to that type of infection, with special attention to Gram-negative bacillary sepsis.

PROTECTIVE ENVIRONMENT

In order to protect the patients during periods of high risk, several programs have been designed to isolate them from the nosocomial flora and/or to suppress their endogenous pathogens. During the last decade a dozen clinical studies have addressed themselves to the investigation of a protected environment (PE) or/and microbial suppression with orally administered prophylactic antibiotics (PA). The technical aspects of the management of these patients which provide adequate isolation and/or consistent microbial suppression have been described extensively in the many reports which form the basis for the present analysis and are not discussed here. We selected, for this review, the seven clinical studies of ANLL available in the literature that are prospective and randomly controlled. Any analysis based on a review of various published series has obvious limitations: variation in age and sex of the patients, the type of leukemia, the chemotherapeutic agents used, and other less apparent factors which may influence clinical responsiveness. Moreover, each of the seven trials employed only a small number of patients, making interpretation of results from individual studies difficult.

The seven studies considered for the present review are indicated in Table 1 (3–9). The first conclusion which appears from these data is the reduced frequency of infection in patients who were treated with PE and PA. This advantage of PEPA could be found in all seven studies. PA was found to be as good as PEPA in reducing the incidence of infection in patients with ANLL in two studies (5,6) and less effective than PEPA in three other (3,4,9). In two studies PA was not found more effective than standard ward care without isolation and microbial suppression (3,4); on the other hand, three studies found PA more effective than standard care (5,6,8). Thus at this stage one cannot make any clear statement about the efficacy of PA when compared to PEPA or to the controls.

PE alone (i.e., without microbial suppression) was evaluated in a controlled fashion in two studies only (4,7). Both trials found PE as good as PEPA in preventing infections in neutropenic patients with ANLL and more effective than standard care. In the EORTC study, PE and PEPA were found particularly effective in preventing infections of the pulmonary tract (7), a finding confirmed in Levine's study as far as PEPA is concerned (3). The observation that PE alone might decrease infection in granulocytopenic patients with ANLL supports Schimpff's finding that hospital-acquired microorganisms are a major cause of infection in these patients (2). In support of this concept are earlier uncontrolled studies indicating that isolated granulopenic patients with leukemia had only minimal acquisition of *Staphylococcus aureus* and Gram-negative bacilli and no infections with pathogens which are spread by the airborne route such as *Aspergillus* sp. (10). More studies are thus indicated to compare further PE and PEPA. One might even ask whether strict reverse isolation in a standard

TABLE 1. *Incidence of infection and remission rate in ANLL adults treated in a protected environment and/or with prophylactic antibiotics*

Study and ref.	Results[a]	
	Incidence of infection[b]	Remission and survival
Levine et al. (3)	PEPA (22) > PA (38) = C (28)	No difference
Yates and Holland (4)	PEPA (28) = PE (22) > PA (28) = C (39)	No difference
Klastersky et al. (5)	PEPA (16) = PA (14) > C (13)	No difference
Schimpff et al. (6)	PEPA (24) = PA (19) > C (21)	Increased survival and remission rates for PE and PA
Dietrich et al. (7)	PEPA (42) = PE (44)[c] > C (51)	No difference
Gaya et al. (8)	PA (46) > C (49)	No difference
Lohner et al. (9)	PEPA (24) > PA (21)	No difference

[a] Only statistically significant differences were taken into consideration.
[b] PE = protected environment. PA = prophylactic antibiotics. C = controls. Numbers in parentheses indicate the number of patients studied.
[c] Difference significant for pulmonary infection only.

hospital room would not be as efficacious as PE (life island or laminar air flow room) where air filtration is an additional protective measure.

The analysis presented here is similar to that made by Levine (11); there is, however, another way to look at the data available in the literature. Since granulocytopenia is such an overwhelmingly important factor predisposing leukemia patients to severe infection, we analyzed the frequency of infection reported in the various series in patients with fewer than 1,000 granulocytes/mm³. These patients can be considered a fairly homogeneous population as far as the risk of infection is concerned. Similarly, since all the patients had some form of ANLL and were treated with modern chemotherapy, they can be considered also as a relatively homogeneous population as far as the outcome of the leukemia is concerned. By combining all the patients with ANLL and fewer than 1,000 granulocytes/mm³ from the various controlled studies available, one can compare the efficacy of PEPA, PE, PA, and standard care on a larger number of patients than those found in individual studies. This type of analysis permits one to express the frequency of infection and the remission rate of leukemia under various conditions of supportive care in a more meaningful fashion.

The infectious morbidity and mortality rates in controls and in patients treated with PEPA, PE, or PA are indicated in Table 2. First, it can be seen that patients treated with PEPA and PE spent more time with a granulocyte count lower than 1,000/mm³ than those treated with PA or controls. This observation might reflect a more aggressive chemotherapy to patients who have been isolated; because chemotherapy of leukemia varied between studies and even within each one of them as time passed, it is possible that isolated patients received more

TABLE 2. *Infectious morbidity and mortality in patients with ANLL treated in a protected environment and/or with prophylactic antibiotics*

Parameter	PEPA	PE	PA	Controls
No. of patients	155	66	140	207
No. of days at risk[a]	4,634	2,022	3,134	3,985
Days at risk/total days	0.64	0.74	0.44	0.50
Mean days at risk per patient	29.8	30.6	22.3	19.2
No. of infections				
Per patient	0.66	0.70	0.92	1.06
Per 1,000 days at risk	22.2	25.2	41.1	53.7
Infectious deaths				
Percent of patients dying[b]	13	—	32	24
No. of deaths per 1,000 days at risk	4.29	—	14.9	11.8

Data computed from a review of seven prospective randomly controlled studies.
See Table 1 for abbreviations.
[a] Days at risk = days spent with WBC < 1,000/mm³.
[b] PEPA/PA: $p < 0.01$. PEPA/controls: $p < 0.01$. PA/controls: not significant.

chemotherapy than others. Nevertheless, severe infections were less frequent among patients in PEPA or PE than in controls or patients treated with PA. This was true whether the frequency of infections per patient or per 1,000 days at risk (days spent with fewer than 1,000 granulocytes/mm^3) was considered. Moreover, the mortality resulting from infection was lower in patients in PEPA (13%) than in those receiving PA (32%) or in controls (24%) ($p <$ 0.01).

Thus this type of analysis clearly confirms the impression already gained from the study of individual investigations that PEPA reduces the morbidity and the mortality from infections in neutropenic patients with ANLL. The rate of infection per patients was reduced from approximately 1.1 to 0.65 in spite of a greater risk in the patients treated in PEPA. Our analysis also suggests the effectiveness of PE; however, only two studies and a limited number of patients are available. On the other hand, it appears clear from this overall evaluation that PAs are not superior to standard ward care for the prevention of morbidity and mortality resulting from infection in leukemic patients. This observation is important since the emergence of antibiotic-resistant strains in patients treated with PA has been reported (5). Such resistant strains can cause severe infection in some patients; in addition, if the patients in whom these strains emerge are not kept isolated, the resistant pathogens can easily spread throughout the hospital. Thus treatment of neutropenic patients with nonabsorbable PA appears not to be warranted on the basis of available evidence, although isolated studies (5,6,8) suggest some efficacy of PA in preventing infection, especially in severely granulocytopenic patients. Recently a controlled study suggested that prophylactic administration of cotrimoxazole not only prevented the occurrence of infection caused by *Pneumocystis carinii*, but also reduced the incidence of bacterial infections in children undergoing maintenance chemotherapy for acute lymphocytic leukemia (12). Other controlled studies by Gurwith and co-workers (13) indicate that cotrimoxazole might reduce the frequency of infections in neutropenic leukemia patients as well. The efficacy of systemic antibiotics in preventing infection in neutropenic patients with ANLL was also studied by Rodriguez and co-workers (14). They found that systemic antibiotics were not superior to nonabsorbable PAs; PE combined with PAs or systemic antibiotics, however, was associated with significant prevention of infection (14). More studies are probably indicated to understand better the possible role of systemic antibiotics in preventing severe infections in neutropenic leukemia patients.

The ultimate goal of the preventive measures against infection in patients with leukemia is an improvement of the rate of complete remission and a prolongation of survival. It can be seen in Table 1 that only one study out of seven demonstrated an improved clinical course of the leukemia itself (6). Schimpff and co-workers (6) speculated that the differences in remission induction and survival might be linked to the form of antileukemic therapy. It is also possible that in Schimpff's study the small size of the sample specimen might have resulted in an uneven distribution of some important prognostic factors, such as age. As a matter of fact, older patients were more numerous (43%) among the controls than in the isolated group (17%).

Isolated patients had an improved remission rate over nonisolated patients, but not prolonged survival, in a prospectively controlled recent study at the M. D. Anderson Hospital in Houston. The authors speculated that unequally effective chemotherapeutic regimens might have been responsible for the difference (14).

Table 3 summarizes the rate of complete remission and the survival at 120 days among the patients included in the seven controlled studies selected for this review (3–9). It appears that the rate of complete remission in PEPA is 59%, whereas it is only 44% in controls ($p < 0.01$). In spite of this increased rate of complete remissions, the survival rate at 120 days was identical in these two groups. Although the median survival could not be calculated accurately for all the studies considered here, we found no difference between the median survival of PEPA patients and controls for whom the calculation could be made: These median survivals were, respectively, 104 and 107 days. Therefore, it appears that the benefit, if any, of PEPA on the course of ANLL is relatively small.

It may be surprising that a technique such as PEPA, which markedly reduces the incidence of infectious morbidity and mortality in granulocytopenic leukemia patients and increases the rate of complete remissions in ANLL, has so little impact on the overall course of the leukemia itself. It must be stressed, however, that many infections in granulocytopenic patients can be controlled effectively with antibiotics and granulocyte transfusions. In a recent large cooperative study it was found that antibiotics alone were effective in 68% of neutropenic patients with Gram-negative septicemia (15). There is also evidence that transfusions of granulocytes can be life-saving in patients with severely depressed bone marrow function (16). Therefore, prevention of the infectious episodes cannot necessarily be expected to influence the overall course of the disease and the survival of the patients.

On the other hand, since the natural history of ANLL is not greatly influenced by a reduction of infectious mortality which results from the use of PEPA or

TABLE 3. *Effect of chemotherapy associated with protected environment and/or prophylactic antibiotics in ANLL patients*

No. of patients	155	66	140	207
Patients achieving complete remission (%)[a]	58.9	53.0	51.3	43.6
Patients surviving 120 days (%)	60.8	63.6	71.0	60.8

Rate of remission and survival were computed from seven prospective randomly controlled studies.

See Table 1 for abbreviations.

[a] PEPA/controls: $p < 0.01$. PE/controls and PA/controls = not significant.

PE, infection is not, and perhaps less so than before, a major factor influencing the survival of patients with ANLL. We found recently that patients with ANLL died as often from hemorrhage (44%) as from infection (44%); lethal extramedullary toxicity from cancer chemotherapy was also a major factor contributing to death (17). Thus in spite of satisfactory control of infectious morbidity and mortality, durable remissions cannot be obtained. The limitation appears to be the lack of adequate chemotherapy, and major efforts are to be made in that direction.

Aggressive bone marrow ablative chemotherapy followed by bone marrow transplantation has been used recently as a successful therapy for ANLL (18). Under these circumstances, because cure appears possible, the protection of the patients in PE with or without PA remains important. Patients transplanted in laminar air flow rooms have significantly less septicemia and major local infections than do patients in a control group, as shown recently by Buckner and co-workers (19). Of the 46 laminar air flow patients, 19 had long-term survivals, whereas only 6 of 44 controls were alive when the study was published. That PE may be useful in bone marrow transplant recipients applies to patients with acute leukemia and to those with anaplastic anemias, 40% of whom can achieve a long-term survival after allogeneic marrow transplantation (20). In addition, there is some indication in animals that PA might be effective in modifying the graft-versus-host disease which is another major complication of transplantation. This might prove to be another area in which PEPA and/ or PE should be investigated.

Intensive chemotherapy of some solid tumors might also benefit from supportive care carried out in protected environments. Good candidates for this type of approach would be tumors which are expected to respond to high doses of chemotherapeutic agents. Along these lines, it should be pointed out that patients with small cell bronchogenic carcinoma who are treated with high-dose chemotherapy have higher response rates than patients treated with a more conventional chemotherapy (21). In that study, the necessity of protected environment was evaluated, but the patients treated with high-dose chemotherapy spent only a few days out of the total course with granulocytopenia and there was no apparent benefit from the protective environment. From experience in acute leukemia, one might have expected a low incidence of infection for this duration of granulocytopenia; therefore, it may be possible to obtain further benefits with still more aggressive chemotherapy administered under protection from PEPA or PE to these patients with small cell bronchial carcinoma. Further studies are certainly indicated in this area. Current studies of intensive chemotherapy in adult and pediatric patients with other solid tumors were reviewed recently by Pizzo and Levine (22). Basically they pointed out a decreased incidence of severe infection among protected patients, with more chemotherapy consequently given to them. It appears also that some patients have profited from this approach as far as survival is concerned. Whether intensive drug schedules will significantly prolong the lives of large numbers of patients with various solid tumors remains to be fully investigated. Protective environment should be studied as a part of these regimens. It remains to be seen whether the limiting factors will be the lack of effective chemotherapy and extramedullary drug toxicity rather than ineffectiveness of support for medullary toxicity.

To conclude, it has become clear after a decade of clinical studies that protection of neutropenic patients with isolation and microbial suppression significantly decreases the infectious morbidity and mortality rates. Patients with ANLL treated in protected environments and with oral nonabsorbable antibiotics (PEPA) have an increased rate of remission. However, in leukemia patients with drug-resistant malignancy, the lack of effective chemotherapy and the extramedullary toxicity of available chemotherapeutic agents reduce the long-term benefit from protection against infection.

It seems likely, however, that a protective environment might prove to be an ideal adjunct to techniques of allogeneic bone marrow transplantation for medullary aplasia and acute leukemia. Protection against infection might also be important for patients who are treated intensively for solid tumors which are likely to respond to available chemotherapy. Under these clinical circumstances protective environment should be studied further.

PROPHYLACTIC TRANSFUSION OF GRANULOCYTES

Another approach to the prevention of infection in myelosuppressed patients might be a prophylactic administration of granulocytes. This hypothesis stems from the well known efficacy of prophylactic transfusions of platelets in preventing hemorrhage in thrombocytopenic patients. Ford and Cullen conducted a clinical trial on 19 patients who had been randomized and among whom 10 received alternate-day transfusions (23). These 10 patients received a total of 82 transfusions (range per patient 1 to 12). Granulocyte transfusions given in this context had no apparent effect on the clinical course of these patients. The number of patients was limited in that study, and in only two cases was death due solely to infection. A much larger number of subjects would be needed to show an effect on the infectious mortality in those patients with leukemia who die for a variety of reasons (17). A larger trial was reported recently by Clift and his co-workers (24); they studied granulocyte transfusions given for the prevention of infection in patients receiving bone marrow transplants (24). This type of prophylaxis was studied in 69 patients receiving transplants for the therapy of hematologic neoplasia or aplastic anemia. Patients were randomized to receive or not to receive granulocyte transfusions when their circulating granulocyte levels fell to less than 200/mm^3 during the period between transplantation and the development of graft function. The transfusions were started on the first posttransplant day after the declining granulocyte count reached 200/mm^3 and were continued daily until the day after the patient was again capable of supporting granulocyte levels of at least 200/mm^3. The mean number of transfusions was 22.2 $\times$ 10^9 for cells obtained by filtration and

14.9×10^9 for granulocytes obtained by continuous flow centrifugation. During the first 21 posttransplant days, there were 2 local infections and no septicemias in 29 transfused patients. Among the 40 controls, 7 local infections and 10 septicemias developed. Prophylaxis of infection was achieved with negligible granuloctye increments; there have been no data to suggest that increments are necessary for effectiveness of granuloctye transfuions in the treatment of infections. Nevertheless, it is difficult to understand how prophylaxis can be achieved without circulating granulocytes. Survival was identical in the two groups of patients (35%), and most patients died as a result of interstitial pneumonia or leukemic relapse. Among the controls, four patients (10%) died as a consequence of bacterial or fungal infection, whereas no mortality caused by infection was observed in the other group.

Another controlled study of the prophylactic use of granulocytes was presented by Mannoni et al. (25). Among 15 patients supported by prophylactic transfusions, only 3 documented infections occurred; whereas among 24 control patients there were 13 documented infections, including 5 cases of pneumonia. The difference between these two groups is highly significant ($p < 0.01$). However, the rate of HLA alloimmunization was very high (8 of 12 patients studied) and made it occasionally difficult to find compatible donors.

It should also be observed that the infections which occurred among the control patients usually could be well managed with antibiotics and therapeutic granulocyte transfusions. It is therefore unclear whether prophylactic granulocytes should be used, as by preventing curable infections they might jeopardize further blood cell support of these patients by allowing the patients to become immunized. It might be surprising that the use of prophylactic granulocyte transfusions has no substantial effect on the survival of the treated group despite significant prevention of infectious morbidity and mortality. The situation is somewhat similar to that observed with the protected environment and prophylactic nonabsorbable antibiotic regimens which are also employed to prevent infection in severely neutropenic leukemic patients. Here also, despite a significant reduction in infectious mortality, there is little improvement in the survival of the leukemic patient.

There are two reasons for the lack of effect on the outcome of the basic disease after preventive measures against infection. First, the effectiveness of therapy of documented infection is considerable: If appropriate combinations of antibiotics are administered early during the course of infection and are supplemented by granulocyte transfusions if bone marrow failure is severe, mortality from infection in neutropenic patients is relatively low. Death from infection usually occurs when the basic disease is unremitting or when there are severe noninfectious complications from the antileukemic therapy. The second reason why prevention of infection does not alter the ultimate course of the neoplastic disease is that the outcome is influenced by factors unrelated to bacterial or fungal infections, among which the relative inefficacy of currently available chemotherapy plays a major role. For example, leukemia patients often die, nowadays, from noninfectious complications such as hemorrhage, toxicity from cytostatic therapy, or extensive tumor (17).

EMPIRIC THERAPY WITH ANTIBIOTICS

When severe sepsis is suspected, initial therapy should provide adequate coverage against all the likely pathogens. In neutropenic patients, infections caused by Gram-negative bacilli are common; however, Gram-positive infections occur as well and usually cannot be distinguished from the former on clinical grounds only. Therefore, both types of infection should be covered by empirical regimens. Unfortunately, this cannot be achieved with a single antibiotic, and the use of combinations of antimicrobial agents is thus mandatory under these conditions. The susceptibility of Gram-positive organisms (e.g., pneumococci or staphylococci) to antibiotics is easily predictable, but the choice of drugs active against Gram-negative bacilli is more difficult and should be based on *in vitro* studies.

As indicated in Table 4, several combinations have been proposed as potentially effective regimens in severe sepsis. From a microbiological point of view, these combinations are not equally effective, but all cover a wide range of pathogens that can be encountered in granulocytopenic patients. Several of these combinations (clindamycin + gentamicin, cephalothin + gentamicin, cotrimoxazole + polymyxin) are inactive against enterococci; cephalothin + gentamicin and cotrimoxazole + polymyxin are also ineffective against *Bacteroides* sp. It must be emphasized, however, that enterococci and *Bacteroides* are rarely implicated as major lethal pathogens in neutropenic patients.

The combination of clindamycin + gentamicin has not been widely used in cancer patients; its main weakness is that clindamycin is devoid of any significant activity against aerobic Gram-negative bacilli, which are the most common pathogens in neutropenic patients. Aminoglycosides are inadequate as the only active agent for bacteremia caused by *Pseudomonas aeruginosa* and presumably other Gram-negative rods in the granulocytopenic patient (26). The poor result attributed to aminoglycosides acting alone is probably related to low blood concentrations and not to any intrinsic effectiveness of these antibiotics. This hypothesis is supported by recent animal data showing that a high dose (7.5 mg/kg) of gentamicin is as effective as the combination of carbenicillin + gentamicin in experimental endocarditis due to *Ps. aeruginosa* (27). Along the same lines, it was recently suggested that the efficacy of aminoglycosides in neutropenic patients can be substantially improved by maintaining high blood levels with continuous infusions (28). In order to maintain these blood levels, one must administer higher doses than those usually used with aminoglycosides. Under these circumstances, favorable responses were reported in 66% of neutropenic patients with Gram-negative infections. It should be stressed that addition of carbenicillin to this form of therapy with aminoglycosides significantly improves the clinical results.

Carbenicillin + cephalothin has a broad spectrum of antimicrobial activity

TABLE 4. Microbiological effectiveness of combinations of antibiotics[a]

Organism	Clindamycin + gentamicin	Carbenicillin + cephalothin	Carbenicillin + polymyxin	Cotrimoxazole + polymyxin	Gentamicin + chloramphenicol	Cephalothin + gentamicin	Carbenicillin + gentamicin
Escherichia coli	+	+	+	+	+	+	+
Staphylococcus aureus	+	+	0	(+)	+	+	+
Klebsiella sp.	+	(+)	+	+	+	+	+
Pseudomonas aeruginosa	+	+	+	+	+	+	+
Proteus mirabilis	+	+	+	+	+	0	+
Streptococcus faecalis	0	+	+	0	(+)	+	+
Enterobacter sp.	+	(+)	+	+	+	+	+
Staphylococcus epidermidis	+	+	(+)	(+)	+	+	+
Serratia marcescens	+	0	(+)	(+)	+	+	+
Streptococcus pneumoniae	+	+	+	+	+	+	+
Bacteroides sp.	+	+	+	0	+	0	+

[a] +: active. (+): active on some strains. 0: not active.

and has been found effective in several clinical trials (29–31) including our own, in which we demonstrated that it was as active but less nephrotoxic than carbenicillin + cephalothin + gentamicin (32). In Gram-negative bacteremia, the rate of favorable response with carbenicillin + cephalothin was found to be close to 55% (29,31,33), which appears lower than the incidence reported for cephalothin + gentamicin or carbenicillin + gentamicin. Bodey et al. (30) found that this type of regimen was not optimal for neutropenic patients, and Gurwith et al. (31) reported that the mortality rate associated with cephalothin + carbenicillin was significantly higher than that observed in patients receiving carbenicillin + gentamicin + methicillin. The major limitation for the use of carbenicillin + cephalothin is the relatively frequent occurrence of pathogens resistant to both carbenicillin and cephalothin in many hospitals. In the recent EORTC trials, 22 of 305 tested bacterial isolates were resistant to both antibiotics in the regimen prescribed (almost always carbenicillin + cephalothin). Therapy with carbenicillin + cephalothin uniformly failed in these patients, i.e., in 6 of 6 patients with Gram-negative bacteremia and organisms resistant to both carbenicillin and cephalothin (15). A similar outcome was not observed when gentamicin was given with either carbenicillin or cephalothin. From these observations comes the impression that, although aminoglycosides alone are not very effective clinically, they may achieve some control of the infection until culture results are available. In the EORTC trial the combination of carbenicillin + gentamicin was found adequate as initial therapy for staphylococcal infections due to penicillinase-producing strains; this observation confirms that gentamicin has a definite antistaphylococcal activity when used alone in infected patients (34). All these data suggest that aminoglycosides are probably an important component of the initial antibiotic regimen.

A carbenicillin + polymyxin regimen has a broad antimicrobial spectrum acting on most common pathogens with the exception of staphylococci. *In vitro,* synergism is less well documented for this combination than for carbenicillin + gentamicin. In addition, clinical experience with this combination is limited to a few studies with relatively low numbers of patients. Favorable results were observed in 15 of 22 cases (68%) (35). These results look better than those obtained with polymyxin alone under similar clinical conditions. Polymyxin alone has proved rather poor therapy for severe infections in neutropenic patients, presumably because high doses cannot be safely administered owing to excessive toxicity. It is therefore unclear whether polymyxin adds to the effectiveness of carbenicillin. Interest for polymyxin has decreased as the newer aminoglycosides have become available. However, polymyxin (and aminoglycosides as well) are synergistic *in vitro* with cotrimoxazole against *Ps. aeruginosa* and other pathogenic Gram-negative rods, e.g., *Serratia marcescens* and *Proteus* sp.

We found cotrimoxazole + polymyxin highly effective for Gram-negative bacteremias in nonneutropenic cancer patients (36). Among 16 such patients with bacteriologically proved Gram-negative septicemia, 13 (81%) responded satisfactorily to the treatment. Little is known about the clinical efficacy of cotrimoxazole alone when administered as empirical therapy in patients with severe underlying disease and suspected sepsis, and this makes the evaluation of its combination with polymyxin difficult. Some data, however, suggest that cotrimoxazole might be effective in neutropenic patients without excessive toxicity (37). As already mentioned, cotrimoxazole alone has been shown to prevent many serious bacterial infections in immunosuppressed patients to whom it had been given as a prophylaxis for *Pneumocystis carinii* infection (12). More studies are probably indicated to investigate the efficacy of combinations of cotrimoxazole + polymyxin (or aminoglycosides) in neutropenic patients. These regimens might prove to be important in those infections caused by microorganisms resistant to the more commonly employed antibiotics.

Gentamicin + chloramphenicol has a very broad spectrum of antimicrobial activity *in vitro*. No extensive experience with that combination is available, however. Gentamicin + chloramphenicol is used occasionally with good results in patients with severe infection not responding to penicillins and/or cephalosporins (38). However, the bone marrow toxicity of chloramphenicol makes it a less desirable candidate than a penicillin or a cephalosporin for therapy of infections in patients with medullary suppression. In addition, it has been reported that gentamicin and chloramphenicol may be antagonistic *in vitro,* and that this antagonism was associated with a decreased survival of neutropenic mice infected with *proteus mirabilis* (39).

Cephalothin + gentamicin (or tobramycin or amikacin) is one of the most commonly employed therapeutic regimens in patients with suspected sepsis, including patients with neutropenia (29,34,40,41). As indicated in Table 5, the rate of favorable response in Gram-negative bacteremia is close to 66%, but it has been shown that this type of combination is definitely more nephrotoxic than either agent employed alone (29,32,34). Although some animal data are not in accord with these findings, another recent prospective randomly controlled trial confirms that cephalothin + an aminoglycoside (gentamicin or tobramycin)

TABLE 5. *Results obtained in cancer patients with Gram-negative bacteremia given cephalosporins + aminoglycosides*

Ref.	Year	Antibiotics	Response in cancer patients with Gram-negative bacteremia	
			No. of patients	% Favorable responses
Klastersky et al. (29)	1975	Cephalothin + tobramycin	19	58
Bodey et al. (40)	1976	Cephalothin + gentamicin	7	71
Hahn et al. (41)	1977	Cephalothin + amikacin	17	65
EORTC (42)	1978	Cephalothin + gentamicin	22	72
Total		Cephalothin + aminoglycoside	65	66

is more nephrotoxic than the use of the aminoglycoside with either carbenicillin or ticarcillin and methicillin (42). In the EORTC trial there was significantly more antibiotic-associated severe nephrotoxicity (defined as a rise in creatinine from normal to >2.5 mg%) among patients who received cephalothin + gentamicin (12%) than those who received either carbenicillin + gentamicin (2%) or carbenicillin + cephalothin (4%). Nephrotoxicity occurred primarily in older patients (>60 years) with a high-normal initial creatinine level. Above age 60 there was a 27% incidence of severe nephrotoxicity (15). These considerations make cephalothin + gentamicin a suboptimal choice for therapy of severe sepsis. If this regimen is chosen for any reason, special attention should be paid to monitoring the blood levels of the aminoglycoside and to adjusting or discontinuing the antimicrobial therapy accordingly.

The combination carbenicillin + gentamicin not only provides complete coverage against most pathogens involved in clinical sepsis in neutropenic patients, but in most studies has also led to adequate clinical results without excessive toxicity (29,33,34,40,43–47). As indicated in Table 6, the rate of favorable responses ranges from 22 to 88%. The overall experience with carbenicillin + gentamicin, available from the literature, indicates a favorable response in 63% of neutropenic patients with Gram-negative septicemia. The adverse effects associated with the use of carbenicillin + gentamicin have been minimal. Nephrotoxicity is usually not a problem, as mentioned earlier; hypokalemia can be safely avoided by administering supplements of potassium salts. The potential adverse

TABLE 6. *Results obtained in cancer patients with Gram-negative bacteremia given carbenicillin or ticarcillin + aminoglycosides*

Ref.	Year	Antibiotics	Response in cancer patients with neutropenia and Gram-negative bacteremia	
			No. of patients	% Favorable responses
Rodriguez et al. (43)	1970	Gentamicin + carbenicillin	15	47
Schimpff et al. (44)	1971	Gentamicin + carbenicillin	26	61
Young (45)	1971	Gentamicin + carbenicillin	15	60
Klastersky et al. (46)	1973	Gentamicin + carbenicillin	11	82[a]
Klastersky et al. (29)	1975	Tobramycin + ticarcillin	15	47
Schimpff et al. (33)	1976	Gentamicin + ticarcillin	9	22
Bodey et al. (40)	1976	Gentamicin + carbenicillin	9	88
Klastersky et al.	1977	Amikacin + carbenicillin	27	70[a]
EORTC (42)	1978	Gentamicin + ticarcillin and carbenicillin	32	75
Total		Aminoglycosides + carbenicillin or ticarcillin	159	63

[a] Some of these patients were not neutropenic.

effect of carbenicillin on the function of platelets has not been demonstrated to be a major concern under clinical conditions so far. Therefore, carbenicillin + gentamicin appears to provide the best overall efficacy as an initial regimen against the more common infectious organisms in neutropenic patients.

Whether a triple drug regimen associating carbenicillin + cephalothin + gentamicin (or another aminoglycoside) would be superior has been explored in several studies (32,48–50). The overall rate of response found with the triple drug combination was 59%, with a range from 45 to 88% (Table 7). These results are comparable to those obtained with carbenicillin + gentamicin or cephalothin + gentamicin, but do not show any superiority. However, if one considers results from individual centers, it appears that the triple combination was superior in studies reported from the BCRC (33,50). Similarly, at the Institut Jules Bordet, the triple combination (carbenicillin + cefazolin + amikacin) proved to be superior (64%) to the combination ticarcillin + tobramycin (47%) (29,49).

A high frequency of nephrotoxicity (17% and 25%, respectively) was observed in two series (32,48) employing a high dosage of cephalothin (9 to 12 g daily). Greene et al. (50) also reported a fairly high incidence of renal dysfunction. This was not the case, however, in our study in which carbenicillin, amikacin, and cefazolin (4 g daily) were used (49). Whether this difference is related to the dosage of the cephalosporin, the type of cephalosporin employed, or the type of aminoglycoside employed remains unclear. Perhaps several factors are involved, but our results suggest that a triple-drug regimen including carbenicil-

TABLE 7. *Results obtained in cancer patients with Gram-negative bacteremia given carbenicillin–cephalosporin–aminoglycoside*

Ref.	Year	Antibiotics	Response in cancer patients with neutropenia and Gram-negative bacteremia	
			No. of patients	% Favorable responses
Greene et al. (50)	1973	Carbenicillin + cephalothin + gentamicin	51	45
Bloomfield and Kennedy (48)	1974	Carbenicillin + cephalothin + gentamicin	9	88
Klastersky et al. (32)	1974	Carbenicillin + cephalothin + gentamicin	19	79[a]
Klastersky et al. (49)	1977	Carbenicillin + cephazolin + amikacin	14	64
Total		Carbenicillin + cephalosporin + aminoglycoside	93	59

[a] Some of the patients were not neutropenic.

lin, a cephalosporin, and an aminoglycoside can be used without excessive fear of nephrotoxicity. The Antimicrobial Therapy Project Group of EORTC is currently exploring, in a controlled fashion, whether a triple-drug regimen (carbenicillin, cephalothin, and amikacin) in which a moderate dose of cefazolin is used would be more active than a regimen associating carbenicillin and amikacin (51). The theoretical advantages of this triple combination are a broader coverage than carbenicillin + an aminoglycoside, especially against *Klebsiella* sp., and a synergistic action of cefazolin and amikacin against *Klebsiella* sp. (52).

It is important to realize that the broadening of the antibacterial spectrum from a qualitative point of view might not be the only advantage in using antibiotic combinations compared with single antibiotics. Interactions between antibiotics may make a combination more active than either drug from that combination being used alone. Such an interaction may be additive or synergistic, although there are no universally accepted criteria to separate the two categories. In our hospital, patients with disseminated cancer are treated at random with gentamicin, carbenicillin, or gentamicin + carbenicillin for bacteriologically proved infections caused by Gram-negative bacilli (46). Favorable results were observed in 13 of 23 (57%) patients who received relatively high doses of gentamicin, in 11 of 22 (50%) of those who were treated with carbenicillin, and in 19 of 23 (83%) who received the combination. These results correlate well with the higher antibacterial activity found in sera of patients who received the combination of gentamicin and carbenicillin as compared to sera of patients treated with gentamicin or carbenicillin alone. When only infections caused by microorganisms fully sensitive to carbenicillin and gentamicin were considered, the respective rates of favorable clinical results for gentamicin, carbenicillin, and the combination of gentamicin + carbenicillin were 57, 64, and 90%, respectively. Of course these studies do not demonstrate *in vivo* synergistic action, but they do indicate that the combination is significantly more effective than either drug alone, in spite of adequate sensitivity of the microorganisms responsible for the infections to each drug alone.

An important question is if the use of synergistic combinations is associated with a better clinical result than that of nonsynergistic associations, and if the former would result in a higher antibacterial activity in the serum of the treated patient. It was shown in our hospital (53) that the bactericidal dilutions of sera in patients treated with synergistic combinations were usually adequate; i.e., these sera were active at a 1:8 dilution whereas sera of most patients who received nonsynergistic combinations were not active at these dilutions. Even more important is the observation that the synergistic combinations were more effective clinically than nonsynergistic combinations (Table 8). Synergistic combinations were associated with a favorable outcome in 80% of the patients, whereas nonsynergistic combinations were effective in only 52%.

The effect of antibiotic synergism on the outcome of Gram-negative sepsis was also studied by Anderson and co-workers (54). In patients with a "nonfatal"

TABLE 8. *Clinical effectiveness and bactericidal activity of serum in patients treated with synergistic and nonsynergistic combinations of antibiotics*

Therapy	No. of patients	Clinical successes		Bactericidal activity of serum	
		No.	%[a]	Trough conc.	Peak conc.
Synergism	100	80	80.0	$\frac{1}{8}$ ($\frac{1}{2} - \frac{1}{16}$)	$\frac{1}{16}$ ($\frac{1}{2} - \frac{1}{64}$)
No synergism	105	52	49.5	$\frac{1}{2}$ ($\frac{1}{2} - \frac{1}{8}$)	$\frac{1}{4}$ ($\frac{1}{2} - \frac{1}{32}$)

[a] $p < 0.01$.

or "ultimately fatal" underlying disease, treatment failure was seen in 25% of those treated with two drugs regardless of whether the combinations were synergistic. However, in patients with "rapidly fatal" underlying diseases and who presented a Gram-negative septicemia, 52% (28/54) responded when treated with the nonsynergistic combination whereas 77% (42/54) treated with synergistic combinations responded. This difference was statistically significant ($p < 0.005$). When the outcome of sepsis in neutropenic patients for all prognostic categories was analyzed, 70% (23/29) of those treated with synergistic combinations responded, whereas only 33% (8/24) of those treated with nonsynergistic combinations did ($p < 0.001$). Recently we studied, in a prospective fashion, the clinical effectiveness of carbenicillin + amikacin versus penicillin + amikacin in Gram-negative infections in nonneutropenic cancer patients. We found that the two regimens were similarly effective but that synergistic combinations (whether penicillin + amikacin or carbenicillin + amikacin) were more often associated with a favorable clinical outcome (75%) than nonsynergistic combinations (41%) (47). These studies are summarized in Table 9. The data obtained in these studies indicate that combination therapy with two antibiotics having synergistic activity *in vitro* might be associated with a more favorable outcome than therapy with single drugs or with nonsynergistic combinations. Lau and co-workers (55) came to the same conclusion in a recently published study comparing the efficacy and toxicity of amikacin/carbenicillin and gentamicin/carbenicillin in leukopenic patients. These observations are not surprising when the considerable potentiation of one drug by the other which occurs *in vitro* in synergistic combinations is taken into account. These reductions of the minimum inhibitory concentration (MIC) to both antibiotics used in synergistic combinations makes it possible to reach higher levels of antibacterial activity in the serum, and presumably in the tissues, of the infected host. The therapeutic value of synergistic combinations and the predictive role of antibacterial activity in the serum have been clearly demonstrated in patients with bacterial endocarditis, and now, as well, in patients with severe infections who have an underlying disease such as cancer (56).

In summary, the main rationale for the use of a synergistic combination of

TABLE 9. *Effectiveness of synergistic and nonsynergistic combinations for Gram-negative septicemia in cancer patients*

Study conditions and ref.	Favorable clinical response to antibiotic combinations	
	Synergistic	Nonsynergistic
Retrospective studies in cancer patients; various infections; various antibiotic combinations (53)	80/100 (80%)	52/105 (49%)
Retrospective study in cancer patients; Gram-negative septicemia; carbenicillin + amikacin (49)	18/24 (75%)	9/22 (41%)
Retrospective studies in neutropenic patients; Gram-negative septicemias; various antibiotic combinations (54)	15/25 (60%)	3/16 (41%)
Total	113/149 (79%)	64/143 (45%)

drugs is to obtain high levels of antibacterial activity in the serum and presumably in the tissues. This high antibacterial activity results from the considerable potentiation of one antibiotic by the other in many synergistic combinations. The magnitude of this potentiation correlates with a favorable outcome, making synergistic combinations more effective *in vivo* than nonsynergistic ones, especially in patients whose natural mechanisms of defense against infection are poor, e.g., neutropenic patients. Therefore, even before knowing the antibiotic sensitivity profile of a specific pathogen, the use of a combination which is synergistic, or which at least has a good chance of being synergistic for a specific organism, can probably be recommended.

OPTIMAL DURATION OF ANTIMICROBIAL THERAPY

Further infection, defined as any infection (other than the initial one) originating either during therapy or within 1 week thereafter, was found in 17% of the neutropenic patients in a recent cooperative EORTC trial (15). Two factors that significantly predisposed to further infection were prolonged antibiotic therapy and persistent granulocytopenia; both factors were independently important. Therefore, it is essential to discontinue antibiotics when no definite evidence of infection has been found after 3 to 4 days of clinical therapy. Rodriguez et al. (38) reported a study in which cancer patients with neutropenia were randomly allocated to continue or discontinue antibiotics 4 days after initiation of carbenicillin and cephalothin therapy if no infection had been demonstrated. They concluded that if after 4 days of therapy no infection is documented and the patient is responding, the antibiotics should be continued for an additional 3 to 5 days. However, for patients not responding after the initial 4 days of therapy, they recommended the addition of gentamicin or a complete change of antibiotic treatment. An alternative approach used successfully at the BCRC is to discontinue antibiotics after approximately 4 days if a repeat history, examination, and laboratory evaluation are unrevealing, the patient is febrile yet appears stable and nontoxic, and all original culture data are noncontributing. This approach has the advantage of eliminating antibiotic pressure likely to favor the emergence of resistant bacteria or fungi. If no infection is documented yet the patient has had an obvious clinical response to antimicrobial therapy, they continue the original antibiotic regimen for approximately 5 more days or a total of about 7 to 10 days of therapy. More recently Pizzo et al. (57) reported preliminary results of a controlled study of the duration of antimicrobial therapy in neutropenic patients who responded to empirical therapy for fever with carbenicillin, cephalothin, and gentamicin. In a group of 17 patients in whom antibiotics were discontinued after 7 days, five new febrile episodes occurred; a bacterial infection could be documented in 3, and 2 patients died of it. On the other hand, in a group of 18 patients in whom therapy had been continued until bone marrow recovery (granulocytes >500/mm³), no febrile episodes and no infections were observed.

These observations suggest that antimicrobial therapy should be continued in severely neutropenic patients who experience a febrile illness until the granulocyte count returns to normal. However, more studies should establish that such a practice will not increase the rate of further infections, especially by fungi, in these patients.

FUNGAL INFECTIONS AND ANTIFUNGAL THERAPY

Fungal infections are being encountered with increasing frequency in neutropenic cancer patients who receive broad-spectrum antibacterial agents (58,59). It seems likely that suppression of the normal body flora can be associated with increased frequency of colonization with fungi and further infection with these organisms (60). There have been several reports of the successful treatment of invasive aspergillosis associated with earlier diagnosis (61,62). Therefore, it has been our policy to start empirical therapy with amphotericin B, 1.2 mg/kg every other day, as recommended by Bindschadler and Bennett (63), in those patients who do not respond to antimicrobial therapy, especially if granulocytopenia is prolonged and if multiple broad-spectrum antibiotic treatments have been given during the past weeks or days. The suspicion of fungal disease is further increased if pneumonia, central nervous system disease, or gastrointestinal tract symptoms or signs develop during antimicrobial therapy for fever in severely neutropenic patients. Obviously, all reasonable procedures to establish the precise diagnosis from the microbiological point of view should be performed prior to the initiation of empirical antifungal therapy. An extensive discussion of fungal diseases which complicate antibiotic therapy in cancer patients is beyond the scope of this review. However, it is clear that more data on the available methods for diagnosing and treating these infections are needed to delineate further areas for clinical investigation.

GRANULOCYTE TRANSFUSIONS

Since platelet transfusions markedly changed the outcome of hemorrhagic complications in thrombocytopenic patients with leukemia, it appeared logical to prevent the consequences of severe neutropenia in these patients by administering transfusions of granulocytes. This approach was also based on animal studies indicating that granulocyte transfusions were beneficial in dogs rendered neutropenic by irradiation or cyclophosphamide (64). Under these experimental circumstances, prevention of naturally acquired septicemia and prolongation of survival after induction of *Pseudomonas* pneumonia have been reported.

Morse et al. (65) and other investigators (66,67) demonstrated that transfusing large numbers of granulocytes from patients with chronic granulocytic leukemia into leukopenic recipients increased the circulating granulocyte count. Some favorable results were noted, but the lack of adequate controls limited the value of these observations. The development of techniques for obtaining large numbers of granulocytes from normal donors (e.g., continuous flow centrifugation and filtration leukophoresis) allowed the realization of controlled studies on the efficacy of granulocyte transfusions in curing or preventing serious bacterial infections in neutropenic patients.

Although several uncontrolled studies reported in the literature suggest that transfusions of granulocytes might be effective in controlling severe sepsis in neutropenic patients (68–71), the present analysis deals only with controlled trials. It has been argued that randomized controlled studies are unnecessary as the high mortality rate of bacterial infections in neutropenics is well documented. However, the use of retrospective controls does not take into consideration changing patterns of infections, emergence of drug-resistant microorganisms, use of new antibiotic combinations, and other possibly not yet recognized factors which might alter survival. Therefore, because so many factors may influence the course of infectious episodes in neutropenic patients, the need for controls is obvious, as pointed out in a recent review by Strauss (72). In addition, the use of controls allows a better evaluation of the natural history of infections in neutropenic patients.

Graw and co-workers (73) reported in 1972 the first controlled study of normal granulocyte transfusion therapy in the treatment of septicemia due to Gram-negative bacteria. Although there was no prospective randomization because transfusions were given on the basis of donor availability, results indicated a better survival (46%) in transfused patients compared to controls receiving appropriate antibiotics alone (29%). When the transfusion recipients were grouped according to the number of transfusions received, a progressive improvement of survival related to the number of transfusions administered was noted, reaching 12 of 12 (100%) in the group receiving four or more transfusions. The survival in this last group was significantly better than that of the control group. Another important finding in that study was the observation that the recovery of neutrophils was progressively lower as the number of mismatched HLA antigen groups increased from zero to three. In addition, the importance of ABO compatibility was clearly shown. The authors suggested also that the time between the onset of infection and the first granulocyte transfusion may be important in determining a successful response. Tolerance to the transfusions was good: No clinical transfusion reactions followed transfusion of compatible cells collected by continuous flow centrifugation. However, despite a careful selection of donors, chills and fever developed after transfusion in most patients receiving cells collected by filtration. Other investigators have reported significant transfusion reactions in patients receiving granulocytes obtained by filtration leukophoresis (68).

The major criticism which can be made of that study, besides the lack of randomization, is the poor survival rate obtained in the control group receiving antibiotics alone. In a recent multicenter cooperative study (15) it was found that, provided the pathogen was susceptible to the antibiotics employed, the rate of response of patients with Gram-negative bacteremia was 88% in those patients whose peripheral granulocyte count rose by more than 100/mm³. The rate of response was only 22% in those patients (7% of all infected granulocytopenic patients) whose granulocyte count did not rise. Since most surviving patients in Graw's study (73), especially in the control group, recovered normal granulopoiesis at the time antibiotics were discontinued, one can wonder whether the patients in that study always received adequate antimicrobial therapy.

Fortuny and co-workers (74) conducted another clinical trial of granulocyte transfusion in patients with acute nonlymphocytic leukemia. Once again, allocation of the patients to the study groups was made on the basis of donor availability. As a consequence, the transfused group was at better risk in terms of previous attempts at remission induction, number of remissions of the leukemia obtained during the febrile episode, and the absolute granulocyte count at the start of the febrile episode. Documented infections responded with the same frequency in the transfused and the control groups (71%). The antibiotics used in Fortuny's study consisted of a carbenicillin, cephalothin, and gentamicin regimen which was associated with a high response rate in granulocytopenic patients with Gram-negative septicemia. The question thus arises as to whether any adjunct therapy can be useful once optimal antimicrobial therapy has been given. However, there is another way to look at these data; they may be interpreted as suggesting that doses of granulocytes in the range of 4 to 7×10^9 are essentially ineffective. It should be stressed, however, that levels in this range have already been used and were considered to be effective (73,75).

Higby and associates (76) reported a comparative clinical evaluation of filtration leukophoresis for granulocyte transfusion therapy. Patients were randomly allocated to receive (or not) granulocytes if an unspecified broad-spectrum antibiotic therapy had been given for 2 days or more and was judged ineffective as evidenced by persisting fever and clinical deterioration. That only patients failing on antibiotics were eligible here might explain why the survival rate to 20 days in the patients who did not receive granulocytes in addition to antibiotics for therapy of documented infections was 14% (1 of 7 patients). In contrast, granulocyte transfusions were associated with 83% survival to 20 days (10 of 12 patients). To analyze the difference between the two groups further, 12 patients were paired on the basis of several characteristics bearing on the outcome of acute leukemia. Five of the six patients in the transfused group survived for 20 days or more and entered complete remission, whereas only two of six patients in the untreated group survived for 20 days and one of these entered complete remission. Although these numbers are too small for meaningful statistical analysis, they suggest nevertheless that the outcome of treatment of leukemia may be influenced favorably in the experimental group. The major problem with Higby's study is the relatively low number of patients with documented infections (i.e., septicemias), making it difficult to appreciate to what extent the infections and their therapy in the two study groups were really comparable.

The next three studies to be analyzed here (16,77,78) have in common a separate analysis of the patients whose granulocyte count returned to normal or at least increased during therapy for infection. In Herzig's study (16) all patients had Gram-negative septicemia and were treated early with cephalothin, carbenicillin, and gentamicin. Granulocytes were randomly added to the antibiotics as soon as the infection was microbiologically documented. Resolution of sepsis was markedly influenced by granulocyte transfusions in patients with no bone marrow recovery. All patients (8/8) not receiving granulocytes died with persistent Gram-negative septicemia. Of 12 patients who received granulocyte transfusions, 8 survived the bout of sepsis. These patients went off the study, and their survival was indistinguishable from that of patients whose peripheral granulocytes returned to normal. The median duration of survival was approximately 3 months; the four patients who died had persistent infection.

Vogler and Winton (77) conducted a randomized trial to determine the efficacy of granulocyte transfusions in neutropenic patients with documented infection not responding to appropriate antibiotic therapy. The survival rate in the control group was only 31%, whereas 59% of the transfused patients survived; the median survival was 22.5 days in the group given transfusions and 7.7 days in the control group. The granulocyte transfusions were most effective in patients with hypocellular marrow who failed to recover during the period of observation. In those patients with bone marrow recovery, 2 of 2 controls and 5 of 6 transfused patients responded to therapy; whereas in those whose bone marrow did not recover, 0 of 11 controls and 5 of 11 transfused patients responded. Once again, mostly patients with persistent granulocytopenia benefited from the granulocyte transfusions. Seventeen leukemic patients became infected and failed to respond to antibiotics during initial therapy to induce remission. Of eight subjects in the control group, seven died during the first 23 days after onset of infection and one, who did not respond to antibiotic therapy during the observation period, eventually had a complete remission. Of nine transfused patients, three died and three eventually had a remission.

Alavi and co-workers (78) evaluated granulocyte transfusions in a prospective controlled randomized study. Patients were admitted to the study as soon as they became febrile; as a result, half the febrile episodes that were evaluated were apparently not due to infection. Among the patients with documented infection, the survival to 21 days was 52% (10/19) among the controls and 78% (11/14) in the transfused patients. Patients with bone marrow recovery during the period of observation were not helped by the transfusions: eight of nine controls and five of six transfused patients survived. On the other hand, in those with no bone marrow recovery, 6 of 8 transfused patients survived whereas only 2 of 10 controls were alive 21 days after onset of treatment. Overall survival was somewhat greater in the transfused group (median 45 days) than in the controls (median 29 days); however, this difference was not statistically significant. For the patients in whom the marrow failed to recover, the median survival was 31 days for transfused patients and 11 days for controls. Thus a prolongation of survival was found in patients without bone marrow recovery; it appeared, however, that the survival advantage did not persist beyond 31 days.

The principal characteristics of the various studies analyzed here are summarized in Table 10. It can be seen that in five of six studies the survival of the patients receiving granulocyte transfusions was better than that of the controls; in two studies (76,77) there was a favorable effect of the transfusions on the course of leukemia, although the number of patients available for analysis is very small. By pooling the two studies, one can observe that 8 of 15 transfused patients went into complete remission whereas only 2 of 14 controls achieved it.

Table 11 summarizes the effect of granulocyte transfusions on the survival of infected granulocytopenic patients. It can be seen that 39% of the controls survived to 21 days after the onset of therapy, whereas 63% of the transfused patients survived. This difference is statistically significant ($p < 0.001$), but it is more striking in those patients whose bone marrow did not recover during the treatment of infection: 61% of the transfused patients survived, but only 7% of the controls ($p < 0.0001$). If one considers only patients in whom bone marrow recovery occurred during therapy, 15 of 17 control patients and 14 of 16 transfused patients survived to 21 days. It is clear from these data that granulocyte transfusions do not add anything to antibiotics once endogenous marrow function recovers.

Granulocyte transfusions appear to prolong survival in infected neutropenic patients with prolonged and severe granulocytopenia. In a recent large cooperative trial, this subgroup of patients with severe infection and persistent granulocytopenia represented only 7% of all infected granulocytopenic patients (15). Thus only a small fraction of febrile granulocytopenic patients appear to benefit from granulocyte transfusions. The definition of such a subgroup is difficult; it was attempted in a recent EORTC protocol of the Antimicrobial Therapy Project Group which considers eligible for granulocyte transfusions only those patients with low granulocyte ($<100/mm^3$) and platelet ($<50,000/mm^3$) counts, high

TABLE 10. Characteristics and results in six controlled trials of granulocyte transfusions

Parameter	Graw (1972)	Fortuny (1975)	Higby (1975)	Herzig (1977)	Vogler (1977)	Alavi (1977)
WBC/mm³ at entry	500	500	500	1,000	300	250
Antibiotics (always given as empirical therapy)	"Appropriate"	Cephalothin + carbenicillin + gentamicin	"Broad-spectrum"	Cephalothin + carbenicillin + gentamicin	Cephalothin + carbenicillin + gentamicin	Cephalothin + gentamicin + carbenicillin or/and other penicillin
Delay between antibiotic therapy and granulocyte transfusions	WBC given as soon as possible after documentation of infection	WBC given if fever persisted 48 hr after onset of antibiotic therapy	WBC given if antibiotic therapy for 48 hr was considered a failure	WBC given as soon as possible after documentation of infection	WBC given if antibiotic therapy for 72 hr was considered a failure	WBC given within 36 hr after onset of antibiotic therapy
Dose of WBC (× 10⁹) and source[a]	CFC: 5,6 FL: 20	CFC: 6,2	FL: 35	CFC: 4/M² FL: 17/M²	CFC: 29	FL: 50
Median No. of transfusions	4	4	4	9	7	7
Survival at 21 days (%)						
Controls	30	71	14	35	31	52
Transfused patients	46	71	83	75	59	78

WBC = white blood cells (granulocytes).
[a]CFC = continuous flow centrifugation. FL = filtration leukopheresis.

TABLE 11. *Survival of neutropenic patients with microbiologically documented infection at 21 days*

Study	Controls			Transfused patients		
	Total no.	No bone marrow recovery	Bone marrow recovery	Total no.	No bone marrow recovery	Bone marrow recovery
Graw et al. (73)	11/37			18/39		
Fortuny et al. (74)	15/21			12/17		
Higby et al. (76)	1/7			10/12		
Herzig et al. (16)	5/14	0/8	5/6	12/16	8/12	4/4
Vogler & Winton (77)	2/13	0/11	2/2	10/17	5/11	5/6
Alavi et al. (78)	10/19	2/10	8/9	11/14	6/8	5/6
Total	44/111 (39.6%)	2/29 (6.9%)	15/17 (88.2%)	73/115 (63.5%)	19/31 (61.3%)	14/16 (87.5%)

$p < 0.001$

$p < 0.0001$

fever ($>39°C$), relatively elevated serum creatinine (>1.0 mg%), and hypocellular bone marrow (79).

Examination of the bone marrow may be important when deciding whether granulocyte transfusions should be initiated in a given patient since there is evidence that patients with a hypocellular marrow benefit most from the granulocyte transfusions. Other tests (e.g., estimation of the granulocyte reserve) might also permit identification of the more favorable prognostic group for which granulocyte transfusions would not be needed.

It is often necessary to make an early decision of whether to transfuse granulocytes to a febrile patient with granulocytopenia as there is often a delay related to the collection techniques and to the recruitment of suitable donors. Among 69 neutropenic febrile patients recently treated at the Institut Jules Bordet, 15 died during the first week of therapy, which was started as soon as fever greater than $38.5°C$ was detected. Among these 15 patients, 10 died from infection; of these, 6 died within 24 hr of the onset of therapy (80). Thus another approach to the management of febrile granulocytopenic patients would be to start granulocyte transfusions as soon as possible after the onset of antibiotic treatment and to discontinue these granulocyte transfusions when there is evidence of bone marrow recovery or if culture results are negative and the patient responds clinically.

When fever and other clinical signs of infection persist in spite of broad-spectrum antimicrobial therapy and if cultures remain negative, a fungal infection must be suspected. Empirical therapy with antifungal agents should then be considered. The importance of granulocyte transfusions under these circumstances has not yet been studied. Some data indicate that fungal infections are not nearly as responsive to granulocyte transfusions as are those caused by bacteria (68), but other observations suggest a possible suppressive effect of the transfusions against fungal infections (78).

CONCLUSIONS

A major effort has been realized during the last decade to prevent and treat infections in granulocytopenic patients. These attempts have usually been successful, and their importance in lessening suffering and creating more patient comfort is beyond evaluation. However, the control of infection in neutropenic patients can have a major influence on the overall survival only in those patients whose underlying disease can be adequately treated; therefore, continuing effort is to be focused there.

REFERENCES

1. Hersch, E. M., Bodey, G. P., Nies, B. A., and Freireich, E. J. (1965): Causes of death in acute leukemia: A ten-year study of 414 patients from 1954–1963. *JAMA,* 193:105.
2. Schimpff, S. C., Young, V. M., Greene, W. H., Vermeulen, G. D., Moody, M. R., and Wiernik, P. H. (1972): Origin of infection in acute non-lymphocytic leukemia: Significance of hospital acquisition of potential pathogens. *Ann. Intern. Med.,* 77:707.
3. Levine, A. S., Siegel, S. E., Schreiber, A. D., Hauser, J., Preisler, H., Goldstein, I. M., Seidler, F., Simon, R., Perry, S., Bennett, J. E., and Henderson, E. S. (1973): Protected environments and prophylactic antibiotics: A prospective controlled study of their utility in the therapy of acute leukemia. *N. Engl. J. Med.,* 288:477.
4. Yates, J. W., and Holland, J. F. (1973): A controlled study of isolation and endogenous microbial suppression in acute myelocytic leukemia patients. *Cancer,* 32:1490.
5. Klastersky, J., Debusscher, L., Weerts, D., and Daneau, D. (1974): Use of oral antibiotics in protected units environment: Clinical effectiveness and role in the emergence of antibiotic resistant strains. *Pathol. Biol.,* 22:5.
6. Schimpff, S. C., Green, W. H., Young, V. M., Fortner, C. L., Jepsen, L., Cusack, N., Block, J. B., and Wiernick, P. H. (1975): Infection prevention in acute non-lymphocytic leukemia: Laminar flow room reverse isolation with oral, non-absorbable antibiotic prophylaxis. *Ann. Intern. Med.,* 82:351.
7. Dietrich, M., Gaus, W., Vossen, J., van der Waaij, D., and Wendt, F. (1977): Protective isolation and antimicrobial decontamination in patients with high susceptibility to infection. *Infection,* 5:1.
8. Storring, R. A., Jameson, B., McElwain, T. J., Wiltshaw, E., Spiers, A. D. S., and Gaya, H. (1977): Oral non-absorbed antibotics prevent infection in acute non-lymphoblastic leukemia. *Lancet,* 2:837.
9. Lohner, D., Debusscher, L., Prevost, J. M., and Klastersky, J. (1979): Comparative randomized study of protected environment plus oral antibiotics versus oral antibiotics in neutropenic patients. *Cancer Ther. Rep. (in press).*
10. Jameson, B., Gamble, D. R., Lynck, J., and Kay, H. E. M. (1971): Five year analysis of protective isolation. *Lancet,* 1:1034.
11. Levine, A. S. (1976): Protected environment–prophylactic antibiotic programs: Clinical studies. *Clin. Haematol.,* 5:409.
12. Hughes, W. T., Kuhn, S., Chaudary, S., Feldman, S., Verzosa, M., Aur, J. A. R., Pratt, C., and George, S. L. (1977): Successful chemoprophylaxis for *Pneumocystis carinii* pneumonitis. *N. Engl. J. Med.,* 297:1419.
13. Gurwith, M. J., Brunton, J. L., Lank, B. A., Harding, G. K. M., and Ronald, A. R. (1979): A prospective controlled investigation of prophylactic trimethoprim/sulfamethoxazole in hospitalized granulocytopenic patients. *Am. J. Med.,* 66:248.
14. Rodriguez, V., Bodey, G. P., Freireich, E. J., McCredie, K. B., Gutterman, J. V., Keating,

M. J., Smith, T., and Gehan, E. A. (1979): Randomization trial of protected environment–prophylactic antibiotics in 145 adults with acute leukemia. *Medicine (Baltimore)*, 57:253.

15. Schimpff, S. C., Gaya, H., Klastersky, J., Tattersall, M. H. N., and Zinner, S. H. (1978): Three antibiotic regimens in the treatment of infection in febrile granulopenic patients with cancer (EORTC International Antimicrobial Therapy Project Group). *J. Infect. Dis.*, 137:14.

16. Herzig, R. H., Herzig, G. P., Graw, R. G., Bull, M. I., and Ray, K. K. (1977): Successful granulocyte transfusion therapy for Gram negative septicemia: A prospective randomized controlled study. *N. Engl. J. Med.*, 296:701.

17. Klastersky, J., Weerts, D., and Gompel, C. (1975): Causes of death in acute non-lymphocytic leukemia. *Eur. J. Cancer*, 11:21.

18. Thomas, E. D., Buckner, C. D., Banaji, M., Clift, R. A., Fefer, A., Flournoy, N., Goodell, B. W., Hickman, R. O., Lerner, G. K., Neiman, P. E., Sale, G. E., Sanders, J. E., Singer, J., Stevens, M., Storb, P., and Weiden, P. L. (1977): One hundred patients with acute leukemia treated by chemotherapy, total body irradiation and allogeneic marrow transplantation. *Blood*, 49:511.

19. Buckner, C. D., Clift, R. A., Sanders, J. E., Meyers, J. D., Counts, G. W., Farewell, V. T., and Thomas, E. D. (1978): Protective environment for marrow transplant recipients: A prospective study. *Ann. Intern. Med.*, 89:893.

20. Storb, R., Thomas, E. D., Weiden, P. L., Buckner, C. D., Clift, R. A., Fefer, A., Fernando, A. L., Glibett, E. R., Goodell, B. W., Johnson, F. L., Lerner, K. G., Neiman, P. E., and Sanders, J. E. (1976): Aplastic anemia treated by allogeneic bone marrow transplantation: A report on 49 new cases from Seattle. *Blood*, 48:817.

21. Cohen, M. H., Creaven, P. J., Fossieck, B. F., Broder, L. E., Selawry, O. S., Johnston, A. V., Williams, C. L., and Minna, J. D. (1977): Intensive chemotherapy of small cell bronchogenic carcinoma. *Cancer Chemother. Rep.*, 61:349.

22. Pizzo, P. A., and Levine, S. A. (1977): The utility of protected-environment regimens for the compromised host: A critical assessment. *Prog. Hematol.*, 10:311.

23. Ford, J. M., and Cullen, M. H. (1977): Prophylactic granulocyte transfusions. *Exp. Hematol.*, 5:S65.

24. Clift, R. A., Sanders, J. E., Thomas, E. D., Williams, B., and Buckner, C. D. (1978): Granulocyte transfusions for the penetration of infection in patients receiving bone marrow transplants. *N. Engl. J. Med.*, 298:1052.

25. Mannoni, P., Rodet, M., Radeau, E., Beaujean, F., and Brun, B. (1972): Granulocyte transfusion: Efficiency of granulocyte transfusions in care of patients with acute leukemia. In: *Blood Leucocytes: Function and Use in Therapy*, edited by C. S. Hogman, K. Lindahl-Kiessling, and H. Wiggel. Almqvist & Wiksell, Stockholm.

26. Bodey, G. P., Middleman, E., Umsawadi, T., and Rodriguez, V. (1972): Infections in cancer patients: Results with gentamicin sulfate therapy. *Cancer*, 29:1697.

27. Archer, G., and Fekety, F. R. (1977): Experimental endocarditis due to Pseudomonas aeruginosa. II. Therapy with carbenicillin and gentamicin. *J. Infect. Dis.*, 136:327.

28. Keating, M. J., Bodey, G. P., Valdivieso, M., and Rodriguez, V. (1979): A comparative trial of three aminoglycosides—a comparison of continuous infusion of gentamicin, amikacin and sisomicin combined with carbenicillin in neutropenic patients with malignancies. *Medicine (Baltimore)*, 58:159.

29. Klastersky, J., Hensgens, C., and Debusscher, L. (1975): Empiric therapy for cancer patients: Comparative study of ticarcillin–tobramycin, ticarcillin–cephalothin and cephalothin–tobramycin. *Antimicrob. Agents Chemother.*, 7:640.

30. Bodey, G. B., Valdivieso, M., Feld, R., Rodriguez, V., and McCredie, K. (1977): Carbenicillin plus cephalothin or cefazolin as therapy for infections in neutropenic patients. *Am. J. Med. Sci.*, 273:309.

31. Gurwith, M., Brunton, J. L., Lank, B., Ronald, A. R., Harding, G. K. M., and McCullough, D. W. (1978): Granulocytopenic in hospitalized patients. II. A prospective comparison of two antibiotic regimens in the empiric therapy of febrile patients. *Am. J. Med.*, 64:127.

32. Klastersky, J., Henri, A., Hensgens, C., and Daneau, D. (1974): Gram negative infections in cancer: Study of empiric therapy comparing carbenicillin–cephalothin with and without gentamicin. *JAMA*, 227:45.

33. Schimpff, S. C., Landesman, S., Hahn, D. M., Standiford, H. C., Fortner, C. L., Young, V. M., and Wiernik, P. H. (1976): Ticarcillin in combination with cephalothin or gentamicin as

empiric antibiotic therapy in granulocytopenic cancer patients. *Antimicrob. Agents Chemother.,* 10:837.

34. Klastersky, J., Hensgens, C., and Daneau, D. (1975): Therapy of staphylococcal infections: Comparative study of cephaloridine and gentamicin. *Am. J. Med. Sci.,* 269:201.
35. Klastersky, J., Cappel, R., Debusscher, L., Daneau, D., and Swings, G. (1971): Use of carbenicillin and polymyxin B for therapy of Gram negative bacilli infections. *Chemotherapy,* 16:269.
36. Gaya, H., and Klastersky, J. (1976): In vitro and in vivo studies with trimethoprim-sulfamethoxazole-polymyxin: sensitivites and synergy; efficacy in Gram negative septicemia. In: *Proceedings of the 16th Interscience Conference on Antimicrobial Agents and Chemotherapy,* Chicago.
37. Israel, L. (1972): Infections au cours des chimiothérapies anticancéreuses: Utilisation de l'association sulfamethoxazole–trimethoprim. *Nouv. Presse Med.,* 1:273.
38. Rodriguez, V., Burgess, M., and Bodey, G. P. (1973): Management of fever of unknown origin in patients with neoplasms and neutropenia. *Cancer,* 32:1007.
39. Sande, M. A., and Overton, J. W. (1973): In vivo antagonism between gentamicin and chloramphenicol in neutropenic mice. *J. Infect. Dis.,* 128:247.
40. Bodey, G. P., Feld, F., and Burgess, M. A. (1976): β-Lactam antibiotic alone or in combination for therapy of Gram negative bacillary infections in neutropenic patients. *Am. J. Med. Sci.,* 271:179.
41. Hahan, D. M., Schimpff, S. C., Young, V. M., Fortner, C. L., Standiford, H. C., and Wiernik, P. H. (1977): Amikacin and cephalothin: Empiric regimen for granulocytopenic cancer patients. *Antimicrob. Agents Chemother.,* 12:618.
42. Wade, J. C., Petty, B. G., Conrad, G., Smith, C. R., Lipsky, I. J., Ellner, J., and Lietman, P. S. (1978): Cephalothin plus an aminoglycoside is more nephrotoxic than methicillin plus an aminoglycoside. *Lancet,* 2:604.
43. Rodriguez, V., Whitecar, J. P., and Bodey, G. P. (1970): Therapy of infections with the combination of carbenicillin and gentamicin. *Antimicrob. Agents Chemother.,* p. 386.
44. Schimpff, S. C., Satterlee, W., Young, V. M., and Serpick, A. (1971): Empiric therapy with carbenicillin and gentamicin for febrile patients with cancer and granulocytopenia. *N. Engl. J. Med.,* 284:1061.
45. Young, L. S. (1971): Gentamicin: clinical use with carbenicillin and in vitro studies with recent isolates of Pseudomonas aeruginosa. *J. Infect. Dis.,* 124:S202.
46. Klastersky, J., Cappel, R., and Daneau, D. (1973): Therapy with carbenicillin and gentamicin for patients with cancer and severe infections caused by Gram negative rods. *Cancer,* 31:331.
47. Klastersky, J., Meunier-Carpentier, F., and Prevost, J. M. (1977): Significance of antimicrobial synergism for the outcome of Gram negative sepsis. *Am. J. Med. Sci.,* 273:157.
48. Bloomfield, C. D., and Kennedy, B. J. (1974): Cephalothin, carbenicillin, and gentamicin combination therapy for febrile patients with acute non-lymphocytic leukemia. *Cancer,* 34:431.
49. Klasterksy, J., Debusscher, L., Weerts-Ruhl, D., and Prevost, J. M. (1977): Carbenicillin, cefazolin and amikacin as an empiric for febrile granulocytopenic cancer patients. *Cancer Treat. Rep.,* 61:1433.
50. Greene, W. H., Schimpff, S. C., Young, V. M., and Wiernik, P. (1973): Empiric carbenicillin, gentamicin and cephalothin therapy for presumed infection. *Ann. Intern. Med.,* 78:825.
51. EORTC International Antimicrobial Therapy Project Group (1977): Protocol for a cooperative trial of empirical antibiotic treatment and early granulocyte transfusions in febrile neutropenic patients. *Eur. J. Cancer,* 13:617.
52. Klastersky, J., Meunier-Carpentier, F., Prevost, J. M., and Staquet, M. (1976): Synergism between amikacin and cefazolin against *Klebsiella:* In vitro studies and effect on the bactericidal activity of serum. *J. Infect. Dis.,* 134:271.
53. Klastersky, J., Cappel, R., and Daneau, D. (1972): Clinical significance of in vitro synergism between antibiotics in Gram negative infections. *Antimicrob. Agents Chemother.,* 2:470.
54. Anderson, E. T., Young, L. S., and Hewitt, W. L. (1978): Antimicrobial synergism in the therapy of Gram negative rod bacteremia. *Chemotherapy,* 24:45.
55. Lau, W. K., Young, L. S., Black, R. E., Winston, D. J., Linner, S. R., Weinstein, R. J., and Hewitt, W. L. (1977): Comparative efficacy and toxicity of amikacin/carbenicillin versus gentamicin/carbenicillin in leucopenic patients. *Am. J. Med.,* 62:959.
56. Klastersky, J., Daneau, D., Swings, G., and Weerts, D. (1974): Antibacterial activity in serum and urine as therapeutic guides in bacterial infections. *J. Infect. Dis.,* 129:187.
57. Pizzo, P. A., Rochibaud, K., Gill, F., Witebysky, F., Levine, A., and MacLowry, J. (1978):

Empiric antibiotic therapy in granulocytopenic cancer patients. In: *Proceedings of the 18th Interscience Conference on Antimicrobial Agents and Chemotherapy,* Atlanta.

58. Bodey, G. P. (1966): Fungal infections complicating acute leukemia. *J. Chronic Dis.,* 19:667.

59. Aisner, J., Schimpff, S. C., and Hahn, D. M. (1976): Fungal infections in patients with cancer: changing frequency associated with broad spectrum antibiotics. *Clin. Res.,* 24:339A (Abstract).

60. Aisner, J., Murillo, J., Schimpff, S. C., and Steere, A. C. (1979): Invasive aspergillosis in acute leukemia: Correlation with nose cultures and antibiotic use. *Ann. Intern. Med.,* 90:4.

61. Pennington, J. E. (1976): Successful treatment of *Aspergillus* pneumonia in hematologic neoplasia. *N. Engl. J. Med.,* 295:426.

62. Aisner, J., Schimpff, S. C., and Wiernik, P. H. (1977): Treatment of invasive aspergillosis: Relation of early diagnosis and treatment to response. *Ann. Intern. Med.,* 86:539.

63. Bindschadler, D. D., and Bennett, J. E. (1969): A pharmacologic guide to the clinical use of amphotericin B. *J. Infect. Dis.,* 120:427.

64. Debelak, K. M., Epstein, R. B., and Anderson, B. R. (1964): Granulocyte transfusions in leukopenic dogs: In vivo and in vitro function of granulocytes obtained by continuous-flow filtration leukopheresis. *Blood,* 43:757.

65. Morse, E. E., Freireich, E. J., Carbone, P. P., Bronson, W., and Frei, E., III. (1966): The transfusion of leukocytes from donors with chronic myelocytic leukemia to patients with leukopenia. *Transfusion,* 6:183.

66. Schwartzenberg, L., Mathe, G., Amiel, J. L., Cattan, A., Schneider, M., and Schlumberger, J. R. (1967): Study of factors determining usefulness and complications of leukocyte transfusions. *Am. J. Med.,* 43:206.

67. Eyre, H. J., Goldstein, I. M., Perry, S., and Graw, R. G., Jr. (1970): Leukocyte transfusions: function of transfused granulocytes from donors with chronic myelocytic leukemia. *Blood,* 36:432.

68. Schiffer, C. A., Buchhlotz, D. H., Aisner, J., Beets, S. W., and Wiernik, P. H. (1975): Clinical experience with transfusion of granulocytes obtained by continuous flow-filtration leukopheresis. *Am. J. Med.,* 58:373.

69. Lowenthal, R. M., Storring, R. A., Goldman, J. M., Buskard, N. A., Grossman, L., Park, T. S., Murphy, B. C., Spiers, A. S. D., and Calton, D. A. G. (1975): Granulocyte transfusions in treatment of infections in patients with acute leukemia and aplastic anemia. *Lancet,* 1:353.

70. Bussel, A., Benbunam, M., and Bernard, J. (1976): Enseignements tirés des transfusions de granulocytes appliquées au traitement des infections compliquant les aplasies induites par les chimiothérapies antileucémiques. *Semin. Hop. (Paris),* 52:105.

71. Vallejos, C., McCredie, K. B., Bodey, G. P., Hester, G. P., and Freireich, E. J. (1975): White blood cell transfusions for control of infections in neutropenic patients. *Transfusion,* 15:28.

72. Strauss, R. G. (1978): Therapeutic neutrophil transfusion: Are controlled studies no longer appropriate? *Am. J. Med.,* 65:1001.

73. Graw, R. G., Herzig, G., Perry, S., and Henderson, E. S. (1972): Normal granulocyte transfusion therapy: Treatment of septicemia due to Gram negative bacteria. *N. Engl. J. Med.,* 287:367.

74. Fortuny, I. E., Bloomfield, C. D., Hadlock, D. C., Goldman, A., Kennedy, B. J., and McCullough, J. J. (1975): Granulocyte transfusion: controlled study in patients with acute non lymphocytic leukemia. *Transfusion,* 15:548.

75. Koza, I., Holland, J. F., and Cohen, E. (1971): Histocompatible leucocyte transfusions during granulocytopenia. *Neoplasma,* 18:185.

76. Higby, D. J., Yates, J. W., Henderson, E. S., and Holland, J. F. (1975): Filtration leukopheresis for granulocyte transfusion therapy: Clinical and laboratory studies. *N. Engl. J. Med.,* 292:761.

77. Vogler, W. R., and Winton, E. F. (1977): A controlled study of the efficacy of granulocyte transfusions in patients with neutropenia. *Am. J. Med.,* 63:548.

78. Alavi, J. B., Root, R. K., Djerassi, I., Evans, A. E., Sluckman, S. J., MacGregor, R. R., Gueery, D., Schreiber, A. D., Schaw, J. M., Koch, P., and Cooper, R. A. (1977): A randomized clinical trial of granulocytes transfusions for infection in acute leukemia. *N. Engl. J. Med.,* 296:706.

79. EORTC International Antimicrobial Therapy Project Group for a cooperative trial of empirical antibiotic treatment and early granulocyte transfusions in febrile neutropenic patients. *Eur. J. Cancer,* 13:617.

80. Stryckmans, P., and Debusscher, L. (1975): Neutrophil collection and transfusion for the treatment of infection in neutropenic patients. *Eur. J. Cancer,* 11:67.

Medical Complications in Cancer Patients,
edited by J. Klastersky and M. J. Staquet.
Raven Press, New York © 1981.

Infections in Patients with Suppressed Cellular Immunity

James C. Wade and Stephen C. Schimpff

Section of Infection Research, Baltimore Cancer Research Program, National Cancer Institute, University of Maryland Hospital, Baltimore, Maryland 21201

The compromised host is an individual with diminished defenses against infections. This increased susceptibility occurs because of reduced or abnormal granulocytes, damaged mucocutaneous barriers, obstructed drainage tracts, reduced antibody production, or deficient cellular immunity. Cellular immunity is important in controlling established infection or preventing reactivation of certain pathogens. Patients with intrinsically impaired cellular immunity (e.g., lymphoma, graft-versus-host disease, DiGeorge syndrome, or malnutrition) or those treated with immunosuppressive agents (e.g., corticosteroids, azathioprine, antithymocyte globulin, or cytotoxic drugs) may become infected with organisms which normally are destroyed by the body's thymus-derived lymphocytes (T-cells) (Table 1). T-cells are found in the blood, thoracic duct, deep cortical

TABLE 1. *Common pathogens: cellular immune dysfunction*

Bacteria	Viruses
Listeria monocytogenes	Cytomegalovirus
Salmonella	Herpes simplex
Mycobacterium tuberculosis	Varicella–zoster
Atypical mycobacteria	
Nocardia asteroides	
Legionella pneumophilia	Protozoa
	Pneumocystis carinii
Fungi	*Toxoplasma gondii*
Cryptococcus neoformans	
Histoplasma capsulatum	Helminths
Coccidioides immitis	*Strongyloides stercoralis*

and peripheral follicular areas of lymph nodes, and periarteriolar region of the spleen. These lymphocytes have a long life and are involved in recognizing and processing antigenic material. Cellular immunity is important in graft rejection, delayed hypersensitivity, and control of certain intracellular pathogens. Discussion of these specific bacterial, viral, fungal, protozoan, and helminthic infections is the purpose of this chapter.

BACTERIA

Listeria monocytogenes

Listeria monocytogenes, a Gram-positive rod that grows well on standard culture media and is often mistaken for a diphtheroid, is the prototype of facultative intracellular pathogens. This organism, with no known natural reservoir, is rarely a pathogen in adults except under circumstances of compromised cellular immunity. Serotypes 1a and 4b most frequently cause infection. Control of this organism depends on a two-cell response: the immunologically committed lymphocyte and the activated macrophage which possesses an enhanced ability to phagocytize and destroy intracellular pathogens. Mackaness (6) further demonstrated this by showing that immunity to *Listeria* could be transferred to unimmunized animals by immune macrophages but not by immune serum. Steroids known to suppress the production of committed lymphocytes (6) also impair resistance to *Listeria* infection.

Listeria infection usually presents as a meningitis or septicemia. Louria et al. (5), in one of the first comprehensive reviews of *Listeria* infections, described 26 cases occurring at the Memorial Sloan-Kettering Cancer Center and reviewed 100 previously reported cases. Among the previously published cases, 78 had meningitis, 12 had primary bacteremias, and 5 had endocarditis. Only one-fourth had easily defined underlying disease. In contrast, 21 of the 26 Memorial Hospital cases had lymphoma, most had undergone irradiation, and 18 were receiving corticosteroids. This and other evaluations indicate an increased incidence and severity of *Listeria* infection in patients with substantial immunosuppression.

Salmonella Species

Salmonella spp., aerobic Gram-negative bacilli acquired by man through the ingestion of contaminated food and water, produce an illness with fever, enteritis, and, rarely, septicemia. Cherubin et al. (7) reviewed all *Salmonella* bacteremias occurring in New York City. A large proportion of these patients with a bacteremia had an underlying illness (lymphoma, carcinoma, sickle cell disease); only 20% had associated gastrointestinal complaints, which is in contradiction to the 60% incidence of enteritis in patients without an underlying disease. This suggests that immunosuppressed patients tend to become bacteremic during *Salmonella* infection even in the absence of overt alimentary canal abnormalities.

A number of investigators have pointed out that *Salmonella* spp., like *Listeria monocytogenes,* are facultative intracellular parasites, and cellular immune macrophages are required for host resistance. Reviews of *Salmonella* infections at major cancer centers show these infections to occur most frequently in patients with lymphoma and lymphocytic leukemia. Wolfe et al. (8) observed that although only 10% of Memorial Sloan-Kettering Cancer Center admissions were patients with lymphocytic leukemia or lymphoma, these patients developed 50% of the *Salmonella* infections. *S. typhimurium* and *S. derby* were the most frequently isolated species, with 35% of these infections having an associated bacteremia. Eighty-five percent of the bacteremic cases had recently received corticosteroids, radiotherapy, or cytotoxic therapy. These reports substantiate the increased susceptibility to bacteremic *Salmonella* infections in patients with cellular immune deficiencies.

Mycobacterium

The mycobacteria include *M. tuberculosis* and the atypical species, such as *M. kansasii, M. intracellulare,* and *M. fortuitium.* Primary infection with *M. tuberculosis* provides the host with persistent immunity, but viable dormant bacilli are harbored within the tubercle and are controlled by activated macrophages. Factors that disturb host immunity allow endogenous reinfection. The more severe the disruption of the immunologic system, the more severe the infection. Kaplan et al. (10), in a review of tuberculosis among cancer patients, found that two patterns of infection occurred: Patients with pulmonary or head and neck tumors most often had their infection present at diagnosis of the neoplasm, whereas patients with cellular immune deficits such as lymphoma developed tuberculosis during or shortly after antincoplastic treatment. The severity and seriousness of the infection was correlated with the degree of immunosuppressive therapy, with dissemination being more frequent among patients who received irradiation, steroids, or cytotoxic agents. Disseminated tuberculosis was associated with a 91% mortality rate in these patients.

At the M. D. Anderson Hospital in Texas, Feld et al. (11) found that atypical mycobacteria were equally as common as *M. tuberculosis. M. Kansasii* and *M. fortuitum* were the most common organisms, and the majority of infections involved the lung.

Nocardia

Nocardia is a Gram-positive, partially acid-fast, branching rod that grows slowly and is easily overgrown by upper respiratory flora. The respiratory tract is the primary portal of entry, although cutaneous inoculation does occur. Infection, either localized or disseminated, has been described in nearly all organs of the body. *Nocardia* infections are divided into primary infections (i.e., the patient has no apparent predisposing cause, with the most frequent infection sites being lung and central nervous sytem) or secondary infections (i.e., the patient has compromised defenses with infection beginning in the lung, becoming locally invasive, and then disseminating to the central nervous sytem and other extrapulmonary sites). The secondary infections are more acute, fulminating, and often rapidly fatal. *Nocardia asteroides* is the predominant species in central nervous system (CNS) and systemic infection, whereas *Nocardia brasiliensis* involves the skin and subcutaneous tissue. The pathologic lesion is one of invasion, necrosis, abscess, and cavity formation. A preponderance of secondary *Nocardia* infections is seen in patients with suppressed cellular immunity. Young et al. (13), reviewing a 10-year period at Memorial Hospital, found only 13 patients with definite infection. Of these, 10 had leukemia or lymphoma, 11 had received corticosteroids, but none were granulocytopenic, suggesting that cellular immune mechanisms were most important. Presant et al. (12), in a review of reported cases, found that symptoms of less than 3 weeks, the presence of steroids, and evidence of dissemination were poor prognostic signs of recovery. Those patients with an underlying illness and being treated with corticosteroids had an 85% mortality rate. Thus *Nocardia* infections, like *Salmonella* and *Mycobacterium* infections, are not only increased in frequency, but are also more severe when associated with compromised cellular immunity.

Legionella pneumophilia

Legionnaire's disease is a recently described polyserotypic bacterial infection caused by *L. pneumophilia*. This Gram-negative bacillus was recovered mainly during epidemics of pneumonia. The organism appears to be spread by an airborne route and frequently is harbored in water, cooling towers, and around recent construction. Those patients in the reported outbreaks frequently have been immunosuppressed. Beaty et al. (14) reported that 39% of their infected patients were immunosuppressed, and all patients of Saravolatz et al. (16) and seven of nine patients of Gump et al. (17) had cell-mediated immune deficits or were receiving immunosuppressive therapy. In the largest reported group from one hospital, Kirby et al. (18) reported a high incidence of Legionnaire's disease in renal transplant patients. Although serum antibody to *Legionella pneumophilia* develops with infection, cellular immune mechanisms have been documented to interact with this organism. The affected patient populations appear to substantiate the role of cellular immunity in host protection and in resolution of established infection.

Recently two new groups of bacteria were described, and it is believed that they represent a new species of bacteria or are closely related to *Legionella.* The organism described by Myerowitz and colleagues (19) is termed the "Pittsburgh pneumonia agent," but was previously recognized as the TATLOCK or HEBA bacillus. The organism described by Rogers et al. (20) is unnamed. Both agents cause a pneumonia in patients with endogenous or pharmacologic immunosuppression and are associated with a high mortality. All of these organisms can be cultured on charcoal–yeast extract agar when incubated in 5% carbon dioxide. Although these organisms have not been completely identified, they may prove to be more commonly recognized in the immunosuppressed host.

FUNGI

Cryptococcus neoformans

Cryptococcus is a yeast-like fungus that has an identifiable mucopolysaccharide capsule, reproduces by budding, and proliferates in avian feces. *Cryptococcus* causes little tissue necrosis and hemorrhage; calcification and fibrosis are not observed. Tissue specimens infected with *Cryptococcus* often show giant cells or macrophages with ingested *Cryptococcus,* suggesting a cellular immune response (23). There is a predilection for *C. neoformans* to infect patients with lymphoma, chronic lymphocytic leukemia, sarcoid, or organ transplants, although Bennett (23) notes that nearly one-third to one-half of patients with meningoencephalitis have no apparent underlying disease. Cryptococcal infections occur primarily as a pneumonic process with dissemination most commonly to the CNS. Schimpff and Bennett (22) evaluated the cellular immune status of 14 patients without clinically detectable underlying illness following complete resolution of disseminated cryptococcosis. Deficits detected included depressed skin test responses, lymphocyte blastogenesis, and leukocyte migration inhibition to whole killed *C. neoformans.* They concluded that *C. neoformans* probably progresses to disseminated infection only in a host who is deficient in cell-mediated immunity. Kaplan et al. (21) studied 46 patients with *Cryptococcus* infection at Memorial Hospital. Forty-one of the patients had an underlying neoplastic illness, Hodgkin's disease and chronic lymphocytic leukemia being the most frequent. Of the infected patients, 80% were receiving corticosteroids, and 75% (28 of 41) of those with an underlying neoplastic disease died from their infection within 60 days. Kaplan also noted that infections by other facultative or intracellular pathogens (e.g., varicella–zoster, *Mycobacterium, Nocardia, Salmonella, Listeria,* or *Pneumocystis*) were frequent and temporally associated with the cryptococcal infection. This again stresses the role of cellular immune mechanisms in the defense against these organisms.

Histoplasma capsulatum

Histoplasmosis is a systemic fungal infection that has global distribution with focal endemic areas. Persistence and growth of the fungus occurs in bird (chickens, starlings) and bat feces. *Histoplasma* is acquired by the respiratory route with the primary focus of infection being the lungs. A mild self-limited course is the general rule, although *Histoplasma* may be fatal when dissemination occurs. Immunity to *H. capsulatum* involves both cellular and humoral components, although antibodies generated during the infection are not protective.

Histoplasmosis is not a frequently reported infection in cancer patients, yet, like those with tuberculosis, patients with cellular immune dysfunction and dormant *H. capsulatum* may experience reactivation with rapid dissemination. The compromised patient with a primary exposure may experience an overwhelming illness with a fatal outcome. Kauffman et al. (25) reviewed *H. capsulatum* infection in 16 immunosuppressed patients; 11 experienced disseminated disease. Davies et al. (26) reported eight cases of *H. capsulatum* with dissemination which occurred in a nonendemic area but in previously exposed, immunosuppressed patients. A similar observation was made by Cox et al. (27) in children with acute leukemia.

Coccidioides immitis

Coccidioides immitis is a highly infectious fungal organism which when inhaled from its soil reservoir causes a primary pulmonary infection. Forty percent of infected individuals experience a self-limited clinical illness, with dissemination occurring in less than 1% of cases. Deresinski and Stevens (28) at Stanford University Medical Center reviewed 44 cases of coccidioidomycosis occurring over 15 years; 13 cases occurred in compromised hosts. Of the 13, 6 had Hodgkin's disease, and 10 of the 13 had received immunosuppressives. Dissemination occurred in 6 of the 13 infections, and 5 of these 6 died. Rutala and Smith (29) reviewed 126 cases of coccidioidomycosis and indicated that 13% occurred in compromised hosts. Dissemination occurred among 50% of the compromised patients compared to 14% in the noncompromised group. The presence of skin test reactivity was a good prognostic indicator, with no correlation possible from serologic reactivity. Cellular immunity is consequently assumed to be the primary mechanism of control, with corticosteroids and immunosuppressives correlating with dissemination.

VIRUSES

Cytomegalovirus

Cytomegalovirus (CMV) is a member of the herpes family and contains a DNA viral genome. Viral replication results in the formation of the characteristic acidophilic, intranuclear inclusion bodies. CMV is a poor interferon inducer and is resistant to its actions. The virus is ubiquitous but can be transferred by blood products (e.g., polymorphonuclear leukocytes, monocytes) and transplanted organs. Few persons during life escape a primary infection, although infection may not be overt. The virus becomes latent following the primary infection, but once the immune system is altered (i.e., decay of immunologic constraints, debilitating disease, immunosuppressive agents) the latent virus reactivates. The relative infrequency of CMV disease in agammaglobulinemic patients suggests that cellular immunity is important. Antibodies are formed in response to CMV infections, but their immune role is unclear since viral excretion continues despite the presence of antibody. Adults experience two types of infection: (a) CMV mononucleosis, characterized by a febrile illness with atypical lymphocytosis, hepatosplenomegaly, but no adenopathy; and (b) CMV infection of target organs, most prominently lungs and liver. The renal, cardiac, or bone marrow transplant recipient is the compromised host most frequently infected by CMV, although CMV remains common in other illnesses with associated cellular immunity dysfunction. Fiala et al. (31) found viruria in 90% of their renal transplant patients, and 96% (24 of 25) of their patients developed a CMV infection within 7 months posttransplantation. Armstrong et al. (34) found a 50% incidence of viremia in their renal transplants. Meyers et al. (30) described CMV pneumonia in 49% of patients undergoing bone marrow transplantation, and Stinson et al. (36) found serologic or autopsy evidence of active CMV infection posttransplantation in 50% (9 of 18) of cardiac transplant patients.

Concurrent infections with CMV and other organisms (*Toxoplasma, Pneumocystis carinii, Candida* spp.) are frequent. The interaction between CMV and *Toxoplasma gondii* was evaluated *in vitro* by Gelderman et al. (35), who showed that human fibroblasts infected with CMV were relatively resistant to *Toxoplasma* superinfection for an initial 2- to 5-day period. However, after the sixth day these CMV-infected cells not only accepted superinfection, but also supported rapid intracellular growth of *Toxoplasma*. Hamilton et al. (32), using a mouse model, found a similar relationship between CMV and *Candida albicans*. These studies suggest CMV enhances susceptibility to certain infecting organisms and may explain the frequently found combination of infections.

Herpes Simplex Virus

Herpes simplex type 1, an intracellular DNA virus, frequently causes a primary childhood illness, becomes latent, and may later reactivate. Although uncommon, a disseminated infection can involve skin, mucous membranes, and, less frequently, the viscera. The immune deficiency responsible for the development of disseminated herpes simplex virus infections is unknown. It may well be a combined effect of humoral and cellular immunity. Corticosteroid impairment of interferon production may be important in decreased host resistance against herpes simplex virus and explain why most visceral herpes has been reported in immunosuppressed patients. Buss and Scharyj (37) evaluated 56 cases of disseminated herpes simplex; 37 had malignant illnesses, especially hematopoietic and lymphoreticular neoplasms, and 41 of the 56 had received corticosteroids. Most infections involved the alimentary or respiratory tract and occurred at sites of previous trauma. The proposed mechanism for this infection is oral virus shedding with secondary infection at traumatized visceral sites and subsequent ulcer superinfection by bacteria or fungi.

Varicella–Zoster Virus

Varicella–zoster is a DNA virus causing varicella (chickenpox) as a primary infection and zoster (shingles) as a secondary infection. Zoster occurs presumably as a result of reactivation of the virus believed to be dormant in the dorsal root ganglion, although controversy exists with regard to zoster occurring as a primary infection. The normal course of varicella in agammaglobulinemic children and the recovery from herpes zoster of hypogammaglobulinemic patients without detectable varicella–zoster antibody are natural evidence that cellular immunity is important in varicella–zoster resistance. There is an increased incidence of zoster in cancer patients, both adults and children. The frequency of infection is highest in patients with Hodgkin's disease. Schimpff et al. (38) found that 15% of Hodgkin's disease patients with herpes zoster experienced dissemination, and another 15% had a mild atypical varicella-form eruption without serious systemic signs or symptoms. They pointed out that the combination of disease anergy and recent irradiation with some additional immune suppression with chemotherapy were the major predisposing factors to infection. As a result, most cases of zoster develop within 6 to 12 months after completion of radiotherapy.

Herpes zoster often involves irradiated or tumor-involved dermatomes. Those patients who experience zoster as a primary infection usually demonstrate an incubation period of 15 to 35 days after exposure. Zoster begins clinically with burning dermatomal pain, followed by the appearance of clear vesicles which progress to pustules. New lesions appear for up to 7 days, and their crusts may persist for weeks. Dissemination, when it occurs, begins within 6 to 10 days of the initial vesicle appearance. Mortality from zoster is low even with dissemination, although the main morbidity is postherpetic neuralgia, superinfection, and neurologic complications.

PROTOZOA

Pneumocystis carinii

Pneumocystis carinii is a protozoan with global distribution but an unknown natural reservoir. Pneumonitis is the only site of the human infection, and considerable evidence suggests that an immunodeficient state provokes the reactivation of latent *P. carinii* organisms. A clinically unrecognized infection likely occurs early in life. This is consistent with the rapidly increasing proportion of the population who with increasing age have demonstrable antibody. The importance of cellular immunity to *P. carinii* pneumonitis is exemplified by the work of Walzer et al. (40), who reviewed the requests for pentamadine to the Center for Disease Control (United States) for presumed or proved *P. carinii* infections. Sixty-nine percent of requests were for patients who had acute or chronic lymphatic leukemia, Hodgkin's disease, lymphoma, and organ transplant as an underlying disease. At St. Jude's Hospital, Hughes et al. (42) demonstrated that the incidence of *P. carinii* pneumonia is increased concurrent with the more intensive immunosuppression used for remission maintenance therapy of acute lymphocytic leukemia. With maintenance regimens containing one or two drugs the incidence was less than 5%; it increased to 20% with three drugs and to nearly 40% with four. *P. carinii* may be the single infecting organism, but frequently there is a polymicrobial pneumonitis with CMV, herpes simplex virus, Gram-negative bacilli, or fungi. The necessity for tissue diagnosis is therefore apparent.

Toxoplasma gondii

Toxoplasma is an ubiquitous protozoan parasite, with the cat being the natural reservoir. The prevalance rate is in excess of 50% in many population groups, and *T. gondii* is capable of living dormantly in multiple tissues for the life of the host. The lymphocyte–monocyte-based system of host resistance is the immune mechanism against *T. gondii*. Vietzke et al. (44) were the first to recognize a distinct syndrome of infection caused by this organism among patients with advanced cancer. In a later literature review, Ruskin et al. (43) found that the majority of *Toxoplasma* cases in compromised hosts occurred in patients with Hodgkin's disease, lymphatic leukemia, non-Hodgkin's lymphoma, and renal transplants, suggesting the importance of cellular immunity. Carey et al. (45) found that of 24 cases of toxoplasmosis 14 patients had an underlying neoplastic illness. Similar findings have been reported by others. Herpesvirus and CMV often coexist with *T. gondii*. Unlike the acute lymphadenitis seen in noncompromised individuals, the CNS is most frequently involved in the immunosuppressed host. Prompt diagnosis is important because specific therapy, when instituted early, is curative.

HELMINTHS

Strongyloides stercoralis

Strongyloides stercoralis is a common parasite in tropical climates, existing in the soil either as rhabdoid or filariform larvae. It infects man by penetrating small cutaneous blood vessels, traveling to the lungs, penetrating the pulmonary capillaries, and entering the alveoli. The larvae move up the respiratory tract, are swallowed, and reach the gastrointestinal tract, where the female invades the mucosa and lays her eggs, which are passed in the stool. Massive invasion of the intestinal tract and lungs have been termed hyperinfection, dissemination, or autoinfection. The exact mechanism of immunity against the helminth is not firmly established, but clinical and experimental evidence suggests that cell-mediated and humoral immunity prevents helminthic hyperinfection. Scowden et al. (46), reporting on five cases of overwhelming *Strongyloides* and reviewing the published literature, described disseminated infection in patients with T-cell defects who were also receiving corticosteroids. Case reviews by other authors substantiated that immunosuppressive therapy is the major predisposing condition to dissemination; in contrast, the nonimmunosuppressed patient only rarely develops massive dissemination after primary infection.

CLINICAL SPECTRUM, THERAPY, AND PREVENTION

The previously described organisms cause variable clinical pictures but often provide characteristic clues helpful in distinguishing or suggesting their presence. Four clinical entities—pneumonitis, meningoencephalitis, hepatitis, and enteritis—are considered. Each of these entities is addressed as to the specific organisms causing infection and the characteristics of those infections.

Pneumonitis (Table 2) is the most common infection caused by the organisms discussed in this chapter. The lung reacts to an insult in only limited ways; consequently, the differentiation between opportunistic infecting agents is difficult without histologic or microbiologic data. Fever and nonproductive cough are universal for each of these organisms, but significant early hypoxia is most suggestive of *Pneumocystis carinii* or viral infection. The roentgenographic picture of an alveolar or miliary process is most frequently seen with the bacterial,

TABLE 2. *Clinical infectious sites of common pathogens in patients with cellular immune deficiency*

Lung
  Mycobacterium tuberculosis
  Atypical mycobacteria
  Nocardia asteroides
  Legionella pneumophilia
  Cryptococcus neoformans
  Histoplasma capsulatum
  Coccidioides immitis
  Cytomegalovirus
  Varicella–zoster
  Pneumocystis carinii
  Strongyloides stercoralis

Central nervous system
  Listeria monocytogenes
  Nocardia asteroides
  Cryptococcus neoformans
  Varicella–zoster
  Toxoplasma gondii

Liver
  Cytomegalovirus
  Toxoplasma gondii
  Strongyloides stercoralis

Alimentary tract
  Salmonella
  Cytomegalovirus
  Herpes simplex
  Strongyloides stercoralis

mycobacterial, and fungal agents, whereas an interstitial picture is characteristic of viral and protozoan infections. Cavitation suggests mycobacterial and *Nocardia* infections but has been described with other bacteria and fungi. Exposure histories, other associated sites of infection, and recognition of concomitant infecting agents are often helpful in the differential diagnosis.

CNS infections (Table 2) appear commonly with five of these organisms: *Listeria monocytogenes, Cryptococcus neoformans,* varicella–zoster virus, *Toxoplasma gondii,* and *Nocardia asteroides.* Headache, fever, and elevated cerebral spinal fluid (CSF) protein are common. *L. monocytogenes, C. neoformans,* and varicella–zoster are more likely to present as a meningitis, a CSF polymorphonuclear pleocytosis differentiating *Listeria* from *C. neoformans* and varicella. Varicella–zoster meningoencephalitis usually is associated with a normal CSF glucose, whereas the glucose is decreased in meningitis caused by *Listeria* and *C. neoformans. T. gondii* and *N. asteroides* usually cause mass lesions; *Nocardia* almost always has other associated sites of infection especially in the pulmonary parenchyma, whereas *T. gondii* may involve mediastinal lymph nodes.

Hepatitis (Table 2) presents difficulties in differentiating CMV from *Toxoplasma,* except in the mononucleosis-like syndrome seen with these two infections: CMV rarely has associated lymphadenopathy, whereas with *Toxoplasma* it is the rule. Hepatitis secondary to *Strongyloides* is always a direct consequence of significant disseminated infection.

Enteritis (Table 2) secondary to herpes simplex virus or CMV takes the form of esophagitis or colitis. These viruses can affect both locations, although herpes simplex is more likely to cause esophagitis and CMV to cause colitis. Both of these infections are frequently polymicrobial in origin. Herpes simplex often is accompanied by obvious oral herpes simplex lesions. With a *Salmonella* infection the enteritis may be minimal, whereas bacteremia with this organism is the most common finding in the immunosuppressed patient. *Strongyloides* causes a frequently severe enteritis, often accompanied by mixed gastrointestinal organism bacteremias and a concurrent pneumonitis.

The diagnostic resources needed vary according to the pathogen and site of infection (Table 3). *Legionella pneumophilia,* coccidioidomycosis, *Toxoplasma gondii,* and cytomegalovirus may be defined using serologic methods. Serum or spinal fluid cryptococcal antigen assay and tuberculin skin testing are helpful for the latter two infections. Nevertheless, definitive diagnosis is dependent on cultural isolation or tissue identification of the organism. As Table 4 demonstrates, a specific diagnosis is mandatory for appropriate therapy because the treatment of each illness is etiology-specific and not always without therapy-related toxicities. Table 4 outlines the current approach to therapy.

The therapy for infections in patients with cellular immune deficiencies is not universally effective, and diagnosis is often difficult. Preventive measures for some of these infections therefore may be more appropriate. A preventive plan must begin by looking at the mode of acquisition and differentiating those infections which are most likely to reactivate with immunosuppression (Table

TABLE 3. Diagnosis of common pathogens in patients with cellular immune deficiency

Pathogen	Serology	Markers	Tissue diagnosis and stain	Exposure history
Bacteria				
Listeria monocytogenes	No	No	Blood/CSF	No
Salmonella	No	No	Blood	±
Mycobacterium tuberculosis	No	+PPD	Acid-fast stain	Yes
Atypical mycobacteria	No	No	Acid-fast stain (≥2+ cultures)	Yes
Nocardia asteroides	No	No	Brown-Brenn	No
Legionella pneumophila	4-fold rise or titer >1:128	No	Culture—blood, lung; direct IF	±
Fungi				
Cryptococcus neoformans	No	Cryptococcus antigen	Blood, CSF; India ink	No
Histoplasma capsulatum	±	No	Giemsa, methenamine silver	Yes
Coccidioides immitis	4-fold rise or titer >1:32	No	Identify spherules with endospores	Yes
Viruses				
Cytomegalovirus	? 4-fold rise	No	Positive tissue culture or blood—not urine	No
Herpes simplex	No	No	Isolation vesicle fluid, inclusions	No
Varicella–zoster	No	Tzanck preparation	Vesicle fluid culture	±Yes
Protozoa				
Pneumocystis carinii	No	No	Tissue; methenamine silver	No
Toxoplasma gondii	2-fold rise IgG; >1:80 IgM	No	Not diagnostic	Yes
Helminths				
Strongyloides stercoralis	No	Eosinophilia	Duodenal/jejunal aspirate	No

TABLE 4. *Therapy for common pathogens: cellular immune dysfunction*

Organism	Therapy: daily dosage and route of administration	Duration
Bacteria		
Listeria monocytogenes	Ampicillin (6–12 g/day ± gentamicin)	2 weeks
Salmonella	Chloramphenicol (500 mg q 6 hr p.o. or i.v.)	14 days
Mycobacterium		
M. tuberculosis	Two antituberculosis drugs, i.e., INH (300 mg/day), ethambutol (15 mg/kg/day), rifampin (600 mg/day)	6–18 months
Atypical mycobacteria	Two to four antituberculous drugs, i.e., INH, ethambutol, rifampin, streptomycin; surgical excision often required	? 2 years
Nocardia asteroides	Trimethoprim/sulfamethoxazole (160 mg/800 mg q 6 hr)	3–12 months
Legionella pneumophila	Erythromycin (500 mg to 1 g q 6 hr)	14 days
Fungi		
Cryptococcus neoformans	Amphotericin B (0.3 mg/kg/day i.v.) + 5-fluorocytosine (37.5 mg q 6 hr)	6 weeks
Histoplasma capsulatum	Amphotericin B (0.6 mg/kg/day i.v.)	Total dose 30–35 mg/kg
Coccidioides immitis	Amphotericin B (0.6 mg/kg i.v.) (miconazole 800 mg q 8 hr i.v.)	Total of 5 g 3–6 weeks
Virus		
Cytomegalovirus	Not available.	—
Herpes simplex virus Disseminated or visceral involvement	Adenine arabinoside[a]	10–14 days[a]
Varicella–zoster		
Varicella-involved viscera	Adenine arabinoside/interferon[b]	
Zoster-disseminated	Zoster immune plasma[c]	
Protozoa		
Pneumocystis carinii	Trimethoprim/sulfamethoxazole (20 mg/kg/100 mg/kg p.o.) (pentammidine 4 mg/kg i.m.)	14 days
Toxoplasma gondii	Sulfonamide/pyrimethamine (1 g q.i.d./75 mg 1st day/25 mg/day p.o.) + folinic acid (6 mg/day)	1 month
Helminths		
Strongyloides stercoralis	Thiabendazole (25 mg/kg q 12 hr p.o.)	2–7 days

[a] Efficacy demonstrated only in herpes simplex encephalitis.
[b] Efficacy suspected but not proved.
[c] Varicella pneumonia.

5). There are no specific preventive measures for *Listeria monocytogenes, Salmo-nella* species, and *Nocardia asteroides. Legionella pneumophilia* appears to have a propensity for epidemic outbreaks which have frequently been linked to contaminated water, cooling towers, and nearby construction. It therefore appears prudent to have immunosuppressed patients avoid previously contaminated areas. The mycobacteria often provide clues to latent infection with positive skin tests or abnormal chest x-rays, which allow selection of patients who are at risk of reactivation. The issue of prophylactic isoniazid for all tuberculin skin test-positive patients receiving immunosuppressive therapy was recently challenged because of the risk of isoniazid hepatotoxicity, especially in older individuals. The American Thoracic Society (9), however, recommends isoniazid therapy for 1 year or continuation until completion of immunosuppressive therapy in patients with positive tuberculin skin tests.

Preventive measures are limited for the fungal infections. The area of viral infections, although ubiquitous, has had some advances. Zoster immune globulin with a titer of >1:256 has been found to be adequate prophylaxis to prevent varicella for exposed individuals without a history of prior varicella infection. An attenuated varicella–zoster vaccine is currently under evaluation. It has been preventive when used in children with leukemia, but to date no data are available regarding prophylaxis against zoster in the immunocompromised patient. The isolation of immunosuppressed patients from other patients with contagious varicella–zoster infection is equally important. The passage of CMV via transplant organs makes donor screening important. Recently Glazer et al. (33) evaluated a live CMV vaccination for renal transplant candidates. They found that their vaccine produced cellular and humoral immunity, was associated with minimal morbidity, and appeared not to reactivate with intense immunosuppression. Although its impact on future renal transplant patients is untested, the concept is exciting. The use of prophylactic interferon as a preventive measure against CMV and herpes simplex viral infections in renal transplantation patients has been tried with a decrease in CMV viremia, although no effect on long-term graft survival was noted. Hughes et al. (41) advanced the prevention of *P. carinii.* They described the elimination of *P. carinii* pneumonia in a group of acute lymphoblastic leukemia patients by treatment with trimethoprim/sulfamethoxazole during susceptible periods. This work seems easily extrapolated to other susceptible patient populations, e.g., organ transplant recipients. Control of *Toxoplasma,* again ubiquitous, requires careful blood screening, an awareness of the passage of infection through granulocyte transfusions, and cautioning of susceptible patients in regard to pet cats and uncooked beef. *Strongyloides stercoralis* infections may be controlled by thiabendazole for patients with an appropriate exposure history and subtle infection clues (e.g., eosinophilia, undiagnosed gastrointestinal symptoms) if diagnosed prior to immunosuppression.

SUMMARY

This chapter outlined the pathogens frequently observed in patients with cellular immune deficiencies. The medical literature can be confusing as to the fre-

TABLE 5. Infection acquisition and prevention of common pathogens in patients with cellular immune dysfunction

| | | Acquisition | | | | | Prophylaxis | |
| | | | | | | | | |
Organism	Reactivation	Person/ person	Food/ water	Airborne	Contact	Biologic	Antimicrobial
Bacteria							
Listeria monocytogenes	No	No	No	No		No	No
Salmonella	No	No	Yes	No		No	No
Mycobacterium tuberculosis	Yes	Yes	No	Yes		No	INH/+PPD
Atypical mycobacteria	Yes	No	No	No		No	No
Nocardia asteroides	No	No	No	No		No	No
Legionella pneumophilia	No	No	No	Yes		No	No
Fungi							
Cryptococcus neoformans	No	No	No	Yes		No	No
Histoplasma gondii	+/−	No	No	Yes		No	Value of prophylactic amphotericin B in immunosuppressed patients is unknown
Viruses							
Cytomegalovirus	+/−	No	No	No	Blood	Vaccine under evaluation	No
Herpes simplex	Yes	No	No	No		No	No
Varicella–zoster	+/−	Yes	No	No		ZIP	No
Protozoa							
Pneumocystis carinii	+/−	?	No	No		No	Trimethoprim/sulfamethoxazole
Toxoplasma gondii	+/−	No	Yes	No		No	—
Helminths							
Strongyloides stercoralis	Yes	No	Yes	No	Soil	No	Thiabendazole prior to immunosup-pressive therapy

quency of these infections, but in the general population infections caused by these organisms are infrequent except for recurrent herpes labialis, childhood varicella, and tuberculosis. These same infections, plus herpes zoster, are most common in the patient with depressed cellular immunity, but the major difference, besides the increase in frequency often related to reactivation of latent organisms, is the increased severity of these infections in the immunocompromised patient. The management of these infections in the compromised host is often frustrating and leaves many physicians with the feeling that the situation is impossible; hence in order to make a rational therapeutic decision and still provide optimal care, one is forced to treat for every conceivable pathogen. An alternative approach is a thoughtful consideration of the patient's underlying immune deficiency and recognition of those infections which are common to that specific deficiency. Appropriate management also requires a thorough diagnostic and microbiologic evaluation followed by the initiation of appropriate therapy. Only limited means of prophylaxis are currently available, but new vaccines may alter this deficiency in the near future.

REFERENCES

1. Ketchel, S. J., and Rodriguez, V. (1978): Acute infections in cancer patients. *Semin. Oncol.,* 5:167–179.
2. Bode, F. R., Pare, J. A. P., and Fraser, R. G. (1974): Pulmonary diseases in the compromised host. *Medicine (Baltimore),* 53:255–293.
3. Iwarson, S., and Larsson, S. (1979): Outcome of *Listeria monocytogenes* infection in compromised and non-compromised adults: A comparative study of seventy-two cases. *Infection,* 7:54–56.
4. Louria, D. B., Le Frock, J. L., Smith, W., and Keefe, M. (1976): *Listeria* infections. *Ann. NY Acad. Sci.,* pp. 545–551.
5. Louria, D. B., Hensle, T., Armstrong, D., Collins, H. S., Blevins, A., Krugman, D., and Buse, M. (1967): Listeriosis complicating malignant disease: A new association. *Ann. Intern. Med.,* 67:261–280.
6. Mackaness, G. B. (1962): Cellular resistance to infection. *J. Exp. Med.,* 116:381–389.
7. Cherubin, C. E., Neu, H. C., Imperato, P. J., Harvey, R. P., and Bellen, N. (1974): Septicemia with non-typhoid salmonella. *Medicine (Baltimore),* 53:365–376.
8. Wolfe, M. S., Armstrong, D., Louria, D. B., and Blevins, A. (1971): Salmonellosis in patients with neoplastic disease: A review of 100 episodes at Memorial Cancer Center over a 13-year period. *Arch. Intern. Med.,* 128:546–554.
9. McConville, J. H., and Rapoport, M. I. (1976): Tuberculosis management in the mid-1970s. *JAMA,* 235:172–176.
10. Kaplan, M. H., Armstrong, D., and Rosen, P. (1974): Tuberculosis complicating neoplastic disease: A review of 201 cases. *Cancer,* 33:850–858.
11. Feld, R., Bodey, G. P., and Groschel, D. (1976): Mycobacteriosis in patients with malignant disease. *Arch. Intern. Med.,* 136:67–70.
12. Presant, C. A., Wiernik, P. H., and Serpick, A. A. (1973): Factors affecting survival in nocardiosis. *Am. Rev. Respir. Dis.,* 108:1444–1448.
13. Young, L. S., Armstrong, D., Blevins, A., and Lieberman, P. (1971): *Nocardia asteroides* infection complicating neoplastic disease. *Am. J. Med.,* 50:356–367.
14. Beaty, H. N., Miller, A. A., Broome, C. V., Goings, S., and Phillips, C. A. (1978): Legionnaires' disease in Vermont, May to October 1977. *JAMA,* 240:127–131.
15. Center for Disease Control (1978): Legionnaires' disease: Diagnosis and management. *Ann. Intern. Med.,* 88:363–365.
16. Saravolatz, L. D., Burch, K. H., Fisher, F., Madhavan, T., Kiani, D., Neblett, T., and Quinn, E. L. (1979): The compromised host and legionnaire's disease. *Ann. Intern. Med.,* 90:533–537.

17. Gump, D. W., Frank, R. O., Winn, W. C., Jr., Foster, R. S., Broome, C. V., and Cherry, W. B. (1979): Legionnaires' disease in patients with associated serious disease. *Ann. Intern. Med.,* 90:538–542.
18. Kirby, B. D., Snyder, K. M., Meyer, R. D., and Finegold, S. M. (1978): Legionnaires' disease: Clinical features of 24 cases. *Ann. Intern. Med.,* 89:297–309.
19. Myerowitz, R. L., Pascolle, A. W., Dowling, J. N., Pazin, G. J., Puerzer, M., Yee, R. B., Rinaldo, C. R., and Hakala, T. R. (1979): Opportunistic lung infection due to "Pittsburgh pneumonia agent." *N. Engl. J. Med.,* 301:953–958.
20. Rogers, B. H., Donowitz, G. R., Walker, G. K., Harding, S. A., and Sande, M. A. (1979): Opportunistic pneumonia: A clinicopathologic study of five cases caused by an unidentified acid-fast bacterium. *N. Engl. J. Med.,* 301:959–961.
21. Kaplan, M. H., Rosen, P. P., and Armstrong, D. (1977): Cryptococcosis in a cancer hospital: Clinical and pathological correlates in forty-six patients. *Cancer,* 39:2265–2274.
22. Schimpff, S. C., and Bennett, J. E. (1975): Abnormalities in cell-mediated immunity in patients with *Cryptococcus neoformans* infections. *J. Allergy Clin. Immunol.,* 55:430–441.
23. Bennett, J. E. (1972): Cryptococcosis. In: *Infectious Diseases,* edited by P. Heoprich, pp. 945–952. Harper & Row, New York.
24. Bennett, J. E., Dismukes, W. E., Duman, R. J., Medoff, G., Sande, M. A., Gallis, H., Leonard, J., Fields, B. T., Bradshaw, M., Haywood, H., McGee, Z. A., Cate, T. R., Cobbs, C. G., Warner, J. F., and Alling, D. W. (1979): Amphotericin B-flucytosine in cryptococcal meningitis. *N. Engl. J. Med.,* 301:126–131.
25. Kauffman, C. A., Israel, K. S., Smith, J. W., White, A. C., Schwarz, J., and Brooks, G. F. (1978): Histoplasmosis in immunosuppressed patients. *Am. J. Med.,* 64:923–932.
26. Davies, S. F., Khan, M., and Sarosi, G. A. (1978): Disseminated histoplasmosis in immunologically suppressed patients: Occurrence in a nonendemic area. *Am. J. Med.,* 64:94–100.
27. Cox, F., and Hughes, W. T. (1974): Disseminated histoplasmosis and childhood leukemia. *Cancer,* 33:1127–1133.
28. Deresinski, S. C., and Stevens, D. A. (1974): Coccidioidomycosis in compromised hosts: experience at Stanford University Hospital. *Medicine (Baltimore),* 54:377–395.
29. Rutala, P. J., and Smith, J. W. (1978): Coccidioidomycosis in potentially compromised hosts: The effect of immunosuppressive therapy in dissemination. *Am. J. Med. Sci.,* 275:283–295.
30. Meyers, J. D., Spencer, H. C., Jr., Watts, J. C., Gregg, M. B., Stewart, J. A., Troupin, R. H., and Thomas, E. D. (1975): Cytomegalovirus pneumonia after human marrow transplantation. *Ann. Intern. Med.,* 82:181–188.
31. Fiala, M., Payne, J. E., Berne, T. V., Moore, T. C., Henle, W., Montgomerie, J. Z., Chatterjee, S. N., and Guze, L. B. (1975): Epidemiology of cytomegalovirus infection after transplantation and immunosuppression. *J. Infect. Dis.,* 132:421–433.
32. Hamilton, J. R., Overall, J. C., Jr., and Glasgow, L. A. (1977): Synergistic infection with murine cytomegalovirus and *Candida albicans* in mice. *J. Infect. Dis.,* 135:918–924.
33. Glazer, J. P., Friedman, H. M., Grossman, R. A., Starr, S. E., Barker, C. F., Perloff, L. J., Huant, E. S., and Plotkin, S. A. (1979): Live cytomegalovirus vaccination of renal transplant candidates: a preliminary trial. *Ann. Intern. Med.,* 91:676–683.
34. Armstrong, D., Balakrishnan, S. L., Steger, L., Yu, B., and Stenzel, K. H. (1971): CMV infections with viremia following renal transplantation. *Arch. Intern. Med.,* 127:111–115.
35. Gelderman, A. H., Grimley, P. M., Lunde, M. N., et al. (1968): *Toxoplasma gondii* and cytomegalovirus mixed infection by a parasite and virus. *Science,* 160:1130–1132.
36. Stinson, E. B., Bieber, C. P., Griepp, R. B., Clark, D. A., Shumway, N. E., and Remington, J. S. (1971): Infectious complications after cardiac transplantation in man. *Ann. Intern. Med.,* 74:22–36.
37. Buss, D. H., and Scharyj, M. (1979): Herpesvirus infection of the esophagus and other visceral organs in adults: Incidence and clinical significance. *Am. J. Med.,* 66:457–462.
38. Schimpff, S. C., Serpick, A. A., Stoler, B., Rumack, B., Mellin, H., Joseph, J. M., and Block, J. (1972): Varicella–zoster infection in patients with cancer. *Ann. Intern. Med.,* 76:241–254.
39. Goffinet, D. R., Glatstein, E. J., and Merigan, T. C. (1972): Herpes zoster–varicella infections and lymphoma. *Ann. Intern. Med.,* 76:235–240.
40. Walzer, P. D., Perl, D. P., Krogstad, D. J., Rawson, P. G., and Schultz, M. G. (1974): *Pneumocystis carinii* pneumonia in the United States: Epidemiologic, diagnostic, and clinical features. *Ann. Intern. Med.,* 80:83–93.
41. Hughes, W. T., Kuhn, S., Chaudhary, S., Feldman, S., Verzosa, M., Aur, R. J. A., Pratt, C.,

and George, S. L. (1977): Successful chemoprophylaxis for *Pneumocystis carinii* pneumonitis. *N. Engl. J. Med.,* 297:1419–1426.

42. Hughes, W. T., Feldman, S., Aur, R. J. A., Verzosa, M. S., Hustu, O., and Simone, J. V. (1975): Intensity of immunosuppressive therapy and the incidence of *Pneumocystis carinii* pneumonitis. *Cancer,* 36:2004–2009.

43. Ruskin, J., and Remington, J. S. (1976): Toxoplasmosis in the compromised host. *Ann. Intern. Med.,* 84:193–199.

44. Vietzke, W. M., Gelderman, A. H., Grimley, P. M., and Valsamis, M. P. (1968): Toxoplasmosis complicating malignancy: Experience at the National Cancer Institute. *Cancer,* 21:816–827.

45. Carey, R. M., Kimball, A. C., Armstrong, D., and Lieberman, P. H. (1973): Toxoplasmosis: Clinical experiences in a cancer hospital. *Am. J. Med.,* 54:30–38.

46. Scowden, E. B., Schaffner, W., and Stone, W. J. (1978): Overwhelming strongyloidiasis: an unappreciated opportunistic infection. *Medicine (Baltimore),* 57:527–544.

Medical Complications in Cancer Patients,
edited by J. Klastersky and M. J. Staquet.
Raven Press, New York © 1981.

Use of Intensive Antineoplastic Therapy in Association with Hematopoietic Reconstitution: Rationale and Results

*Ross A. Abrams, **Arthur S. Levine, and †Albert B. Deisseroth

*Section on Hematology/Flesh Oncology, Medical College of Wisconsin, Milwaukee, Wisconsin 53226; and **Infectious Disease and †Experimental Hematology Sections, Pediatric Oncology Branch, National Cancer Institute, National Institutes of Health, Bethesda, Maryland 20205

Myelosuppression is the most frequent dose-limiting toxicity acutely encountered when cytoreductive agents are used in the management of neoplastic disease (54). The clinical correlates of profound, sustained pancytopenia—infection and hemorrhage—are well defined, as is their management in cytopenic patients. Over the past 20 years, the ability of patients to tolerate the hematopoietic toxicity of antineoplastic therapy has been improved by the development of platelet and granulocyte support as well as by the use of empiric antibiotic regimens (33,34,36,50). Studies have been undertaken to define the role and importance of regimens incorporating protected environments, nonabsorbable antibiotics, and topical antiseptics in decreasing the exposure of cytopenic patients to exogenous and endogenous microflora (49). Finally, efforts have been made to improve the therapeutic index of myelosuppressive, antineoplastic regimens through the use of pharmacologic rescue (8) and improved sequencing and timing when administering chemotherapeutic agents (31).

In the oncologic setting, these modalities are used either to protect endogenous hematopoietic function against therapeutic injury or to support patients through periods of inadequate hematopoietic function until endogenous recovery occurs. Unfortunately, the intensity of regimens that can be safely administered is still limited by hematopoietic toxicity despite optimal use of blood component and antibiotic therapies (35), an impression further confirmed by the limitations of these modalities in managing severe aplastic anemia (40). Thus the ability to reconstitute hematopoietic function through the use of stem cell infusions in order to accelerate hematopoietic recovery from treatment-induced myelosuppression is obviously a desirable objective.

The technical capability to reverse potentially lethal hematopoietic injury when induced in the management of malignant disease has been substantially advanced by the development of methods for bulk collection and infusion of bone marrow cells (69), as well as by advances in transplantation biology, cryopreservation techniques, and in vitro methods for growing and quantifying hematopoietic stem cells (6,7,37,39,42,45,47,51,58,63,74). These methods are being applied to the use of allogeneic, autologous, and syngeneic stem cells to permit the safe administration of intensive and ablative levels of therapy. In this chapter we attempt to review the therapeutic rationale for utilizing intensive treatment regimens and the recent progress achieved in the field of clinical oncology by combining intensive therapy with hematopoietic reconstitution.

CLINICAL RATIONALE FOR INTENSIVE
AND ABLATIVE THERAPIES

In this discussion, we use the term "hematopoietically ablative therapy" to refer to myelosuppressive therapy producing such severe damage to endogenous hematopoietic stem cells that spontaneous hematopoietic recovery cannot be expected. The concept of "hematopoietically intensive therapy" is broader and more difficult to define. Pragmatically, any treatment producing sufficient myelo-suppression to be routinely associated with fever or infection at times of therapy-induced leukopenia and granulocytopenia may be considered intensive; however, unless such therapy produces profound leukopenia ($<1,000/mm^3$) and granulo-cytopenia ($<500/mm^3$) that is sustained for a minimum of 14 to 21 days, it is probably not sufficiently "intensive" to require the use of hematopoietic reconstitution *(vide infra)*. In the literature, authors may refer to a spectrum of therapeu-tic intensity ranging from only slightly more myelosuppressive than commonly used outpatient regimens [such as CMF (cyclophosphamide/methotrexate/5-fluorouracil) for breast cancer and CVP (cyclophosphamide/vincristine/pred-nisone) for lymphoma] to combined modality regimens producing sustained, profound myelosuppression of up to several weeks' duration before the appear-ance of endogenous hematopoietic recovery.

For hematopoietic reconstitution to be of clinical value to a patient undergoing hematopoietically intensive therapy, the following criteria should be fulfilled:

1. The treatment utilized must produce profound myelosuppression that is sustained for at least 2 to 3 weeks. Otherwise, hematopoietic recovery from endogenous stem cells will be more rapid than any recovery potentially produced by infusion of exogenous stem cells.

2. The patient's prognosis in the absence of intensive therapy must be suffi-ciently limited to warrant the risks of the treatment.

3. The malignancy in question must exhibit a substantial increase in clinical response as therapy is escalated beyond conventional dose levels.

Assessment of factors 2 and 3 requires knowledge of diagnosis, extent of metastatic dissemination, performance status, prior treatment and response to prior treatment; an awareness of underlying medical conditions; and an under-standing of the clinical biology of the tumor in question.

4. The patient should have a reasonable chance of surviving the obligate period of hematopoietic hypoplasia (minimum of 2 to 3 weeks) that ensues

during the interval between administration of severely myelosuppressive therapy and recovery of peripheral blood leukocyte, granulocyte, and platelet counts. This estimate should be based, in part, on the patient's condition and in part on the level of hematopoietic and other forms of supportive care available.

5. Nonhematopoietic, organ system toxicity must be acceptable and manageable.

6. There must be an appropriate source of reconstituting hematopoietic stem cells (HSC) capable of producing reliable immunohematopoietic recovery. The HSC, if autologous, should be free of contaminating tumor cells and, if allogeneic, of sufficient genetic compatibility with the recipient to result in either minimal, or at least manageable, graft-versus-host disease (GVHD).

WHEN IS HEMATOPOIETIC RECONSTITUTION NECESSARY AFTER INTENSIVE MYELOSUPPRESSIVE THERAPY?

Restoration of hematopoietic function through the use of exogenously administered hematopoietic stem cells might logically be considered when endogenous hematopoietic recovery is not expected; when spontaneous recovery will occur only after prolonged delay; or when hematopoietic "reserve," as judged by the inability of peripheral blood counts to recover after the administration of subsequent nonintensive therapy, is markedly impaired.

The ability of bone marrow to recover from acute chemotherapeutic insult is generally underestimated. For example, Ettinger et al. (21) observed well-tolerated levels of hematopoietic suppression followed by prompt recovery in previously untreated patients with small cell carcinoma of the lung who were given two doses of cyclophosphamide 60 mg/kg either on days 1 and 2 or on days 1 and 8 of each treatment cycle. In spite of the fact that no exogenous HSC were used to effect hematopoietic reconstitution, these patients experienced granulocytopenia ($\leq 1,000/mm^3$) on only about 10 days per cycle and were able to tolerate additional cycles of combination chemotherapy and repeated cycles of high-dose cyclophosphamide. This result is entirely consistent with clinical earlier work by Buckner et al. (10), recent animal studies (60), and work at the National Cancer Institute utilizing an intensive regimen incorporating cyclophosphamide 180 mg/kg and BCNU (BACT) 200 mg/m² (3,5). In all of these studies, hematopoietic toxicity after doses of cyclophosphamide as high as 120 to 240 mg/kg was found to be substantial, but the dose-limiting toxicity appeared to be myocardial damage rather than hematopoietic aplasia. Our own experience with BACT in the treatment of undifferentiated lymphoma is illustrative of this principle of therapy. Although patients receiving BACT chemotherapy (BCNU 200 mg/m², cyclophosphamide 180 mg/kg, cytosine arabinoside 800 mg/m², and 6-thioguanine 800 mg/m²) followed by infusion of cryopreserved, autologous marrow cells recovered leukocyte and granulocyte counts statistically more rapidly than patients receiving BACT without marrow infusion, the absolute differences in days to recovery were small (days to leukocytes $\geq 1,000/mm^3$: 23 versus 13; days to granulocytes $\geq 500/mm^3$: 25 versus 21), and there was no difference in the incidence of bacterial sepsis between the two groups. Thus although it is unquestionably true that the BACT study was of substantial importance in helping to demonstrate that infusions of autologous marrow, even though cryopreserved, would accelerate hematopoietic recovery in patients exposed to intensive therapy of this magnitude, it also demonstrated the difficulty of designing intensive regimens whose primary toxicities are limited to myelosuppression. In fact, in the BACT study the dose-limiting toxicity was myocardial—not hematopoietic—as 4 of the 22 patients studied died shortly after therapy with left ventricular failure and/or refractory ventricular arrhythmias.

Following infusion of autologous or allogeneic bone marrow cells, a minimum of 14 to 21 days is generally required before sustained leukocyte and granulocyte recoveries are observed (5,16,70). Even regimens incorporating substantial doses of phase-specific and/or cycle-specific agents that are specifically intended to render the marrow profoundly hypoplastic (e.g., those used in the treatment of acute nonlymphocytic leukemia) are usually associated with the onset of hematopoietic recovery within 14 to 21 days—if adequate cytoreduction is achieved among the malignant cell population.

At present, the efficacy of exogenous hematopoietic reconstitution has been most clearly demonstrated in association with regimens incorporating large, single doses of total body irradiation (TBI). Based on animal studies in dogs (4) and primates (71) and clinical experience in humans (2), spontaneous hematopoietic recovery from surviving endogenous stem cells is not expected following acute exposure to doses of TBI in excess of 500 to 1,000 rads. Doses of TBI in this range have now been used clinically in association with high-dose cyclophosphamide prior to infusing syngeneic (22,23), allogeneic (70), and autologous (18,29) marrow cells. In addition to providing sustained cytoreduction of neoplastic cells, TBI in combination with high-dose cyclophosphamide has produced adequate immunosuppression to permit proliferation and engraftment of infusions of allogeneic marrow cells (70).

High-dose nitrosourea therapy may also be used to induce apparently irreversible marrow aplasia, a model studied in dogs by Abb et al. (1). Autologous stem cell reconstitution has been used in this setting to permit the testing of tumor response patterns to BCNU when delivered at doses taken to the limits of nonhematopoietic toxicity (48) among patients with neoplasms considered refractory to more conventional management.

Convincing demonstration of the efficacy and need for hematopoietic reconstitution following intermediate levels of intensive therapy has been difficult to obtain. However, using a regimen incorporating 150 rads TBI fractionated over 5 weeks followed by treatment with cyclophosphamide (80 mg/kg), doxorubicin (70 mg/m²), vincristine (4.0 mg/m²), and imidazole carboximide (750 mg/m²), we found that autologous cryopreserved marrow results in a 3- to 4-week acceleration of hematopoietic recovery among patients with Ewing's sarcoma (Abrams et al., *unpublished observation*). Interestingly, in this patient population accelerated hematopoietic recovery was also associated with improved ability subsequently to tolerate maintenance chemotherapy.

Recently Parker et al. (43) suggested that adequate cytoreductive therapy may be necessary in the autologous setting—not only for allowing objective demonstration of accelerated hematopoietic recovery, but also for creating sufficient "marrow space" to allow exogenously infused hematopoietic cells preferentially to repopulate the marrow. The concept of marrow "space" being necessary to permit engraftment and proliferation of infused hematopoietic stem cells has been considered for some time by investigators in this field (70). In the treatment of acute leukemia with intensive regimens supported by allogeneic marrow infusion, recipient preparation has been based on providing adequate marrow "space," sufficient immunosuppression to prevent host rejection of the infused cells, and adequate cytoreduction of malignant cell populations. Experience thus far has demonstrated that either high-dose cyclophosphamide (e.g., 50 mg/kg $\times$ 4 doses) or TBI (e.g., 800 to 1,000 rads) suffices for creating marrow space and immunosuppression, but a durable period of control of leukemia can be achieved only through utilizing a combination of TBI and cyclophosphamide (70).

WHAT ARE THE THEORETICAL AND PRACTICAL CONSIDERATIONS THAT HELP DETERMINE WHEN INTENSIVE/ ABLATIVE THERAPIES SHOULD BE UTILIZED?

Hematopoietically ablative therapy is associated with significant patient morbidity and some degree of nonhematopoietic toxicity *(vide infra)*. Moreover, although hematopoietic reconstitution may be achieved by infusion of hematopoietic stem cells, there is at present no way to prevent or rescue cumulative toxicity to other vital organs such as the heart and lungs. Thus it is unlikely that many patients could routinely be expected to undergo multiple rounds of truly ablative therapy. These considerations suggest that ablative therapies should be reserved for only those patients who are likely to derive substantial benefit from them, and that the use of ablative therapies should be timed in the patient's course to allow maximal therapeutic gain. If autologous cells are to be used to effect hematopoietic reconstitution, their collection should be timed to minimize the risk of contamination by residual tumor cells.

The extent to which a given experimental treatment is found or hoped to be beneficial is usually comparative and based on anticipated results with other available therapeutic options. For an unproved treatment of uncertain value but obvious morbidity, therapeutic risk is not balanced by potential therapeutic gain until all standard treatment options are fully exhausted. For this reason, initial trials utilizing ablative theapy and hematopoietic reconstitution have been performed on patients with advanced illness refractory to other treatments (19,22,67). Although this approach has been appropriate and ethically necessary, one should not infer either that intervention with ablative therapy should be reserved for "end stage" patients with malignancy or that such timing represents the optimal moment for intervention of this nature.

When seeking to determine criteria for selecting patients and timing for ablative therapy, we can be guided by studies utilizing *in vitro* and *in vivo* (animal) tumor models. A number of workers have sought to define the determinants of malignant cell kill in response to therapeutic intervention and the circumstances under which cure of experimental tumors may be expected (9,20,55, 56,59,73). These efforts, taken collectively, support the following conclusions:

1. For neoplastic cells susceptible to the cytocidal effects of a given therapy, a definite dose-response curve may be defined. In some instances, a doubling or tripling of drug dose may increase tumor cell kill by one or more logs (i.e., a geometric increase in dose may lead to an exponential increase in cell kill).

2. Cell kill after chemotherapy is more analogous to first-order kinetics than to zero-order kinetics. That is, a given dose of drug (or constant level of therapeutic intensity) tends to kill a constant fraction of cells present rather than a constant number. Recently this concept was re-evaluated by Shackney et al. (57) and Norton and Simon (41). Both of these groups suggest that the log kill achieved at a given level of therapeutic intensity may vary with the tumor burden remaining at any point in time. Using different approaches, these groups suggest that under certain circumstances, for a constant level of therapeutic intensity, fractional cell kill may actually increase as the tumor burden is reduced from clinical to subclinical levels.

3. For many drugs there is limited differential toxicity between proliferating tumor cells and proliferating normal cells (e.g., hematopoietic, gastrointestinal). This was elegantly demonstrated in an *in vivo* model by Rosenoff et al. (52). In clinical practice, one kind of "working" definition of drug resistance is that within dose range limitations imposed by normal tissues a given therapy fails to produce clinically adequate reduction in tumor cell numbers.

4. Host survival from a given point in time may be correlated with tumor cell burden at that point in time.

5. The presence of a single, viable neoplastic cell may ultimately lead to tumor proliferation and dissemination, and finally to host death.

Once the efficacy of hematopoietic reconstitution following intensive/ablative therapy has been reliably established, these principles suggest that the optimal time for utilizing intensive/ablative therapy would coincide with the period of lowest tumor burden that can be achieved through the use of less-toxic forms of regional and systemic therapy. Such timing would perforce offer the additional advantage of coinciding with relief of symptoms and organ dysfunction previously related to the presence of a large tumor burden. Under such circumstances, performance status and physiologic reserve should improve, truly, helping to make the toxicity of intensive therapy more manageable.

The flow and development of this theoretical construct has now begun to converge and interdigitate with the progress of clinical oncology. As reviewed by Zubrod (76), the development of chemotherapeutically induced cures in the management of human neoplasia has occurred in a stepwise progression beginning with the ability to produce convincing partial responses and progressing to the ability to produce complete responses as therapeutic improvements are delineated. Cures, when they occur, are then found among those patients who have experienced a sustained complete response. Efforts at quantifying tumor burden (55) suggest that the number of tumor cells present in a host with disseminated neoplasm is about 10^{10} to 10^{11}. If so, a 99.9% reduction in tumor cell number would leave a residual tumor burden of 10^7 to 10^8 cells (i.e., 10 million to 100 million residual tumor cells). This remaining tumor burden, although substantial in absolute terms, might not be clinically detectable and would thus be consistent with achievement of "complete" response. Thus in the short term at the clinical level, it may not be possible to differentiate a complete response with many residual tumor cells present subclinically from a total response with no residual tumor cells remaining. However, over time these types of "complete" response distinguish themselves. In the latter case, one observes continued disease-free survival; in the former case, therapeutic resistance ultimately develops (59) followed by recurrence and progression.

Among the 10 or so tumors that can be reliably brought to complete remission (CR) status by standard therapies, there are those associated with a substantial percentage of cure [e.g., Burkitt's lymphoma (75), acute lymphocytic leukemia (38), gestational choriocarcinoma (30)] and others that almost invariably are associated with disease recurrence and progression after CR [e.g., acute myeloblastic leukemia (24) and extensive small cell carcinoma of the lung (12)]. Patients with tumors in these latter categories would consequently be likely to benefit from the application of ablative therapies with hematopoietic reconstitution early in their courses shortly after CR status has been achieved. In contrast, for patients with Burkitt's lymphoma, gestational choriocarcinoma, or acute lymphoblastic leukemia in first remission, the risks of ablative therapy could not be justified for patients in CR since many will never relapse even without more aggressive treatment. Since this conceptual model has now been clinically tested with encouraging results in the setting of acute myelogenous leukemia (25,32), it is appropriate to review some of the trials and results that led to current levels of clinical success.

RESULTS OF STUDIES INVOLVING ABLATIVE THERAPY AND HEMATOPOIETIC RECONSTITUTION IN THE MANAGEMENT OF HUMAN NEOPLASIA

Initial studies involving intensive therapy and hematopoietic reconstitution were designed to demonstrate whether such efforts were technically possible and of benefit to patients for whom other therapeutic alternatives were either unavailable or previously exhausted. This early work has been reviewed in detail

(16,17,28,70). Studies are now available involving late-stage patients with acute nonlymphocytic leukemia, acute lymphocytic leukemia, chronic myelogenous leukemia (accelerated phase), Burkitt's lymphoma, anaplastic carcinoma of the nasopharynx, malignant glioma, small cell carcinoma of the lung, melanoma, and selected pediatric malignancies (3,5,11,14,18,19,25,29,32,44,48,67,70).

The most common diagnosis among patients treated in this manner is acute leukemia in relapse, predominantly either acute nonlymphocytic leukemia or acute lymphocytic leukemia. In 1977 Thomas et al. (65) reviewed their experience in 100 patients with acute leukemia who received allogeneic bone marrow following ablative therapy with various regimens incorporating TBI and high-dose (120 mg/kg) cyclophosphamide. Even though this patient population consisted of individuals with multiple leukemic relapses for whom conventional levels of antineoplastic therapy held little promise of response or improvement, there were 13 long-term (>11 months postablative therapy) disease-free survivors and 4 long-term survivors who had experienced leukemic relapse. Six patients died acutely (3 to 17 days after marrow infusion), and overall survival at 1 year was approximately 25%. Of the 83 patients who died, only 26 demonstrated recurrent or residual leukemia. The remainder of those who died succumbed primarily to respiratory failure (interstitial pneumonia) in association with either moderate to severe GVHD (26 patients), respiratory failure (interstitial pneumonia) with minimal GVHD (8 patients), or GVHD with infection (8 patients). This experience supports several substantial conclusions:

1. All of these patients had progressive leukemia following therapy of standard intensity, yet in the vast majority remission did occur in response to ablative therapy. Thus therapeutic resistance in these patients was relative rather than absolute.

2. Hematopoietic reconstitution as judged by rising granulocyte counts was observed in 91 of 94 patients surviving more than 13 days. Thus the hematopoietic reconstitution was extremely reliable.

3. The mortality due to the nonhematopoietic toxicity of this treatment regimen as judged by interstitial pneumonia and GVHD was greater than the mortality due to recurrent leukemia. Importantly, clinical condition at the time of ablative therapy correlated significantly with survival.

4. Finally, the data suggest that a small fraction of these patients have been cured of their "refractory leukemia."

These results encouraged the study of leukemic patients earlier in the course of their illness. Thomas et al. have now reported their findings with marrow transplantation for acute nonlymphoblastic leukemia (ANLL) in first remission (66) and acute lymphoblastic leukemia (ALL) in remission following prior relapse (68). Of 19 ANLL patients, 12 (63%) are in remission and off therapy more than 1 year, confirming the theoretical model and the conclusions discussed in the first part of this chapter. Moreover, these results have been extended to the setting of chronic myelogenous leukemia (CML) (23). Four patients with chronic phase CML have now been placed into sustained disease-free remission through the use, early in their illness, of ablative therapy (TBI + dimethylbusulfan + cyclophosphamide) and syngeneic (identical twin) hematopoietic reconstitution. It is unclear, however, whether their CML will yet recur.

Efforts in patients with nonleukemic neoplasms resistant to standard therapy have resulted in some cures (3,22) and in some unsustained partial and complete responses (14,18,29,32) following autologous or syngeneic hematopoietic reconstitution. The principles demonstrated in the setting of acute leukemia are likely to be applicable to these settings as well. For the present, however, the application of these principles is impaired by our inability to produce complete responses for many solid neoplasms and, in those cases where many CRs are obtained (e.g., Burkitt's lymphoma), the difficulty encountered in identifying those CR patients who are likely to suffer relapse. These problems await continued therapeutic advances at the level of nonintensive therapy and improved methodologies for identifying subclinical tumor burdens.

TECHNICAL CONSIDERATIONS IN THE USE OF ABLATIVE THERAPY AND HEMATOPOIETIC RECONSTITUTION

As the previous discussion suggests, morbidity and mortality following ablative therapy are multifactorial and depend in large part on the genetic source of the hematopoietic stem cells used for reconstitution, the cytoreductive regimen employed, and the clinical condition and prior management of the patient population in question.

As has been alluded to previously, hematopoietic stem cells suitable for effecting hematopoietic reconstitution may be collected autologously (self), syngeneically (identical twin), or allogeneically (usually HLA matched at A, B, and D loci). The number of cells required is of the order of magnitude of 1.0 to 2.0×10^8 nucleated bone marrow cells per kilogram of recipient (69). This dose has been associated with a high rate of engraftment in all three settings described (16,17,70) and can generally be obtained by collecting 10 ml of bone marrow per kilogram of recipient. This bulk collection of bone marrow constitutes an operative procedure with attendant need for anesthesia, sterility, and in some cases red blood cell transfusion (69).

Syngeneic cells represent the theoretically ideal source of hematopoietic stem cells for this use. They have the dual advantage of being free of contaminating tumor cells and genetically identical with the hematopoietic cells of the recipient. The latter attribute minimizes the risks of host rejection of the infused cells and of GVHD. Although syngeneic donors are found with low frequency (approximately 1 in 300), the incidence of malignancy in the general population is substantial, and patients with chemotherapeutically responsive hematopoietic and nonhematopoietic neoplasms having healthy identical twins are encountered. Such individuals should have the advantage of consultation with a transplant center early in the management of their illness. The availability of identical twin donor–patient pairs has permitted key clinical experiments in the management of hematopoietic neoplasms with ablative therapy (22,23). It is likely that continued utilization of such donor–patient pairs will be important in allowing ground-breaking research into the management of patients with selected nonhematopoietic neoplasms with ablative therapies.

Autologous hematopoietic stem cells have the advantage of genetic identity with the patient and are obviously more frequently available than syngeneic cells. Unfortunately, many of the neoplasms for which ablative therapy is appropriately considered are either hematopoietic or subject to hematogenous dissemination. Under these circumstances, the risk of tumor cell contamination—even if marrow cells are collected at times of CR—may be substantial. Although experience with Burkitt's lymphoma (3) has shown that the use of autologous marrow infusions may be associated with long-term remission, experience with acute leukemia has been far less encouraging in this regard (18). The other major problems associated with the use of autologous marrow cells are those of collection and cryopreservation. The bony pelvis is the most readily available source of bone marrow for collection. When the pelvis has been compromised by clinically evident tumor and/or radiotherapy, bone marrow collection may be impossible. In addition, the patient must be a candidate for general or at least regional anesthesia and be able to tolerate intraoperative management involving aspiration of 10 cc of bone marrow fluid per kilogram and appropriate fluid and packed red blood cell replacement. Finally, the cells must be preserved in a viable state prior to use. For short periods (hours) some workers have used simple refrigeration at 4°C (43). However, for viability to be maintained for weeks to months, cryopreservation in a frozen state is required. The details and complexity of cryopreservation are reviewed elsewhere (16), but this technique is associated with risk of lost viability.

Allogeneic marrow is the most frequently utilized source of reconstituting hematopoietic stem cells. Allogeneic sources are free of tumor, may be collected when needed, and generally are used without need for cryopreservation. However, the potential difficulties that arise from the genetic heterogeneity that perforce exists between donor and recipient—even when matching at HLA loci A, B, and D is accomplished among sibling donor–recipient pairs—are substantial and include graft rejection or failure, acute and chronic GVHD, acute and chronic immunosuppression, and interstitial pneumonitis (70). The presence of GVHD, especially when severe, may be correlated with immunosuppression and interstitial pneumonitis (65). Understanding GVHD has progressed from canine studies (63), which suggest that prior alloimmunization, resulting from transfusion exposure before transplantation, is an important factor in the development of GVHD after allogeneic marrow infusion. It has been suggested that GVHD may have an antitumor effect against leukemia (72), but the overall importance of this phenomenon is not clear. The elucidation of the mechanisms and components of this fascinating syndrome of aberrant immunity should substantially advance our understanding of basic immunobiology.

ACUTE NONHEMATOPOIETIC TOXICITIES
OF INTENSIVE THERAPY

Glode (27) recently reviewed the significant nonhematopoietic toxicities that may be seen following intensive therapy. In addition to interstitial pneumonitis, these include gastrointestinal, urologic, cardiac, and metabolic abnormalities. The potential significance of these toxicities is underscored by the four cardiac deaths that occurred among 22 patients receiving high-dose cyclophosphamide and BCNU (BACT) (3); the four cardiac deaths seen among 10 patients receiving high dose regimens of varying combinations of velban, adriamycin, cyclophosphamide, and TBI (26); and the five acute cardiopulmonary deaths seen among 21 leukemic patients treated with TBI and piperazinedione (19). Even when not directly lethal, toxicities such as mucositis or chemical cystitis can greatly compromise natural anatomic barriers to bacterial invasion and severely complicate the management of neutropenic patients. When doses of agents well beyond the usual pharmacologic levels are employed, previously unappreciated toxicities may occur. Phillips et al. (48) observed clinically significant pulmonary, hepatic, and central nervous system abnormalities following infusion of BCNU in total doses of 1,200 mg/m^2 over a 3-day period. These results emphasize the importance of designing ablative regimens to have toxicities focused solely on hematopoiesis and of proceeding cautiously and logically in their design.

LONG-TERM CONSIDERATIONS REGARDING THE USE OF
INTENSIVE COMBINED MODALITY THERAPIES WITH
HEMATOPOIETIC RECONSTITUTION

As mentioned above, in the past, patients with neoplastic disease were generally not considered candidates for intensive or ablative levels of therapy until far along in the course of their illness. Then, in a setting usually defined by progressive malignancy, diminishing numbers of therapeutic options, declining performance status, and dismal prognosis, intensive therapy was attempted in the hope of achieving dramatic response but with limited overall expectations for either sustained complete response or long-term survival. Under such circumstances, concerns beyond the immediate, acute realities have been limited.

With increasing experience and confidence *vis-à-vis* the technical demands of using intensive therapies and reliably effecting hematopoietic reconstitution, it is likely that utilization of these techniques will be considered earlier in the course of patient management—as has already occurred in the setting of acute leukemia—and that an increased number of these patients will survive for periods ranging from months to years after undergoing such treatment. To what extent these patients will then be at risk for the development of second malignancies (46,53) or delayed toxicity in normal organs (64) is unknown. However, such phenomena have been observed among patients treated aggressively, even though not to hematopoietically ablative levels, and are clearly of concern. Whether the risk of development of leukemia as a second malignancy can be delayed or decreased by combining intensive therapy with hematopoietic reconstitution, either autologous or nonautologous, is not known.

Encouragingly, we observed that, following intensive combined modality therapy incorporating TBI and systemic chemotherapy, patients undergoing hematopoietic reconstitution were better able to tolerate maintenance chemotherapy—in terms of doses and frequency of administration—than similarly treated patients managed without hematopoietic reconstitution (1a). Whether this evidence of sustained, posttreatment improvement in hematopoietic status will have broad, long-range importance or perhaps decrease the potential risk for developing leukemia as a second, treatment-related neoplasm is at present speculative.

SUMMARY AND CONCLUSIONS

In our opinion, current experience with intensive/ablative therapies and hematopoietic reconstitution supports several important conclusions. There is no longer any question that appropriately collected and processed stem cell populations, whether syngeneic, autologous, or allogeneic, are capable of effecting full hematopoietic recovery, even after therapies that would otherwise be hematopoietically lethal. The combined methodologies of ablative therapy and hematopoietic reconstitution have allowed clinical investigators successfully to apply principles learned from tumor cell growth kinetics, cellular pharmacology, and clinical observation to the needs of patients with disseminated neoplasms. This has resulted in long-term disease-free survival in patients who would otherwise have succumbed. The application of ablative therapy must be on a highly selective basis, incorporating an understanding of therapeutic principles and the potential for nonhematopoietic toxicity. The results achieved serve to emphasize the importance of defining clinical and preclinical models for developing and testing in a rational manner the principles, concepts, and methodologies that are needed effectively to advance our ability to treat neoplastic disease.

Thus in addition to its role in other hematologic and immunologic settings (13,15,61,62), the use of hematopoietic reconstitution in association with intensive antineoplastic therapy has achieved an established and developing role in medical oncology.

REFERENCES

1. Abb, J., Netzel, B., Rodt, H., and Thierfelder, S. (1978): Autologous bone marrow grafts in dogs treated with lethal doses of 1-(2-chloroethyl)-3-cyclohexyl-1-nitrosourea. *Cancer Res.*, 38:2157–2159.
1a. Abrams, R. A., Glaubiger, D., Simon, R., Lichter, A., and Deisseroth, A. B. (1980): Results with autologous cryopreserved marrow in patients with Ewing's sarcoma. *Lancet (in press).*

2. Altman, P. L., and Katz, D. D., editors (1977): *Human Health and Disease,* p. 357. Federation of American Societies for Experimental Biology, Bethesda, Md.
3. Appelbaum, F. R., Deisseroth, A. B., Graw, R. G., et al. (1978): Prolonged complete remission following high dose chemotherapy of Burkitt's lymphoma in relapse. *Cancer,* 41:1059–1063.
4. Appelbaum, F. R., Herzig, G. P., Graw, R. G., et al. (1978): Study of cell dose and storage time on engraftment of cryopreserved autologous bone marrow in a canine model. *Transplantation,* 26:245–248.
5. Appelbaum, F. R., Herzig, G. P., Ziegler, J. L., et al. (1978): Successful engraftment of cryopreserved autologous bone marrow in patients with malignant lymphoma. *Blood,* 52:85–89.
6. Ashwood-Smith, M. J. (1964): The preservation of bone marrow. *Cryobiology,* 1:61–63.
7. Bach, F. H. (1978): Cellular immunogenetics of HLA: Quantitative crossmatches for LD and CD determinants. *Transplant. Proc.,* 10:63–66.
8. Bertino, J. R. (1977): Rescue techniques in cancer chemotherapy: Use of leucovorin and other rescue agents after methotrexate treatment. *Semin. Oncol.,* 4:203–216.
9. Bruce, W. R. (1967): The action of chemotherapeutic agents at the cellular level and the effects of these agents on hematopoietic and lymphomatous tissue. In: *Canadian Cancer Conference,* edited by J. F. Morgan et al., pp. 53–64. Pergamon Press, Oxford.
10. Buckner, C. D., Rudolph, R. H., Fefer, A., et al. (1972): High dose cyclophosphamide therapy for malignant disease. *Cancer,* 29:357–365.
11. Buckner, C. D., Stewart, P., Clift, R. A., et al. (1978): Treatment of blastic transformation of chronic granulocytic leukemia by chemotherapy, total body irradiation, and infusion of cryopreserved autologous marrow. *Exp. Hematol.,* 6:96–109.
12. Bunn, P. A., Cohen, M. H., Ihde, D. C., et al. (1977): Advances in small cell bronchogenic carcinoma. *Cancer Treat. Rep.,* 61:333–342.
13. Camitta, B. M., Thomas, E. D., Nathan, D. G., et al. (1979): A prospective study of androgens and bone marrow transplantation for treatment of severe aplastic anemia. *Blood,* 53:504–514.
14. Clifford, P. (1961): Nitrogen mustard therapy combined with autologous marrow infusion. *Lancet,* 1:687–690.
15. Cline, M. J., Gale, R. P., Steihm, E. R., et al. (1975): Bone marrow transplantation in man. *Ann. Intern. Med.,* 83:691–708.
16. Deisseroth, A., and Abrams, R. A. (1979): The role of autologous stem cell reconstitution in intensive therapy for resistant neoplasms. *Cancer Treat. Rep.,* 63:461–471.
17. Dicke, K. A., Lotzva, E., Spitzer, G., and McCredie, K. B. (1978): Immunobiology of bone marrow transplantation. *Semin. Hematol.,* 15:263–282.
18. Dicke, K. A., Spitzer, G., Peters, L., et al. (1979): Autologous bone marrow transplantation in relapsed adult acute leukemia. *Lancet,* 1:514–517.
19. Dicke, K. A., Spitzer, G., Zander, A. R., et al. (1979): Autologous bone marrow transplantation in relapsed adult leukemia and solid tumors. *Transplant. Proc.,* 11:212–214.
20. Drewinko, B. (1975): Cellular chemotherapy in the design of clinical trials. In: *Cancer Chemotherapy—Fundamental Concepts and Recent Advances,* pp. 63–77. Year Book, Chicago.
21. Ettinger, D. S., Karp, J. E., Abeloff, M. D., et al. (1978): Intermittent high dose cyclophosphamide chemotherapy for small cell carcinoma of the lung. *Cancer Treat. Rep.,* 62:413–424.
22. Fefer, A., Buckner, C. D., Thomas, E. D., et al. (1977): Cure of hematologic neoplasia with transplantation of marrow from identical twins. *N. Engl. J. Med.,* 297:146–148.
23. Fefer, A., Cheever, M. A., Thomas, E. D., et al. (1979): Disappearance of Ph'-positive cells in four patients with chronic granulocytic leukemia after chemotherapy, irradiation, and marrow transplantation from an identical twin. *N. Engl. J. Med.,* 300:333–337.
24. Gale, R. P. (1979): Advances in the treatment of acute myelogenous leukemia. *N. Engl. J. Med.,* 300:1189–1199.
25. Gale, R. P., Feig, S., Opelz, G., et al. (1976): Bone marrow transplantation in acute leukemia using intensive chemoradiotherapy (SCARI-UCLA). *Transplant. Proc.,* 8:611–616.
26. Gale, R. P., Graze, P. R., Wells, J., et al. (1979): Autologous bone marrow transplantation in patients with cancer. *Exp. Hematol.,* 7(Suppl. 5):351–359.
27. Glode, L. M. (1979): Dose limiting extramedullary toxicity of high dose chemotherapy. *Exp. Hematol.,* 7(Suppl. 5):265–278.
28. Graze, P. R., and Gale, R. P. (1978): Autotransplantation for leukemia and solid tumors. *Transplant. Proc.,* 10:177–184.

29. Graze, P. R., Wells, J. R., Ho, W., et al. (1979): Successful engraftment of cryopreserved autologous bone marrow stem cells in man. *Transplantation,* 27:142–145.
30. Hammond, C. B., Borchert, L. G., Tyrey, L., et al. (1973): Treatment of metastatic trophoblastic disease: Good and poor prognosis. *Am. J. Obstet. Gynecol.,* 115:451–457.
31. Hedley, D. W., McElwain, T. J., Millar, J. L., and Gordon, M. Y. (1978): Acceleration of bone marrow recovery by pretreatment with cyclophosphamide in patients receiving high dose melphalan. *Lancet,* 4:966–977.
32. Kaizer, H., Levinthal, B. G., Wharam, M. D., et al. (1979): Cryopreserved autologous bone marrow transplantation in the treatment of selected pediatric malignancies: A preliminary report. *Transplant. Proc.,* 11:208–211.
33. Klastersky, J. (1979): Combinations of antibiotics for therapy of severe infections in cancer patients. *Eur. J. Cancer,* 15:3–13.
34. Klastersky, J. (1979): Granulocyte transfusions as a therapy and a prophylaxis of infections in neutropenic patients. *Eur. J. Cancer,* 15:15–22.
35. Levine, A. S., and Deisseroth, A. B. (1978): Recent developments in the supportive therapy of acute myelogenous leukemia. *Cancer,* 42(Suppl.):833–894.
36. Lister, T. A., and Yankee, R. A. (1978): Blood component therapy. *Clin. Haemotol.,* 7:406–432.
37. Lowenthal, R. M., Park, D. S., Goldman, J. M., et al. (1976): The cryopreservation of leukemic cells: Morphological and functional changes. *Br. J. Haematol.,* 34:105–117.
38. Mauer, A. M. (1978): Treatment of acute leukemia in children. In: *Clinics in Haematology, Vol. 7: Acute Leukemia,* edited by J. V. Simone, pp. 245–258. Saunders, London.
39. Mazur, P. (1970): Cryobiology: The freezing of biological systems. *Science,* 168:939–949.
40. Najean, Y., and Pecking, A. (1979): Prognostic factors in acquired aplastic anemia: A study of 352 cases. *Am. J. Med.,* 67:564–571.
41. Norton, L., and Simon, R. (1977): Tumor size, sensitivity to therapy, and design of treatment schedules. *Cancer Treat. Rep.,* 61:1307–1318.
42. Opelz, G., Gale, R. P., Feig, S. A., et al. (1978): Significance of HLA and non-HLA antigens in bone marrow transplantation. *Transplant. Proc.,* 10:43–46.
43. Parker, L. M., Takvorian, T., Hochberg, F. H., and Canellos, G. P. (1979): BCNU and autologous bone marrow reinfusion: Dose-dependent creation of marrow space. *Blood,* 54(Suppl. 1):229a (abstract).
44. Parkman, R., Rappeport, J., Geha, R., et al. (1978): Complete correction of the Wiskott-Aldrich syndrome by allogeneic bone marrow transplantation. *N. Engl. J. Med.,* 298:921–927.
45. Pegg, D. E. (1964): Freezing of bone marrow for clinical use. *Cryobiology,* 1:64–71.
46. Penn, I. (1976): Second malignant neoplasms associated with immunosuppressive medications. *Cancer,* 37:1024–1032.
47. Perkins, H. A. (1979): Concise review: Current status of the HLA system. *Am. J. Hematol.,* 6:285–292.
48. Phillips, G. L., Fay, J. W., Herzig, G. P., et al. (1979): Intensive 1,3-bis(2-chloroethyl)-1-nitrosourea (BCNU) autologous bone marrow transplantation therapy of refractory cancer: A preliminary report. *Exp. Hematol.,* 7(Suppl. 5):372–383.
49. Pizzo, P. A., and Levine, A. S. (1977): The utility of protected environment regimens for the compromised host: A critical assessment. In: *Progress in Hematology, Vol. 10,* edited by E. B. Brown, pp. 311–332. Grune & Stratton, New York.
50. Pizzo, P. A., Robichaud, K. J., Gill, F. A., et al. (1979): Duration of empiric antibiotic therapy in granulocytopenic patients with cancer. *Am. J. Med.,* 67:194–200.
51. Quesenberry, P., and Levitt, L. (1979): Hematopoietic stem cells. *N. Engl. J. Med.,* 301:755–760, 819–823, 868–872.
52. Rosenoff, S. H., Bull, J. M., and Young, R. C. (1975): The effect of chemotherapy on the kinetics and proliferative capacity of normal and tumorous tissues in vivo. *Blood,* 45:107–118.
53. Rosner, F. (1976): Acute leukemia as a delayed consequence of cancer chemotherapy. *Cancer,* 37:1033–1036.
54. Rubin, P., and Scarantino, C. W. (1978): The bone marrow organ: The critical structure in radiation–drug interaction. *Int. J. Radiat. Oncol. Biol. Phys.,* 4:3–23.
55. Schabel, F. M. (1975): Concepts for systemic treatment of micrometastases. *Cancer,* 35:15–24.

56. Schabel, F. M. (1975): Animal models as predictive systems. In: *Cancer Chemotherapy—Fundamental Concept and Recent Advances,* pp. 323–355. Year Book, Chicago.
57. Shackney, S. E., McCormack, G. W., and Cuchural, G. J. (1978): Growth rate patterns of solid tumors and their relation to therapy. *Ann. Intern. Med.,* 80:107–121.
58. Shlafer, M. (1977): Drugs that modify cellular responses to low temperature (cryoprotectants). *Fed. Proc.,* 36:2950–2959.
59. Skipper, H. E. (1979): Historic milestones in cancer biology: A few that are important in cancer treatment (revisited). *Semin. Oncol.,* 6:506–514.
60. Storb, R., Buckner, C. D., Dillingham, L. A., and Thomas, E. D. (1979): Cyclophosphamide regimens in rhesus monkeys with and without marrow infusion. *Cancer Res.,* 30:2195–2203.
61. Storb, R., Prentice, R. L., and Thomas, E. D. (1977): Treatment of aplastic anemia by marrow transplantation from HLA identical siblings. *J. Clin. Invest.,* 59:625–632.
62. Storb, R., and Thomas, E. D. (1978): Marrow transplantation for treatment of aplastic anemia. In: *Clinics in Haematology, Vol. 7: Aplastic Anemia,* edited by E. D. Thomas, pp. 597–610. Saunders, London.
63. Storb, R., Weiden, P. L., Deeg, H. J., et al. (1979): Rejection of marrow from DLA-identical canine littermates given transfusions before grafting: Antigens involved are expressed on leukocytes and skin epithelial cells but not on platelets and red blood cells. *Blood,* 54:477–484.
64. Tefft, M., Lattin, P. B., Jereb, B., et al. (1976): Acute and late effects on normal tissues following combined chemotherapy and radiotherapy for childhood rhabdomyosarcoma and Ewing's sarcoma. *Cancer,* 37:1201–1213.
65. Thomas, E. D., Buckner, C. D., Banaji, M., et al. (1977): One hundred patients with acute leukemia treated by chemotherapy, total body irradiation, and allogeneic marrow transplantation. *Blood,* 49:511–533.
66. Thomas, E. D., Buckner, C. D., Clift, R. A., et al. (1979): Marrow transplantation for acute nonlymphoblastic leukemia in first remission. *N. Engl. J. Med.,* 301:597–599.
67. Thomas, E. D., Buckner, C. D., Fefer, A., Neiman, P. E., and Storb, R. (1978): Marrow transplantation in the treatment of acute leukemia. In: *Advances in Cancer Research, Vol. 27,* edited by G. Klein and S. Weinhouse, pp. 269–279. Academic Press, New York.
68. Thomas, E. D., Sanders, J. E., Flournoy, N., et al. (1979): Marrow transplantation for patients with acute lymphoblastic leukemia in remission. *Blood,* 54:468–476.
69. Thomas, E. D., and Storb, R. (1970). Technique for human marrow grafting. *Blood,* 36:507–515.
70. Thomas, E. D., Storb, R., Clift, R., et al. (1975): Bone marrow transplantation. *N. Engl. J. Med.,* 292:832–843, 895–902.
71. Van Bekkum, D. W. (1978): The rhesus monkey as a preclinical model for bone marrow transplantation. *Transplant. Proc.,* 10:105–111.
72. Weiden, P. L., Flournoy, N., Thomas, E. D., et al. (1979): Antileukemic effect of graft versus host disease in human recipients of allogeneic marrow grafts. *N. Engl. J. Med.,* 300:1068–1073.
73. Weiden, P. L., Storb, R., Deeg, H. J., and Graham, T. C. (1979): Total body irradiation and autologous marrow transplantation as consolidation therapy for spontaneous canine lymphoma in remission. *Exp. Hematol.,* 7(Suppl. 5):160–163.
74. Weiner, R. S., Richman, C. M., and Yankee, R. A. (1979): Dilution techniques for optimum recovery of cryopreserved bone marrow cells. *Exp. Hematol.,* 7(Suppl. 5):1–6.
75. Ziegler, J. L., Magrath, I. T., and Olweny, C. M. (1979): Long survival of Burkitt's lymphoma in Uganda. *Proc. Am. Soc. Clin. Oncol.,* 20:430 (abstract).
76. Zubrod, C. G. (1975): Heath Memorial Award Lecture: contributions of chemotherapy to the control of cancer. In: *Cancer Chemotherapy—Fundamental Concepts and Recent Advances,* pp. 7–17. Year Book, Chicago.

Subject Index

Subject Index